# After We Die

NORMAN L. CANTOR

# After We Die

*The Life and Times
of the Human Cadaver*

Georgetown University Press | Washington, D.C.

**Library of Congress Cataloging-in-Publication Data**
Cantor, Norman L.
After we die : the life and times of the human cadaver / Norman L. Cantor.
p. cm.
Includes bibliographical references and index.
ISBN 978-1-58901-695-8 (hardcover : alk. paper)
1. Dead bodies (Law)   2. Human body—Law and legislation.   3. Dead—
Legal status, laws, etc.   4. Burial laws.   5. Offenses against the person.
6. Sacrilege.   I. Title.
K564.H8C36 2010
393—dc22
2010012452

∞This book is printed on acid-free paper meeting the requirements of the American National Standard for Permanence in Paper for Printed Library Materials.

15  14  13  12  11  10       9  8  7  6  5  4  3  2
First printing

Printed in the United States of America

*For Tamar, again*

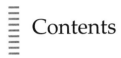# Contents

# Part II | Disposition of Human Remains

*Chapter 4*

## Decomposition of the Body and Efforts to Slow Its Disintegration   75

*Chapter 5*

## Final Disposal of Human Remains   91

*Chapter 6*

## Eternal Preservation of the Deceased: Literally and Figuratively   119

# Part III | The Multiple Roles of a Cadaver

# Part IV | Abuses of the Cadaver: What Does Decency Demand?

No matter how healthily you eat,
how much you deny your sedentary desires in the name of fitness,
no matter how many sacrifices you make to the great god of
   longevity,
you are going to die.

> Simon Critchley, "How to Make It in the Afterlife"

I knew that everybody had to die sometime,
but I always felt that an exception would be made
in my case.

> William Saroyan

# Introduction

My stepbrother died in 1973 at age thirty-nine. He was a flamboyant criminal trial lawyer and, true to his character, he left unusual instructions for his funeral arrangements. He wanted a New Orleans–style funeral in Trenton, New Jersey. His widow was to wear white. During the wake in the funeral home, a Dixieland band was to play jazz. On the day of the burial, the band was to lead the procession out of the funeral home.

My stepfather, a traditional Italian *padrone di casa*, was scandalized. He objected strenuously to his son's unconventional funeral arrangements. The widow, my stepsister in law, wanted to fulfill her late husband's wishes. After soul-searching and counsel, the widow and the father agreed to implement all of my stepbrother's instructions. A Dixieland band provided the loud background music for the otherwise somber wake and funeral procession. I didn't like Dixieland jazz, but I certainly admired my stepbrother's characteristic flair, as well as his determination to leave his signature on the disposal of his remains. The recollections of that funeral, and of its star, are indelible.

That intrafamily disagreement over funeral arrangements tweaked my law-related curiosity. As a then young lawyer interested in medico-legal matters, I wondered who had legal control in such a funeral controversy. Who would have had the ultimate say if the deceased's widow and father hadn't reached an accommodation? And no matter who was ultimately responsible, was there a legal duty to follow the decedent's instructions, no matter how bizarre? If there was such a duty, did that mean that cadavers have rights? What other rights could a cadaver have—beyond having its predecessor's wishes carried out? If cadavers have rights, who enforces them?

Twenty-nine years later, in July 2002, another funeral controversy rekindled my interest in the issues surrounding the disposition of corpses. Ted Williams, one of the all-time greats of major league baseball, died at age eighty-four. There was no memorial service. His son, John Henry Williams, arranged to have his father's corpse frozen in dry ice and flown to the Alcor Life Extension Foundation in Scottsdale, Arizona. Alcor, a cryonics facility, would arrange to have the body permanently frozen, ready for restoration whenever science mastered the technique of revivifying and restoring dead human beings. John Henry purportedly wanted to give his father "a new chance at life."[1]

Ted Williams's daughter, Bobby Jo Ferrell, went to court to try to prevent the cryonic disposition that her brother was arranging. She relied on a 1996 will in which Ted Williams had asked to be cremated, with his ashes to be scattered over the Florida Keys, where he had spent so many happy times fishing. Ms. Ferrell believed that her father had never wanted to be frozen. She claimed that her brother only wanted to preserve her father's DNA in order to sell it to baseball fan parents who dream of having sons capable of batting .400 in the major leagues.

Al Cassidy, the executor of Ted Williams's will, was happy to be guided by a court as to what to do in the face of the family dispute. He waited for a judicial hearing. John Henry, acting together with another sibling, Claudia Williams, produced a handwritten scrap of paper on which Ted Williams had in 2001 purportedly indicated a wish for a cryonic disposition. After a handwriting expert verified Ted Williams's signature on the note, Al Cassidy entered into a court-supervised agreement that allowed the body to be permanently frozen at Alcor. Bobby Joe Ferrell relented, not because she thought that her father had really wanted to become a frozen remnant (a corpsicle), but because she had no more money to contest the case. No one else sought to rein in John Henry Williams.

Ted Williams's corpse (or at least its head) is now suspended in a large metal cylinder at Alcor.[2] Far from the Florida Keys, he hangs in company with four or five other human remains suspended in the same cylindrical container in the same highly chilled atmosphere. In all, there are ninety-eight permanent residents at Alcor.

Many things about the story of Ted Williams's remains caught my attention. I wondered why I cared about the disposition of those remains. Death is death whether the body is buried, reduced to ashes, or frozen stiff. Yet my strong feeling was that the remains of Ted Williams should have been scattered over his beloved Florida Keys. I love warmth and sun and a tropical climate. I hate cold and ice. To me, Ted Williams would somehow *feel* better far from the Alcor freezer; I strongly identified his corpse with his former persona and its sensibilities. On the other hand, if a corpse could feel extreme temperature, had Ted really thought about being reduced to ashes at 1800 degrees Fahrenheit?

The Ted Williams story retriggered thoughts about related legal or quasi-legal issues. Which of the several interested parties really controlled the disposition of the corpse? The executor responsible for implementing the will? The son and daughter who believed that their father wanted to be frozen? The daughter who believed that he wanted to be cremated, as stated in his will? And even if someone could reliably discern Ted Williams's wishes, would those wishes be binding on the responsible parties? My stepbrother's wishes were modest, involving unusual accoutrements of an otherwise conventional cemetery burial. What if Ted Williams had indeed wanted cryonic disposition but his descendants believed that it was a futile waste of money, or sacrilegious, or just undignified? Would the responsible parties still be bound to implement his wishes even if the wishes were burdensome? What if Ted had wanted to have his corpse shot into space? In short, I continued to wonder about the legal principles governing the disposition of a human corpse, especially the question of self-determination concerning one's earthly remains. Can a corpse have legal rights? Is a corpse legally entitled to have prior instructions carried out? Or do the descendants of the deceased have their own right to govern the disposition of the human remains?

My research on cadavers was driven by more than jurisprudential questions. On a practical level I also wanted to know what range of dispositions is open to the persons who control the fate of human remains. This, in turn, meant learning what physical consequences accompany each means of disposal—including sepulture, cremation, cryonic freezing, and mummification. Somehow it matters whether a buried corpse retains its shape and form or is transformed into a moldy, shapeless, shrunken mass. Is corporeal disintegration inevitable, and at what pace does it occur? What is left after decomposition? Some people believe that the fate of human remains is irrelevant to a now-dead person, so they are indifferent about postmortem bodily transformations. I am not one of them. Somehow it mattered (and still matters) to me whether my cadaver would stay pristine after being laid to underground rest.

In writing this book I learned, as expected, a lot about both the physical fate of human remains and the legal rules that govern a cadaver's disposition. The surprising lesson, though, was the extent to which custom and law attribute a quasi-human status, a sort of quasi-personhood, to the cadaver. That finding led to the book's subtitle, *The Life and Times of the Human Cadaver*. The tendency of custom and law to give quasi-human status to the cadaver is reflected in various ways in the chapters. People's attribution of human feelings and/or a live presence to the cadaver (sometimes via a connected soul or spirit) is described in chapter 2. The law's bestowal of enforceable legal rights upon the cadaver is considered in chapter 3. The intimate association between a cadaver and its predecessor also accounts for the common expectation of dignified and respectful treatment of a cadaver.

The dignity and respect that a cadaver's quasi-personhood entails are suffused with human values, but they are different from the level of dignity accorded to the living. Chapters 9–12 examine the boundaries of what I label "postmortem human dignity." They discuss the extent to which postmortem human dignity limits the choices of both the person trying to shape his or her own postmortem fate and the people ultimately responsible for the disposal of the corpse. Surely a person can donate his or her body to scientific research aimed at human betterment, but can a person agree to becoming fodder for military or police units interested in measuring the effects of new weapons on human flesh? Can a person agree to have his or her corpse dehydrated, plasticized, and hung in a public exhibition? In other words, when does the exploitation of a cadaver become an intolerable offense to postmortem human dignity? A British surgeon named Richard Selzer once dictated: "Upon the wall of some quiet library ensconce my skull. Place oil and a wick in my brain-pan. And there let me light with endless affection the pages of books for men to read." He had a noble goal, but was Richard Selzer entitled to have a part of his corpse serve as a handy reading lamp? Or is it intrinsically undignified to make utilitarian, everyday uses of something as sacred as human remains?

Is it conceivable that people have unfettered control over the postmortem disposition of their own bodies and body parts? Aren't there some uses of human remains that are inherently repulsive and intolerable—such as necrophilia, cannibalism, other forms of ingestion? In 2007 Keith Richards, of Rolling Stones fame, said (though he later claimed that he was joking) that he had mixed his father's ashes with cocaine and snorted them. He was quoted: "I couldn't resist grinding him up with a little bit of blow. My Dad wouldn't have cared."[3] Does it matter whether a survivor who ingests part of a cadaver does so for therapeutic purposes, for titillation, or for symbolic absorption of the positive attributes of the deceased?

In the absence of premortem consent, can the corpse be exploited for reasons of medical knowledge, crime investigation, education, or public health? Could government confiscate body parts needed for transplantation to critically ill or injured people? Can entrepreneurs display cadavers in traveling exhibits aimed at educating the public or in works of art aimed at entertaining viewers? Is it acceptable to make a corpse a parent, as by extracting semen from a male cadaver or forcing a female cadaver to gestate a fetus to term?

Beyond the bestowal of various protections and rights, the quasi-human nature of the cadaver emerges in additional ways in this book. One is the tendency of people to seek perpetuation of their persona or memorialization of their lives by means of treatment of their remains. People sometimes seek to immortalize themselves by physical preservation of their remains, by expression in epitaphs, or by physical monuments (see chapter 6). Another human phenomenon that carries over to the postmortem context is socioeconomic differentiation. Cadavers, like living persons, have suffered racial and economic disadvantage in the accoutrements of funerals, in the locus of final disposal, and in the use (or nonuse) of grave markers (see chapters 5 and 6).

As I contemplated writing a book about the legal status of cadavers, I thought that many potential readers might share my fascination with people's postmortem fate. After all, under the constraints of today's medical science, every one of us will become a corpse. In 2010, it is projected, 7,200 deaths will occur in the United States every day. Therefore, many moribund patients and concerned loved ones will be deliberating the fate of human remains.

Of course there were contraindications about the breadth of the reading public's interest in cadavers. Despite the inevitable postmortem fate lying ahead of them, many people have a strong aversion to considering their own mortality. They prefer not to deal with the dying process, death, or disposition of human remains. Only about 20 percent of people sign advance medical directives covering the treatment or nontreatment of serious conditions they may face after they lose the mental capacity to make their own medical decisions. Only about 40 percent prepare a last will and testament governing the postmortem disposition of their property, even though that disposition may strongly affect estate taxes and other matters of survivors' well-being. A much smaller percentage of people leave instructions about the ultimate disposition of their corpses.

People also tend to have a strong aversion to a human corpse. This phenomenon seems to stem from more than natural revulsion at the sight and smell of putrefaction. The mere presence of a cadaver tends to cause extreme awe and discomfort. Survivors generally hasten to call a funeral director to collect a deceased's body and remove it to a funeral home. In May 2006, residents of an apartment house in Zurich complained bitterly that corpses were occasionally transported in a closed body bag in their building's elevator. (The corpses were being transported from an apartment owned and used by Dignitas, a Swiss group that assists suffering, seriously ill people to commit suicide.) No resident suggested that the odor or noise was disturbing or that the elevators were overcrowded. Some residents just couldn't stand the fact that a human cadaver might share the same elevator during descent to the ground floor. The expelled suicide-assisting organization ultimately found refuge adjacent to a house of prostitution, where the neighbors did not complain about nearby cadaver traffic.

The common aversion to corpses seemed to bode ill for sales of a book about the physical disintegration, assorted uses and abuses, and legal status of the human cadaver. A ray of light suddenly appeared for books about cadavers in January 2007 upon the untimely death of celebrity Anna Nicole Smith and the controversy about disposition of her corpse. Ms. Smith had never definitively expressed her wishes about the disposition of her remains. The executor of her estate (her former lawyer, lover, and putative father of her only living child) insisted that she wanted to be buried next to her beloved deceased son in the Bahamas. Supposedly Ms. Smith had even bought a double burial plot at the time she buried her son. Ms. Smith's estranged mother, her only adult kin, claimed that Ms. Smith should be buried in a family plot in her native Texas. Both sides conceded that—at least at one point in her life—Ms. Smith had expressed a wish to be buried near Marilyn Monroe in Los Angeles.

There it was—grist for the mill of this book. If only the book had been published by January 2007! What a chance to do the cable network shows! What an opportunity to become a high-paid legal consultant to one of the hard-pressed lawyers struggling to cope with the unfamiliar law of human remains! (A Florida appellate court ultimately upheld, as conforming to Ms. Smith's wishes, her burial in the Bahamas next to her deceased son.[4])

Yet it really did not matter to me that this 2007 media frenzy over a celebrity's cadaver generated great public interest in the disposition of human remains. I couldn't help writing a book about cadavers. I can't claim, as my Hoboken neighbor Mark Leyner did in a book called *Why Do Men Have Nipples?*, that even as a child I subscribed to the *Journal of the American Society of Investigative Pathology*. Nonetheless, my curiosity about corpses, along with my legal inquisitiveness, were driving me to explore the world (or afterworld) of cadavers. Issues such as the moral limits of self-determination in cadaver disposal were spurring my passion for cadavers (as a literary topic).

A word about terminology. The dead human has many names and nicknames—"corpse," "cadaver," "remains," "body," "stiff," "newly dead," "neomort," "loved one," "deceased," "departed," and "decedent," among others. Similarly, euphemisms are frequently used to ease the harshness of some of the terminology relating to dead humans. Polite people talk about "passing away" rather than "croaking." Some people prefer to say "recovery" of human organs for transplant rather than "harvesting." A pathologist may refer to the material oozing from a decomposed brain as "frothy purge." I do not subscribe to such delicacy. I use a variety of terms interchangeably to refer to the dead human—

usually "body," "cadaver," "corpse," or "remains." Occasionally I use more unsavory words, such as "cremains," as applied to human ashes. I mean no disrespect to the departed. I just prefer the freedom to use a variety of terms to describe the dead humans who occupy these pages. As a conciliatory gesture to the editors, though, I will henceforth refrain from using the term "corpsicle" in the context of cryonics.

The words "coffin" and "casket" are used interchangeably here. A coffin was originally a narrow, six-sided, wooden receptacle, wide at the shoulders.[5] That version of a burial container "nicely corresponded to the shape of the human form before the advent of the junk food era."[6] Starting in the 1850s, burial practice moved to the rectangular, hinged-cover box known as a "casket."[7] I use "coffin" and "casket" interchangeably, as is frequently done in modern parlance.

# Part I
# Status and Rights of the Cadaver

> As virtuous men pass mildly away,
> And whisper to their souls, to go,
> Whilst some of their sad friends do say,
> "The breath goes now," and some say, "No."
>
> John Donne, "A Valediction: Forbidding Mourning"

## Chapter 1

# When Does a Person Become a Corpse?

Important consequences hinge on when a person becomes dead, that is, reaches the point at which a moribund human officially qualifies as a corpse. The first impact is upon potential medical or quasi-medical intervenors. Doctors, nurses, and emergency personnel must decide whether to start pounding the flaccid body in an effort to resuscitate a person who is experiencing or has lately experienced cardiac arrest. Pathologists must determine whether the body will be dismantled and minutely examined—that is, whether an autopsy will be performed in order to seek information about the cause of death. (Even with sophisticated diagnostic tools, physicians are often uncertain about the physiological cause of the now-dead person's demise. An autopsy might provide important information about disease processes leading to better treatments, prevention, or cure of various diseases or conditions.) Medical personnel must also know whether it is permissible to open the inert body surgically and remove tissue for transplantation to desperately ill individuals or to exploit the body for general research and educational benefit. All utilizations of human remains are supposed to await an accurate pronouncement of death.

Death also determines when a body can be readied for ultimate disposition. When can a funeral director come and take the body away? When can a death certificate be prepared, and should the county coroner or medical examiner be notified in order to investigate a homicide or a suspicious death? Can the body now be embalmed? Should a memorial service or some other form of commemoration be prepared? Can final disposal of remains occur—whether by burial, cremation, or other means? Can the corpse's estate—meaning all property belonging to the deceased—be distributed? The determination of death also fixes the legal status of life insurance, Social Security and other survivors' benefits, personal credit, and marriage. The time of death can even determine the level of crime committed in the context of possible homicide. In *People v. Dlugash*, Melvin Dlugash fired four small-caliber bullets into Michael Geller after an accomplice, Joe Bush, had fired three large-caliber bullets into Geller.[1] Mr. Dlugash, despite having fired a bullet into the victim's brain, could only be convicted of *attempted* murder, not murder, because the prosecution could not show that Geller was still alive when Dlugash fired.

### Recognizing the Permanent Cessation of Breathing

Although we all know (or should know) that sooner or later we will become corpses, we do not necessarily know by what criteria that status will be measured. Nor do we know whether the prevailing criteria are dependable. Can we be sure that the determination of death will be made accurately? Can we avoid premature disposal of our bodies?

For millennia determination of death was an uncertain task, and live persons were sometimes treated as corpses. The legendary feather in front of the nose or mirror in front of the mouth did not always detect flickering life. John Donne's poem quoted above reflects the uncertainty of declaring death as late as the nineteenth century: "The breath goes now, and some say 'no'." An anonymous Victorian limerick goes:

> There was a young man at Nunhead
> Who awoke in his coffin of lead;
> "It was cozy enough"
> He remarked in a huff,
> "But I wasn't aware I was dead."

During the eighteenth and nineteenth centuries in the United States there were many tales of pallbearers tripping and falling, jarring the coffin, and prompting a vigorous reaction from the occupant. In 1894 Eleanor Markham "died" and her body was being carried to the cemetery in a coffin. A pallbearer sensed movement within the coffin. When the coffin was opened, Eleanor admonished: "My God! You are burying me alive!" There were even stories of putative corpses popping the top off their coffins after they had been lowered into a grave.

Other nineteenth-century misdiagnoses of death surfaced at the moment of autopsy. In May 1864 an autopsy was scheduled for a New York man who had died suddenly for unexplained reasons. With the first incision the "corpse" sat up and grasped the doctor's throat. The man recovered fully but the doctor died of apoplexy. In 1906 an Iowa man was undergoing an autopsy. When his chest was opened and the heart was touched, it began to beat at a normal rate. The man recovered. These were just some of the instances in which an autopsy revived the putative corpse instead of discovering a cause of death.

Sometimes the coffin occupant's activity came too late to avoid permanent disposal. On some occasions when a body was being disinterred (perhaps because of a descendant's decision to change the place of burial), corpses were found in positions that indicated that they had died of suffocation in their graves. Premature burial was signaled by signs of futile struggle and disarray of the body. For example, a body might be found sprawled outside of a coffin but still within its locked mausoleum. Or an exhumed body might be found in a very different position than at burial, with the shroud torn and apparent unexplained flesh wounds.

No doubt some of the reports about premature burial were erroneous. A contorted face observed at exhumation might well be attributable to rigor mortis or to other natural degeneration. Damage to corpses and coffins was "not incompatible with putrefactive postmortem changes or with wounds inflicted by rodents."[2] Noises and even movements of a coffin could be attributed to the gases that emerged during the course of bodily decomposition.[3] Yet books published in 1895 and 1905 purported to document hundreds of cases of premature burials or narrow escapes.

How could so many mistakes about pronouncing death occur? During much of the nineteenth century certification of death by a physician was not a prerequisite to disposition of a corpse. Sometimes an undertaker (who might be the same cabinetmaker who had made the coffin) or a lay relative claiming to have experience in assessing death would pronounce death. Numerous conditions might prompt such a lay observer to conclude mistakenly that death had occurred. Deathlike trances

or paralysis could stem from shock, apoplexy, epilepsy, coma, or cata-
lepsy, among other conditions. A heartbeat could be so feeble as to be
inaudible.

From the later nineteenth century on, people relied more and more
on physicians to pronounce death. In 1866 F. I. A. Boole, a lay health
inspector in Brooklyn, New York, was caught selling blank burial certificates that were used by murderers to conceal their crime. That was
an impetus for public authorities to require a physician's certification
of death in order to keep more careful track of who died, when, and
why.

Physicians themselves constantly sought improved techniques to
achieve accurate pronouncement of death. In 1784 a Belgian physician
suggested administration of tobacco smoke enemas, which was a technique adopted by the Dutch for a short period. There was no physiological rationale for the enema procedure unless the "pain and indignity of
having a blunt instrument violently thrust up one's rear passage might
have had some restorative effect."[4] During the nineteenth century physicians and others continued their search for more reliable indices of death.
In 1867 a British medical journal collected 102 suggestions for ways to
measure death more accurately. The most helpful tool turned out to be
the stethoscope. When it was introduced in the 1840s, the stethoscope
was a primitive and insensitive instrument made of wood. By 1883,
though, the considerably improved stethoscope made absence of a heartbeat a much more reliable index of death than previously.[5]

Whatever the actual number of deaths from premature burials, the
widespread perception in nineteenth-century America was that steps
could and should be taken to avoid that dismal fate. A variety of techniques were designed to prevent premature burial and accompanying
asphyxiation. The wake ritual meant "staying awake with the deceased
to make sure he or she was in fact dead."[6] Another nineteenth-century
technique for avoiding premature burial was to administer enough noxious stimuli to the putative corpse to wake any slumbering body. These
stimuli included needles jammed under toenails or into muscles, bugles
blasted into ears, wiry brushes rubbed over the body, boiling wax poured
on the forehead, and sharp objects shoved up the nose.[7] Another tool
was a pair of sharp tongs used to pinch the nipples of both male and female bodies. Some people placed provisions in their will that dictated

taking a precautionary step before burial, whether an incision, amputation of a finger, or application of boiling water. The writer Hans Christian Anderson, who died in 1875, had habitually kept a note by his bed that said "am merely in suspended animation."[8] But just in case his persistent optimism turned out to be misplaced, he also instructed that his veins be opened before burial.

Not surprisingly, extreme stimuli aimed at preventing premature burial sometimes proved counterproductive. One nineteenth-century Virginia family observed a custom in which the head of the family would plunge a knife into the newly dead relative. In 1850 the ritual caused such a pierced relative to scream and then die from the knife wound. Another counterproductive technique was to sever the neck arteries to ensure that the dead body stayed dead.

In ancient times, premature disposition of a body was also a concern. Romans and Greeks who disposed of corpses by burial believed that putrefaction was the only sure index of death, so they waited three or four days to make sure that the decay process had begun. As late as the nineteenth century, people in Europe and the United States used a similar technique—waiting for decomposition and stench to prove death. The Germans developed "waiting mortuaries," buildings where bodies were kept above ground in open coffins until unmistakable decay occurred. In the meantime, each corpse's hand was attached by string to a signal bell. Such mortuaries—featuring rows of putrefying corpses exposed to paying visitors—existed in Denmark and Austria in the second half of the nineteenth century.[9] Some American cemeteries of that period had "waiting houses" where corpses could be lodged for several days before burial.

Despairing of the existing capability of definitively pronouncing death, nineteenth-century inventors took numerous steps to allow false-positive cadavers to escape their premature underground home. The first step was to try to permit any awakened cadaver to signal from the grave. Pipes or tubes sometimes connected the buried coffin to the air above ground. Ropes were strung from the interior of the coffin (tied to the head, hands, and feet) to bells or rescue flags above ground. Of course, a rope would only be useful if a cemetery attendant happened to pass during the brief period when the awakened victim could still make sounds or movements.

The next step was to produce "security coffins" to keep the buried victim alive while facilitating escape from premature burial.[10] These inventions included devices for longer, more comfortable underground subsistence as well as for better communication. Some security coffins supplied light, a heater, and a telephone. In 1868 the New Jerseyan Franz Vester designed a coffin with a partial flip-open lid that led into a square shaft that further led to ground level.[11]

The notion of security coffins persisted for a surprisingly long time. Between 1868 and 1925, twenty-two American patents were issued for such devices. In 1899 a Russian nobleman presented his version of a security coffin during a lecture to the Medico-Legal Society of New York. The society was impressed enough to express its worry about premature burial and to endorse the Russian's escape coffin.[12] In the 1960s a wealthy Arizonan built a huge vault in a churchyard for his crypt. When he died in 1969 the steel doors to the vault were opened for several hours every night for twelve weeks. Onlookers gathered every night, to no avail. An attempted resurgence of security coffins, which featured a food locker, ventilating fan, chemical toilet, and shortwave radio, failed in the 1970s.

By the twentieth century the hazard of premature pronouncement of death was markedly reduced. State laws required physicians, rather than undertakers or embalmers, to certify death. Physicians were confident of their ability to verify corpsehood, and they scoffed at claims that people were still being buried alive. Also, starting in the 1880s, embalming became a frequent part of a funeral process. Draining blood from the body and substituting chemical preservatives ensured that those supposed cadavers were indeed dead.

All of this did not mean that mistakes in pronouncing death no longer occurred. Even in late-twentieth-century America, occasional reports surfaced of discoveries that death had been pronounced prematurely. In 1993 emergency medical service (EMS) personnel, as well as a medical examiner, declared a forty-year-old New Yorker dead following her severe drug overdose. Two hours later, as an autopsy was about to begin, she sputtered and regained consciousness.[13] A similar mistake by paramedics and a medical examiner occurred in 2001 in Massachusetts. This time the apparently overdosed corpse was heard rustling in a body bag at a funeral home.[14] Nursing home patients still occasionally "come to life" during or after transportation to a funeral home.[15]

## An Alternative to Heart Stoppage as the Definition of Death

The traditional measure of death—permanent cessation of heart and lung function—has served as a valid criterion to this day. Yet in the 1960s, with accurate medical assessment of cardiopulmonary death pretty much assured, a new issue emerged in pronouncing death. Medical technology had become capable of artificially sustaining heartbeat and breathing after a person's brain had completely ceased to function. Medical science, thanks to new immunosuppressive drugs, had also become capable of transplanting lifesaving organs from a newly dead person into a critically ill recipient. The problem was that an organ could be transplanted legally only after death had occurred, yet mechanical maintenance of heartbeat and breathing obstructed a declaration of death during the time that transplantable organs were still usable.

In the early 1960s transplant surgeons using traditional cardiopulmonary criteria were uncertain about when death could officially be declared for people who were attached to ventilators. If the surgeons kept insensate and brain-dead persons attached to machines until all breathing stopped, the vital organs deteriorated in the mechanically preserved body. Cell degeneration begins quickly after death and can impair or destroy harvestable organs and tissue.[16] Even if a dead donor's body is refrigerated, eyes must be removed within two hours of death; bones and heart valves within four hours; and blood vessels within six hours.

No one in the 1960s wanted to abandon the requirement that death be pronounced accurately before organ harvest. The "dead donor" principle was salutary in assuring potential donors that their death would not be declared prematurely by physicians just to facilitate organ recovery. By barring removal of vital organs until death, medical personnel could reassure donors that transplant would occur only when the donor had expired—that is, when he or she was totally immune to pain, unable to sense any surgical removal process, and incapable of recovery. But sole reliance on cardiopulmonary criteria for pronouncing death was wasting organs capable of salvaging potential recipients' lives. Physicians were understandably hesitant to salvage organs by detaching ventilators while the body still appeared to be functioning. They feared that they would be declared murderers if they removed a vital organ and detached machinery that was pumping blood and oxygen into a pink, ostensibly throbbing body. (Indeed, a number of criminals sought—unsuccessfully—to avoid homicide charges by claiming that the killer was not the accused who had delivered the vicious blows, but rather the physician who had disconnected the insensate crime victim from the life-extending medical machinery.)

By the late 1960s physicians were determined to end the approach to organ harvesting (from brain-devastated sources) that resulted in the unnecessary death of thousands of potential donees awaiting transplantation while suitable organs deteriorated in a brain-dead donor's still pink and warm body. They argued that death should be pronounced, and donated organs removed, at the point that the entire brain (including the lower part controlling only autonomic functions like regulation of body temperature) had permanently ceased to function. The thesis was that death meant the end of coherent function of the human organism as a whole. That point was reached, they said, upon cessation of all brain function even if a ventilator might be able temporarily to maintain respiration and blood circulation in what was essentially a dead body.

In 1968 a special Harvard University committee announced reliable ways, including the use of electroencephalograms (EEG), to measure the total cessation of brain activity. The formulation of reliable measurement criteria for whole-brain death allowed surgeons to harvest organs promptly after pronouncement of death according to the new criteria. Whole-brain death allowed pronouncement of death and efficient organ removal while the dead donor was still connected to machines that pumped oxygen to organs still fresh for transplantation.

State courts and legislatures quickly adopted whole-brain death as an alternative way to measure the death of a human organism. By 1981 the Uniform Declaration of Death Act (UDDA), a model law aimed at guiding future state legislation, approved whole-brain death as an acceptable alternative definition of death. The UDDA gave impetus to the movement to accept whole-brain death. This effectively meant that 98 percent of Americans would still have their deaths determined according to the traditional definition—permanent cessation of heart and lung function. A small percentage, those whose end-of-life care included maintenance on a ventilator, might have their deaths declared according to the Harvard whole-brain death criteria.

Physicians have largely (though not unanimously) accepted whole-brain death as an alternative way to measure a human being's demise. A problem of acceptance may arise for nonmedical people because a brain-dead body that is still connected to machines does not look dead; its heart beats, blood circulates, and respiration continues. Resistance to disconnecting a respirator may therefore come from family members who cannot accept that their pink, warm loved one with a still-heaving chest is now a corpse. The patient's representative (the next of kin is usually the patient's legal surrogate) may refuse to authorize detachment of medical machinery and disposition of the body. In most hospitals today, medical staff members try to explain gently to the resisting family that their loved one is in fact dead. Most families end up accepting the reality of death, sometimes taking time to say goodbye before the ventilator is disconnected from the still heaving body. If that acceptance does not come, hospital personnel typically explain that hospitals are health institutions rather than mortuaries, and that if the family does not arrange for disposition of their loved one's body, the hospital will detach the ventilator within a certain number of hours. That proclamation usually persuades still-resisting family members to start the process of disposing of the corpse.

Sometimes, though, an inconsolable family still believes that their heaving loved one, though totally and permanently lacking brain function, is alive and able to recover. They doggedly insist that the ventilator be kept in place, and they threaten to go to court or to the media to claim that the hospital's unauthorized detachment of a ventilator will kill their loved one—that is, will constitute homicide. The hospital knows that the "patient" is a corpse and that the hospital is no longer obligated to continue medical intervention. But the hospital also knows that a local newspaper headline saying that the hospital is killing a family's loved one despite the family's vigorous objections will harm the hospital's community relations. The hospital may therefore accommodate the family by keeping the corpse attached to a ventilator until the family arranges to preserve the ventilator-assisted body elsewhere—usually at a family member's home. The corpse then leaves the hospital still attached to machinery. Eventually, though, even machines cannot keep the heart pumping.

Occasionally the family's insistence on ventilator maintenance of their brain-dead loved one leads to litigation. Surprisingly, some judges do not have the courage to disappoint the overwrought family members. One such incident occurred in Utah in October 2004. Jesse Koochin was then a six-year-old with end-stage cancer and was being cared for at Primary Children's Medical Center in Salt Lake City. After the hospital's physicians pronounced Jesse dead by brain-death criteria, Jesse's father, Steve Koochin, insisted that "life support" be maintained because Jesse had previously recovered miraculously from what had seemed to be a fatal coma. Steve Koochin went to court to keep the hospital from discharging Jesse. Even though a Utah statute allowed a declaration of death according to "accepted medical standards," and even though whole-brain death is widely accepted as an alternative measurement of death, the judge issued an order that precluded detachment of life support and allowed an ambulance to remove Jesse for additional tests at home. Four and a half weeks later, his artificially maintained heart completely stopped responding.

Though physicians have accepted total brain death as a measure of death, some philosophers and bioethicists have been less satisfied.[17] They question the key assumption that total cessation of brain function and death of the whole human organism are virtually simultaneous. A twentieth-century limerick, though probably not composed by a bioethicist, expresses a similar theme:

> In our graveyards with winter winds blowing
> There's a great deal of to-ing and fro-ing,
> But can it be said
> That the buried are dead
> When their nails and their hair are still growing?

Forensic anthropologists dispute whether hair grows after death. They contend that it only appears to grow when the surrounding tissue shrinks. Nonetheless it has become plain that some lifelike events go on even after a person's brain has totally ceased to function. That is, the human biological organism, with its billions of cells, continues to live in some ways after total brain death.[18] The heart may continue to beat for as long as 20 minutes after a ventilator is stopped in a person whose brain has totally ceased to function. Sperm live on and can be harvested for up to forty-eight hours. Continued muscle reflexes may cause a corpse's hand to twitch or an eye to wink. The stomach may continue to digest. Hormone secretion and regulation of body temperature may continue. Total brain death still allows homeostatic functions like metabolism of food and excretion to be possible, at least with mechanical assistance.[19] Indeed, a pregnant corpse is capable of gestating a fetus and giving birth—in one instance, 107 days after brain death—with the help of continuing ventilator maintenance. In short, a corpse may temporarily continue to perform certain bodily functions even while its brain is totally and permanently inert.

The continuing cellular, hormonal, and electrical functions after total cessation of brain function prompt some bioethicists and philosophers to question whether total brain death is an accurate alternative definition of death.[20] They fear that a brain-death measure of death will be viewed simply as a gimmick to promote organ transplant programs. Despite these hesitations, the reality is that total brain cessation will continue to serve well as an alternative measure of death along with cessation of cardiopulmonary function. Given the complexity of the human organism and its 100 billion cells, there is no way to fix a *moment* of death. Time of death has always been an arbitrary point "within an overlapping segment of decreasing vital functions" and increasing cell death.[21] Death can be broadly defined as the permanent cessation of the integrated functioning of the human organism as a whole. Total cessation of brain function serves as a reasonable determinant of the permanent end of integrated bodily function. It is an operational definition of death that sufficiently mirrors human experience and understanding, despite the temporary persistence of some activities (such as digestion) beyond the end of brain, heart, and lung function. The end of life may have to be redefined at some future point—especially if stem cell manipulation becomes capable of restoring dead tissue—but the current alternative definitions seem intuitively correct and adequate for contemporary societal needs.

At various points in the 1980s and 1990s there was a philosophical push to redefine death according to a different element of brain function. The central notion was that the essence of life—awareness, knowledge, memories, and emotions—is contained in the upper brain. If the upper brain, the neocortex, permanently stops working, a person is insensate and can no longer relate to his or her environment. Therefore, the argument went, a human organism lacking neocortical function should be deemed dead even if the remaining brain stem could still control breathing, blood pressure, and body temperature. This approach meant that humans in a permanently unconscious state, totally lacking neocortical function and hence any ability to relate consciously to their environment, should be considered dead. Under a neocortical definition of death, a person could not insist in advance on being medically maintained on life support despite loss of upper brain function, nor could a surrogate insist on maintaining such life support. Also under this approach, the famous cases of Karen Ann Quinlan, Mary Beth Cruzan, and Teresa Schiavo would never have occurred. Opposition to detaching any of them from "life support" machinery would have been nonsensical, because these permanently vegetative (unconscious) people were already dead according to a neocortical definition of death.

This proffered redefinition of death—loss of upper brain function—has never been widely accepted and probably never will be. A human without neocortical function cannot think or feel, but the body can still cough, blink, swallow food, breathe spontaneously, and have circadian rhythms—all based on brain stem function. The body looks, feels, and sounds like that of a living person. The upper-brain-dead body would be subject to treatment like any other human corpse. That would permit organs to be harvested for donation and even gifting of the body or its parts for research and education. Before final disposal of a corpse with lower brain activity, some affirmative act to end spontaneous breathing might have to take place. Such acts to permanently still the very humanlike body and then bury it would be distasteful, if not repulsive, to many people. Today thousands of families continue to sustain permanently unconscious patients either by medical machinery or by artificial nutrition and hydration.[22]

As noted above, an upper-brain-based definition of death has never prevailed. Instead a permanently unconscious human body (with some remaining brain stem function) is still deemed to be a live person. Of course, status as a live person does not mean indefinite maintenance of ventilation or any other critical medical procedure. A permanently vegetative person is an extremely debilitated and diminished human who is almost always dependent on medical machinery to maintain life. That

life-sustaining medical intervention is controlled by a conscientious surrogate seeking to do what the now incompetent person would want to
be done if he or she was capable of deciding for him- or herself. Using
that approach, a surrogate can and usually does dictate removal of further life support from the permanently unconscious person. The surrogate knows that the vast majority of persons do not want to be preserved
artificially in a permanently insensate state. The vast majority of persons
regard a permanently unconscious existence as intrinsically undignified
or gratuitously burdensome for loved ones and prefer to be removed
from life support. This common preference is reflected in numerous
surveys and polls of persons who are asked to contemplate their own
postcompetence medical fates. Therefore, the surrogate's good-faith pro-
jection of the unconscious patient's wishes would normally result in a
decision to withdraw life support. A sensible surrogate decision maker
would insist on extended medical intervention for a permanently unconscious person only upon some indication that the person would prefer
that course.

The only deviation from this framework (in which a permanently
unconscious person is still a live person) surfaced for a brief period in
1995. It concerned anencephalic infants—babies who are born without
any upper brain function and who are unable to experience or interact
with the world around them. Though unaware of their environment,
anencephalic infants can still breathe, suck, excrete, and flail their arms.
They do not look or act like corpses ready for burial. In 1995 the American Medical Association's (AMA) Council on Ethics and Judicial Affairs
(CEJA) recommended in a report that anencephalic infants be treated as
a unique species without any interest in further life; their vital organs
would be subject to immediate harvesting for transplantation to save
other fatally stricken infants even though that surgical intervention
would end their permanently unconscious but live existence. However,
harvesting of vital organs from unconscious anencephalic infants actually constituted the killing of one person in order to save the life of another, which is a violation of the dead donor rule. In December 1995
CEJA shelved its proposal, saying that more had to be learned about the
diagnosis of anencephaly and the precise level of consciousness, if any,
of such infants. The anencephalic infant continues to be treated as a live
person. As in the case of other permanently unconscious persons, it may

be appropriate to end artificial life support and let anencephalic patients die, but it is not appropriate to treat them as already existing corpses whose vital organs can be immediately removed.

### Does Cessation of Heartbeat Have to Be Irreversible?

Bioethicists have recently made another fuss—in the context of organ recovery—about the appropriate moment for declaring death. This pending controversy relates to dying patients who are not connected to ventilators and whose deaths will be declared (and their organs harvested where appropriate consent has previously been secured) by traditional cardiopulmonary criteria. The claim (by a few bioethicists) is that current protocols for pronouncement of death preceding such organ recovery violate the dead donor rule—that is, that transplant surgeons might be killing organ donors by premature initiation of transplant procedures.

The background for this controversy is that organ procurement in the United States—relying primarily on cadavers pronounced dead by whole-brain criteria—has not supplied enough transplant organs to meet the critical demand.[23] Thousands of potential organ recipients die each year awaiting transplants. If organ harvest can take place promptly following cessation of cardiopulmonary function, many more potential organ donors become available. This organ-recovery technique is known as donation after cardiac death (DCD). These new potential organ transplant sources are sometimes called non-heart-beating donors (NHBD). To procure healthy organs following cardiopulmonary death, the surgical removal process must begin as soon as possible after death to limit ischemia and attendant organ deterioration.

The pending controversy surrounding DCD involves how quickly to begin the surgical procedure for organ removal. It is easy enough to determine when the moribund potential donor's heart has stopped. The issue is how long to wait before beginning surgery to see if spontaneous resumption of heart function might take place. American transplant centers wait between two and five minutes after measuring cessation of heartbeat to begin the transplant process. A 1997 protocol from the Institute of Medicine (IOM) declared five minutes to be the appropriate waiting time. Some transplant centers do wait for five minutes. However, a

2000 report from the IOM endorsed a shorter two-minute waiting period.[24] Protocols that guide the University of Pittsburgh and the Cleveland Clinic—famous centers for organ transplantation—prescribe a two-minute wait. Yet some critics insist that a two-minute wait is inadequate to rule out spontaneous regeneration of heart function and that an inert person whose heart might resume beating spontaneously is not yet dead.[25] For them, starting to harvest a vital organ two minutes after heartbeat and respiration have ceased can be viewed as a killing (if in fact the patient's heart might have revived on its own). Surgeons might be accused of actively causing death in violation of the dead donor rule by initiating a transplant procedure.

This criticism of DCD organ transplantation is unconvincing to me. It is unclear to what extent, if any, autoresuscitation after two minutes of heart stoppage is possible. At least one source contends that spontaneous resuscitation has never occurred more than sixty-five seconds after cardiac death.[26] But even if spontaneous regeneration of the heartbeat might occur more than two minutes after cessation, that should not necessarily preclude a valid medical pronouncement of death.

Irreversible cessation of heartbeat is not a prerequisite for a reasonable medical determination of death. The mere possibility of a later regeneration of heart function has never prevented a declaration of death—without regard to the matter of organ transplantation.[27] Many waning, terminally ill patients have Do Not Resuscitate (DNR) orders in place, which dictate that when their hearts stop beating, no further medical intervention takes place even if cardiopulmonary resuscitation (CPR) could have restored their heartbeat for a considerable period. In other words, completely irreversible heart stoppage has not been a precondition to a declaration of death. Patients and/or surrogates (in conjunction with physicians) may determine whether to take resuscitative steps to reverse an initial heart stoppage. And attending physicians do not have to wait for more than two minutes to pronounce death. "Outside the setting of organ donation, death is routinely, legitimately, and legally certified with the timescale of two minutes."[28]

Keep in mind that no single moment defines death and that medical determinations of death represent efforts to define the demise of the human organism as a whole. Even total brain death leaves certain homeostatic functions still possible, including metabolism of food; recall that a brain-dead pregnant woman can still, with mechanical assistance, gestate a fetus. Yet organ removal following total brain death is customarily deemed to be entirely appropriate.

Keep in mind also what is foregone when death is pronounced two minutes after heart failure. In the context of a terminal patient and DCD, physician conduct after two minutes of heart stoppage foregoes the possibility, probably slight at most, of brief restoration of heartbeat in a status that is dismal and unwanted by the patient/beneficiary. After cessation of blood flow accompanying heart stoppage, the brain sustains damage. Any dying patient who regained consciousness spontaneously after two minutes without heart function would likely survive only briefly and would be in a highly debilitated mental condition.[29] So the typical moribund patient would not want any regeneration—spontaneous or otherwise—of heart function more than two minutes after heart failure. And it is of little interest to the potential organ donor that some flicker of life might have rekindled (and then sputtered out) if only the transplant surgeon had waited another three minutes. It is reasonable to believe that the donor patient (or patient's representative) prefers the prompt action (organ removal) that will promote the success of the intended transplant.

It can be argued that undertaking a surgical process to remove a vital organ is a different form of conduct precluding heart regeneration than failure to undertake CPR. An affirmative act by a transplant surgeon ensures that spontaneous resumption of heartbeat will not take place. Yet the performance of such an affirmative act might not be a significant distinction for purposes of legal and moral responsibility in the case of a moribund patient.

Under current principles that govern end-of-life medical intervention, physicians who act in conjunction with patients and/or patients' representatives are entitled to take a variety of steps that hasten death (and forego extendable life). One example is authorized withdrawal of life-sustaining mechanical intervention, such as a respirator, that precipitates a patient's prompt demise. Another example is authorized administration of palliative substances, such as opioids or sedatives, that risk depressing respiration and thus accelerating death. Physicians are entitled to administer necessary analgesics to a moribund patient even though such an affirmative act might in fact accelerate a suffering patient's death. As a result of medical administration of palliative substances, "some patients who might have survived actually die."[30]

I suggest that a moribund patient's actual or putative wishes also govern decisions concerning possible resumption of heart function. This goes well beyond the DNR order already mentioned. Suppose that a moribund patient was seeking cryonic disposition of his corpse and had therefore ordered that his body be frozen two minutes after initial cessation of heart function. I am unaware of judicial precedent, but such conduct seems lawful to me, even if there was a chance that the heart (absent freezing) would have resuscitated spontaneously. Another instance of a justified medical step that possibly could foreclose extension of a life is a variation on the palliative conduct just mentioned. Suppose that a dying patient who has refused all nutrition and hydration also seeks a sedative to prevent discomfort during the dying process. Such a palliative step is almost surely lawful even though it renders the patient unable to change her mind and to request life-extending intervention. In short, a variety of circumstances permit a patient (or a patient's representative) to take steps that risk accelerating death. I suggest that another justified circumstance is a prompt declaration of death (that might prevent spontaneous, temporary heart regeneration) in order to improve the lifesaving chances of a scheduled organ transplant.

Death by cardiac criteria (as used in DCD protocols for organ transplant) do not seem to me to be incompatible with the dead donor rule. The rationale for that rule is to reassure potential organ donors that their death will not be declared prematurely. A potential donor (patient or family member) should not be daunted by a prospective declaration of death that precludes a tiny chance of temporary maintenance of a highly distasteful physical state.

In sum, a person becomes dead upon the occurrence of either of two related phenomena. Either the heart and lungs permanently cease to function or the entire brain becomes permanently inert. Both phenomena are reliable indices of the demise of a human organism as a whole, and both can be accurately measured. In either case, a corpse—a former person—then exists. Having defined corpsehood, our enterprise continues by examining the social and moral status of the corpse—the relation between human remains and the living world.

> A corpse in some respects is the strangest thing on earth. A man who but yesterday breathed and thought and walked among us has passed away. Something has gone. The body is left still and cold, and is all that is visible, to the mortal eye, of the man we knew.
>
> *Louisville Ry. v. Wilson*, 51 S.E. 24 (Ga. 1905)

> The mortal remains signify the history of that life in all its connections, especially with those to whom the person now dead was closely attached.
>
> Gilbert Meilander, Medical College of Wisconsin Listserv, 2006

*Chapter 2*

# The Human Nature of a Cadaver

Some people say that they don't care what is done with their corpse. After all, it is just inanimate waste—crow bait or fly bait, depending on how much shelter is provided to the cadaver.[1] Tell those people that their corpse will be tied to a jeep and dragged naked through the streets with a sign giving their name, after which their remains will be fed to the local farm animals. See if they are still indifferent to their postmortem treatment!

The vast majority of people seem to care whether their remains will be mutilated, desecrated, or treated with honor and respect. Yet how can posthumous events—including those involving mistreatment of human remains—harm or benefit the dead? The live person no longer exists and can no longer sense any violations of the corpse's integrity. One funeral director insists: "The central fact of my business [is] that there is nothing, once you are dead, that can be done *to you* or *for you* or *with you* or *about you* that will do you any good or any harm."[2] Why then do most people care so much about their postmortem treatment?

Dead people have a variety of personal interests that can be affected by posthumous events. While harm to a person's interests is ostensibly sensed only while the person is still alive, and while a decedent's interests may be asserted only by live persons such as an executor of a will or

*28*

a surviving relative, American culture and law rightly recognize post-mortem interests and even legal rights belonging to the corpse itself. (The next chapter focuses on those legal rights.) Social solicitude for these postmortem interests flows from the close association, both literally and figuratively, between the human decedent and his or her postmortem successor—that is, the cadaver.

Perhaps the most obvious surviving interest is fulfillment of a decedent's wishes. In essence, a person's interest in self-determination extends to prearranging events that will only occur postmortem—an interest I call "prospective autonomy." This autonomy interest is recognized in the venerable tradition enforcing a person's premortem wishes (as expressed in a will) in the postmortem disposition of that person's property. People frequently leave testamentary instructions about the disposition of their property in the hope and expectation that these instructions will be implemented, and every state maintains a probate system for such implementation. Prospective autonomy applies as well to issues affecting the fate of human remains, including means of disposition. (Recall the putative wishes of Ted Williams and Anna Nicole Smith regarding disposal of their remains.) As chapters 3, 7, and 9 explain, prospective autonomy influences the fate of human remains not just as to mode and place of disposal, but also as to utilization of cadaver parts for research, teaching, transplantation to needy recipients, or even reproduction.

The postmortem interests and rights of a cadaver extend well beyond fulfillment of the decedent's instructions or preferences. Even if a decedent expresses no wishes about postmortem treatment, his or her cadaver receives a variety of entitlements and protections. Chapter 3 describes entitlement concepts such as decent disposal of a cadaver, quiet repose, and postmortem human dignity. "Corpses may still be honored or outraged, exalted or vilified, reverenced or debased."[3]

Before we examine the scope of postmortem protections, however, let us consider the humanlike attributes that have earned a quasi-human protected status for cadavers. The human associations of the cadaver start with its physical and temporal connection to a decedent; the cadaver represents the continuing embodiment of a particular human being. People who have died "were loved, are loved, were bodies, are bodies."[4] The cadaver is the vessel that held a unique person and is still the most tangible manifestation of its human predecessor. "Everything tangible that is human is present in our cadavers. Their dead body parts are structurally identical to our living ones. Our cadavers are undeniably human."[5] Additional commonalities between cadavers and their predecessors contribute to the quasi-human stature accorded to cadavers.

## Appearance and Identity

In external appearance as well as in material composition, a fresh corpse looks very much like its human source. At death, skin tone changes somewhat as cessation of blood flow in capillaries creates a paler appearance. As blood settles downward in the corpse, its underside also becomes mottled in red and purple shades. Such discoloration, however, is later eliminated in the embalming process (which includes draining blood from the body). Even weeks and months after death, the face of an embalmed corpse is readily identifiable as that of its predecessor.[6] Medical students dissecting a corpse in an anatomy lab acknowledge the humanity of their charge by affectionately attaching a name or nickname. Only toward the end of a months'-long dissection process does the face become unidentifiable.[7]

Survivors recognize the remaining human aura of the recently deceased and continue to identify the cadaver with its predecessor persona, the deceased. D. Gareth Jones and Maja I. Whitaker comment: "We consider that a person and his body are inseparable. . . . While this applies supremely during life, some very important aspects of identity continue following death. . . . While the body retains a recognizable form, even in death, it commands the respect of identity."[8] The cadaver's continuing identification with the deceased helps explain the phenomenon of viewing the corpse, whether in private or at an open-casket wake. The viewing of the corpse, with its face and hands exposed, has long been an important "ritual moment" in the disposal of the dead.[9] The function of a viewing is apparently to facilitate leave-taking—"closure" in modern parlance.[10] "A brief, intimate moment with the dead—looking at the face, touching the casket, being in the presence of the corpse for a short time— is an ingrained ritual gesture that brings meaningful . . . order out of the chaos of death."[11] Mourners sometimes say that "because [the loved one] looked dead, I was ready to let go."[12] Of course, the degree of "viewing" varies widely according to ethnic, family, or religious traditions, but an open-casket wake is not unusual. Even when no public display of the cadaver is anticipated, some family member may want to view and/or touch the remains, either as a parting gesture or as confirmation that death has occurred and mourning is appropriate.

Given the continued identity of a cadaver, a funeral director is sensitive to preserving its human appearance. This is so even with violent crime or accident victims. If trauma has mangled or badly disfigured a corpse, the first task of a mortuary may be to restore the contours and image of a human body. Large holes (from a gunshot or car part) are filled with wax or cloth, and the areas are shaped to their former contours.[13] Missing body parts are replaced by shaping clay, plaster, wax, or wire mesh; these "prostheses" can be colored to match the body or covered by clothing. A jaw can be reconstructed with wax and plaster of paris. Missing ears are replaced with replicas. A decapitated head is restored to its rightful place secured by a stick sharpened on both ends and by stitches sewn between the reconnected parts. Some cadavers, whose circulatory systems have been wrecked by fire or trauma, are beyond repair and beyond arterial embalming; they can only be combined with preservative chemicals in a body bag.[14]

Especially when an open-casket wake or funeral is contemplated, efforts are made to maximize the cadaver's aesthetic appeal. Part of a funeral parlor's function (as fans of *Six Feet Under* are well aware) is to restore a "peaceful, pleasant appearance."[15] A prolonged dying process or virtually any terminal condition may have created a gaunt facsimile of the original person's face. The embalmer (or an associate) then works to create "the sculptured image of a living human body who is resting in sleep."[16] The embalming process is detailed in chapter 4. Suffice it to say here that the restoration effort involves the use of cosmetics, putty, ice packs, gravity, and prosthetics. The end product is less discolored, less wrinkled, and more healthily tinged than the original cadaver. It may not be true that the deceased "never looked better," as is sometimes exclaimed in front of an open casket, but the deceased almost certainly looks younger, less wan, and less shriveled than at the moment of death. The serene, peaceful expression may or may not be natural, but the appearance following restoration certainly reinforces the human aura of a corpse.

## Sentience and Feelings of the Corpse

The humanlike nature of a cadaver is reflected in the common phenomenon of attributing human feelings and reactions to it. Especially in the period soon after death, when the corpse still bears a striking resemblance to the living person, it is easy to continue identifying the body with its former occupant even to the point of attributing to it continued physical and emotional awareness. This powerful tendency to anthropomorphize the cadaver is expressed in many ways.

Often observers at a viewing treat the decedent's remains as capable of physical and emotional feelings. At an open-casket wake, many people approach the exposed cadaver. Kissing the departed is a frequent gesture. Some people caress and speak soothingly to the laid-out corpse. Others lower their voices in the presence of the body, as if not to wake or disturb it. Conversations with the corpse may continue for some period, including at the graveside, as the mourners find it difficult to treat the remains as mere inanimate matter. Eulogies at funerals or memorial services are often addressed not only to the mourners but also to the recently departed. "You will be missed," the speaker intones toward the casket.

Anthropomorphization of a cadaver extends to physical pain. Observers' attribution of pain to the corpse may go on "as if the remnant of the body in continuing to occupy space/time continues to suffer in space/time."[17] When a surviving family member is asked to grant permission for an autopsy (involving making incisions, taking tissue specimens, and thoroughly probing the corpse), a not unusual response is that the decedent has "suffered enough." Or a family granting permission for an autopsy may ask the pathologist to "be gentle." A similar aversion to surgically opening and probing a corpse may inhibit organ donation. Some people contemplating their own postmortem organ donation express antipathy to being cut up after their death on the basis that the experience will somehow be painful. And some survivors in control of a corpse's fate may share that assumption and therefore withhold consent for organ transplant.

Fledgling medical students can be subject to the tendency to attribute pain to a human cadaver. In an anatomy lab, the initial dissector may be "surprised when the body does not flinch or cry out when cut."[18] Fellow students observing the process may have an urge to place a hand on the cadaver's arm and reassure the prone figure that the incisions will hurt only for a while.[19]

The tendency to attribute pain and other feelings to the corpse often surfaces in the context of final disposition of human remains.[20] When cremation emerged as an American mode of body disposal in the late nineteenth century, mourners witnessing the process screamed in vicarious pain and horror as their loved one was placed on the red-hot burners.[21] The tendency to think about a human corpse as a sentient entity also applies to modes of disposition other than cremation. That is, people's varied preferences for the mode of disposition of their remains are often guided by projected visions of the comfort of the cadaver. Assessment of belowground burial may be influenced by thoughts of the coldness of the grave or the presence of maggots or other disturbances to the physical integrity or restfulness of the body. A common attitude is that foul weather will cause underground suffering.[22] The tendency toward the use of an aboveground mausoleum is inspired in part by negative images of the consequences of belowground burial. A coffin may be selected for its thick interior padding, as if comfort matters to the corpse. One man demands to be buried on his right side because he always sleeps most comfortably in that position. Another dictates that he be buried naked and face down—the way he sleeps best.[23] A woman once dictated that she be buried with a television set pretuned to her favorite station. (If her corpse was going to be animated enough to enjoy watching television, couldn't it change the channel itself?)

Just as people attribute physical pain and suffering to human remains, they also attribute emotional reactions. Survivors who consider the means of disposal may speculate about the corpse's prospective response to its resting place.[24] A family choosing a cemetery plot may note how much "Dad will love the view of the mountains from here" or may worry that "Mom will be upset" if she is buried next to one of her hated relatives. "We still endow a lifeless corpse with the capacity for feeling hurt."[25] If cadavers are deemed to be capable of experiencing their posthumous treatment, it is no wonder that live people associate cadavers with humanity and care so much about that treatment.

## The Quasi-Human Spiritual Connections of Human Remains

A common religious or cultural precept is that a cadaver and/or its resting place have a role in perpetuating a spiritual presence that succeeds and stays with the human remains for a period. Many religions believe in "a strong tie between body and personality/soul for an undefined period of time after death."[26] Beliefs vary as to how long a spiritual presence is deemed to remain with the corpse. Rabbinic lore contends that the soul remains associated with the cadaver for three days.[27] The precise linkage between body and spirit may also be murky. It is not clear whether a spiritual presence hovers nearby or is somehow embedded in the physical remains.

The precise form or duration of the spirit–body linkage does not matter. The idea that a personal spiritual force stays for a period with human remains helps account for people's special solicitude toward a cadaver and attribution of a quasi-human status to the remains. At one stage of British jurisprudence in the Middle Ages, an accused murderer was brought close to the victim's body in the hope that the corpse (or its lingering spiritual presence) would exhibit some reaction incriminating the accused.[28] The soul or spirit may be metaphysical or fleeting in nature, but it and its associated human remains still relate to a particular human being and may help humanize and create solicitude toward a cadaver. People may not be sure about the composition of a returning spirit, but even if it is not formed from human materials, it is likely to be projected as bearing the physical appearance of the departed. That is, the physical characteristics of the decedent (in the minds of survivors) likely shape any "imaginary personal identity in the afterlife."[29] This link in appearance to a spiritual successor may reinforce a tendency to attribute personalized, humanlike qualities to a cadaver.

Some religions posit ultimate reanimation and/or reembodiment of a human cadaver—a belief that the life of the body "can somehow persist or be restored."[30] For such believers, maintenance of posthumous bodily integrity is important because mutilation of the corpse may cause disability or disfigurement in the next cycle of existence. Orthodox Jews, for example, believe in revivification upon the future coming of a messiah. For them, bodily integrity of the corpse is important for reawakening in bodily form. They therefore have a strong aversion to cutting a corpse

open. Numerous New York cases deal with Orthodox Jews seeking judicial intervention to prevent an autopsy or to collect damages for
unauthorized removal of body parts from a decedent. Other religions,
including Hinduism and Greek Orthodoxy, share this aversion to
autopsies.[31]

According to some religious or cultural beliefs, the bodily integrity
of a corpse may be important not for reappearance on earth but rather
for entry into an entirely different domain. Many who believe in an afterlife in a different world care mightily about the disposition of the
corpse, both while still in its initial resting place and while undergoing
an anticipated voyage or transition to a supernatural setting. The ancient
Egyptians believed that after death the spirit of the deceased would return to reclaim the body and then journey with it to an unworldly domain. It was important to preserve a cadaver's image so that the spirit
would recognize its body at the time of rendezvous.

For cultures that view the body or spirit as embarking on a journey
to a new domain—whether to a heavenly abode, a spiritual world inhab-
ited by ancestors, an earthly reincarnation, or a new world in which the
dead are ultimately resurrected—the dead have continuing needs. Not
surprisingly, then, many cultures over time have placed provisions in
tombs, burial chambers, mausoleums, graves, or caskets as needed to
sustain the body or soul on its journey.[32] Supplying "grave goods" is a
practice at least eight thousand years old.[33]

Food is an obvious need for long-distance travelers, and many cultures provided nutritional sustenance for the dead on their expected
journeys.[34] Egyptian tombs contained grain stores; other peoples merely
filled their corpses' mouths with grain. Still other peoples anticipated a
certain amount of initiative on the part of the departed. Fishing gear
(bone hooks but not spinning reels) has been found in Siberian graves
seven thousand years old and with Chilean mummies five thousand
years old.[35]

A traveling spirit requires more than food. Some cultures provided
coins so that the dead travelers could pay off anyone who sought to
obstruct their journey. The Chinese placed a coin in the corpse's mouth,
as did pre-Christians providing fare for Charon, the boatkeeper at the
River Styx. Some cultures supplied the corpse's grave with a walking
stick. Russians provided a certificate of good conduct to facilitate entry

to heaven.[36] All these items were intended to facilitate the postmortem journey.

Other items were supplied upon burial in order to assure the protection, happiness, and quality of existence of the departed body or spirit upon reaching the next world.[37] Furniture, jewelry, tools, medications, pets, and weapons all fall into this category (though some of the items would also be useful during the journey to the afterworld). Sometimes companionship was provided. Females were thought to be useful to males' comfort in the afterworld to provide company, perform chores, and provide sexual gratification. The Romans provided one dead woman for every ten dead soldiers.[38] Comanche Indians buried a dead warrior's favorite wife and favorite horse with him. Until 1829 in India, a Hindu wife was supposed to be part of her husband's funeral pyre, even if that had to be accomplished by force.[39] (This "suttee" practice was sometimes rationalized as sparing the widow her inevitable desolation or as alleviating her son's financial burden.)

American practice has never provided much in the way of accompaniment or material accessories in crypts or caskets. No one can be killed in order to facilitate another person's postmortem comfort. Murder is murder even if the motive is to provide companionship or comfort for a deserving cadaver. Occasionally devastated surviving spouses or loved ones have committed suicide and have been buried next to their mate, but that is hardly the same as homicide in order to meet a deceased person's supposed postmortem needs. Nor is personal wealth commonly interred with its owner (though it may not be unusual to bury someone wearing jewelry). A testamentary directive to inter expensive jewelry or other valuables would not be enforceable. Such dictates are deemed to violate public policy because they might lead to the desecration of cemeteries. On occasion, burying valuables with a corpse led to spoliation of graves and was abandoned as a futile enterprise. In short, the popular admonition that "you can't take it with you" is essentially accurate according to American custom.

This is not to say that Americans never provide accessories to the dead. Usually, though, this is done as a sentimental gesture—burying the deceased with some formerly meaningful object—rather than as outfitting the corpse for the next world. Ulysses Grant had his horse buried with him. People have been buried seated in their car or in a coffin within a buried car. People have specified that they be interred with a television or a stocked bar to ward off anticipated boredom.[40] Survivors have been known to place a provolone cheese in the casket of their beloved cheese-loving departed — presumably as a sentimental gesture.[41]

Sentimental survivors often slip a teddy bear or some other keepsake into the coffin of a loved one. They should be careful in stowing items. On one occasion, bereaved golfing friends of a now-deceased golfer lifted the coffin cover and surreptitiously slipped in a couple of golf balls. When attendants later lifted the coffin, they were shocked to hear something bouncing around inside. They lowered the casket, opened it, and found the offending balls. This resulted in embarrassment and delay in the trip to the cemetery.[42] To avoid such mishaps, casket companies provide drawers for sentimental items like golf balls, cigars, rosaries, or cell phones.[43]

The Christian image of an eternal afterlife in heaven entails, for many believers, a need for posthumous bodily integrity. Early Christians believed that the soul or spiritual self would eventually reunite with the corporeal being in some heavenly state.[44] Bodily integrity would apparently facilitate this reunion of soul and body. Between the sixteenth and twentieth centuries, anatomists who dissected bodies for ostensibly worthwhile purposes like medical education were reviled by many Christian observers who believed that anatomists were destroying the integrity of human remains destined for a better fate.

Christian attitudes toward the sanctity of a cadaver have varied over time. Some sects viewed bodily remains as inconsequential to a postmortem spiritual domain.[45] In America, the Puritan colonists did not put much emphasis on the continuation of physical remains. For them the cadaver was essentially a "meaningless husk" to be disposed of quickly because divinely restored bodies would be sufficient for any heavenly sojourn, regardless of their postmortem physical condition.[46] Postcolonial Protestants in the United States, though, generally did feel extreme solicitude for a corpse in the belief that the soul would later be reunited with a miraculously reanimated physical body.[47]

Religious solicitude for a cadaver's continuing well-being in an afterlife does not account fully for people's widespread preoccupation with postmortem bodily integrity. Religious belief in an afterlife tends to accept a divine power to reconstitute a disintegrated human form in due time. Even a corpse pulverized in an inferno like that of 9/11 could, according to most religious precepts, be reconstituted by miraculous intervention. Nonetheless, intuition or instinct perhaps tells people that postmortem re-formation of a humanlike form is easier if corporeal integrity is present. At a ceremony I attended honoring a departed colleague, the person interring the ashes employed a container (rather than mingling the ashes with dirt) expressly to facilitate any conceivable reincarnation.

One does not have to be religious to wonder about an afterlife and to be concerned about the continuing status and integrity of human remains. Though organized religion may be declining in America, belief in life after death remains robust. For most Americans, "the cemetery is not the end of the line; it is the gateway to some other realm, however ill-defined."[48] "Afterlife beliefs lie just beneath the skin of many avowed secularists."[49] The fate and status of a corpse and/or its spirit are, after all, a subject of human uncertainty. No one knows whether there is a postmortem future for the body and the soul. Many people, even skeptics, would still like to think that there is a chance for some sort of afterlife. This uncertainty and ambivalence surrounding the cadaver help impel protection of a cadaver's well-being. Gary Laderman comments: "[A corpse's] uncertain status—as an empty container for the newly departed spirit, as an evocative representative of the lost loved one, as a highly charged object of reflection and remembrance, and as a decomposing, unstable cadaver—contributes to the deliberate, careful handling by the living survivors."[50]

Another concomitant of uncertainty about the postmortem status of human remains (and a possible spiritual presence) is fear and awe. Part of this dread may relate to offensive smells, putrid emanations, and even contagion.[51] (Before the development of antiseptics, putrefying human remains did cause infections.) Further fear relates to the possibility of unfriendly influences from the grave.[52] This fear stems from the ancient belief that a person's spirit is present at the grave and is ready to wreak havoc if the remains are not treated properly. Horror movies have, for many decades, played on phobias about cadavers by portraying zombies, ghosts, vampires, or other fearful manifestations of the dead. If the dead can return, an inscrutable power is lodged in the cadaver. Survivors who anticipate interaction with the departed have an incentive to cater to the assumed needs of the corpse in order to ensure that the spiritual force remains positive and friendly. In short, fear of cadavers and their humanlike emanations plays a role in shaping some attitudes toward the dead, including the attribution of quasi-human status.

## Preoccupation with the Decedent's Image and Identity

Even if one's belief structure rejects any postmortem spiritual presence within or about a cadaver, there is another enduring, intangible humanizing element surrounding a cadaver. Survivors retain a lasting memory picture—a human image—drawn from a decedent's lifetime behavior, beliefs, and character. The association of that retained image with the cadaver helps explain why people care so much about the fate of its remains. It also helps explain how cadavers have earned a quasi-human status.

An enduring image is a legacy of a decedent no less than the instructions and distributions contained in a will. Every human constructs a personal identity and an image that are projected to the world. Part of that personality and image is visual—stemming from the person's physical appearance and actions. Part of that image is emotional—involving impressions and feelings associated with the character and conduct of the deceased. Religious beliefs are part of that character image, along with various other beliefs associated with the person.

For many people, a lifetime image is cultivated at least in part in contemplation of making a postmortem mark on the world. The intention is to construct a favorable memory picture that will endure postmortem and be appreciated by survivors. Defilement of a corpse or any denigration of the personal identity and character associated with that corpse can taint a lifetime's image. This preoccupation with lifetime image explains why my stepbrother prescribed a funeral that would be fully "in character." Even if cadavers cannot sense the actual violation of a lifetime's legacy, their image and identity are things they have worked to establish that can be harmed. Postmortem harm to the reputational interests of the corpse is no less than that which would exist if the deceased's property were distributed in a way that was contrary to the deceased's preferences.

Harm to the memory picture that a decedent has constructed is most obviously experienced by survivors. Friends, family, and well-wishers of the late person are angered by what they perceive as insults to the departed. For example, desecration of a loved one's grave typically provokes outrage about the offense to remains held sacred by the survivors. Witness the strong reactions of surviving family members to the revelation in 2009 that cemetery workers in Alsip, Illinois, had systematically moved and dispersed human remains in order to resell the original cemetery plots.[53]

Any postmortem betrayal of the deceased's lifetime beliefs also provokes survivors' upset. For example, in *Lott v. State of New York*,[54] a hospital mixed up the corpses of two patients—one Jewish and one Catholic—so that the corpse of an Orthodox Jewish woman ended up embalmed, lying in an open coffin with a crucifix and rosary draped on her body. The Jewish family expressed shock and upset and recovered damages for emotional harm due to the gross violation of the deceased's religious heritage. The Catholic family was extremely disturbed to receive a strange woman's corpse wrapped in a shroud; they also recovered damages.

The harm to the deceased person's image and identity from posthumous mistreatment extends beyond the realm of the shocked survivors. Any treatment of a corpse that violates the religious or personal precepts of the decedent constitutes a harm of sorts to the decedent's personal interests. People while still alive certainly care about their prospective legacies, including their posthumous image and reputation. There may be uncertainty that postmortem fate can actually be experienced, but the postmortem interest of the deceased in preserving their memory picture is harmed by any betrayal of their beliefs. Ms. Lott's family objected that the handling of her corpse according to the rites of another religion violated her religious preferences, not just their own. Arguably, someone who believes passionately in integration is injured by burial in a segregated cemetery.

Public authorities have long sought to exploit the common human preoccupation with postmortem images and events. Governments sometimes made the disposition of wrongdoers' corpses distasteful and dishonorable in an effort to deter undesirable conduct. The underlying assumption was that people cared so much about their life image as reflected in their corpse's treatment, or so much about projected disturbance to their corpse's repose, that they would conduct their lives in such a way as to avoid that fate. As it was widely believed that denigration of corpses could be experienced in the afterlife, it is not surprising that public authorities thought that the miscreants themselves (or at least their spirits) could be punished by public humiliation of their human remains.[55]

In the context of criminal sentencing, many countries for centuries used the disposition of the criminal's corpse as one element of punishment—as an expression of public outrage and as a glaring warning to prospective wrongdoers. It was not enough to publicly execute a criminal (sometimes by horrific means, such as drawing and quartering by horses pulling in opposite directions). In England, starting in the Middle Ages, the corpses of executed prisoners were publicly gibbeted. This involved treating the body with tar to slow the rotting process and then suspending it in an iron cage to decay gradually and be picked apart by birds of prey and insects. Some gibbeted bodies hung for years until they were reduced to skeletons.

In 1752 England added public dissection as another possible mode of postmortem degradation of the corpses of executed criminals. After being removed from the gallows, the corpse of the executed criminal was turned over to a "surgeon" for public dissection and anatomizing. This process entailed publicly slicing open, disemboweling, and dismembering the corpse. Dissection was supposedly an important learning tool for students of anatomy, including artists, physicians, and surgeons, who could view actual physical specimens rather than drawings or facsimiles. At the same time, the anatomizing created a disgusting and degrading public spectacle. The stench of the body spilling excretions, internal organs, and possibly contagious fluids added to the revulsion from this profanation of human remains. In 1784 Massachusetts made public dissection of the corpse a possible means of disposition for slain duelists, not just executed criminals. The duelist's cadaver could either be buried without a coffin (but with a stake driven through its heart) or delivered to a surgeon for dissection and anatomizing. In 1789 New York State law gave sentencing judges discretion to add dissection to any death sentence.

A similar effort to deter lifetime conduct by mistreatment of a corpse concerned the disposition of suicides' corpses. Suicide was an abominable act according to British and European tradition. In England the primary deterrent to suicide was the Crown's expropriation of all property owned by the late suicide. Another disincentive was denial of an honorable burial. Until 1823 the firm custom in England was to refuse burial in consecrated grounds (churchyards) and to bury the suicide's corpse at night at a crossroad with a stake driven through the heart. (The purpose of the stake was to disable the prospective spirit; the burial at a crossroad was done to confuse the spirit if it managed to rise.) After 1823 the consequence of suicide was both forfeiture of all property to the Crown and handing over of the corpse to a medical school for dissection. That practice continued for fifty years.

Some authorities envisioned other mistreatments of cadavers as timely deterrents. In Russia in the early eighteenth century, Peter the Great had the head of an unfaithful mistress immersed in a jar of alcohol and placed in his bedroom as a not so subtle message to other mistresses.[56] He did the same with the head of his wife's lover, though the final resting place for that head was presumably her bedroom, not Peter's.

We cannot know or measure the deterrent effect of the distasteful disposition of corpses on some wrongdoers. But in the context of disposition of the corpses of suicides, there are stories about purported impacts. Supposedly waves of suicide were countered and successfully quelled in both England and France by the public announcement that, following suicide, the corpse would be dragged naked through the streets. If true, these stories demonstrate that the messages flowing from undignified disposition of corpses can indeed create enough anxiety to affect the conduct of the living.

The harm of postmortem degradation can extend beyond injury to a decedent's image and character. I have pointed out the uncertainty surrounding the postmortem fate of a human soul or spirit. While emotional harm from injury to a corpse's lifetime image is most obviously felt by the survivors, at least some people believe that a spiritual presence associated with a corpse is aware of offense to that image and actually experiences injury. This possible impact further explains why mistreatment of a corpse could deter proscribed behavior.

## The Benefits of Having a Quasi-Human Nature

The humanlike attributes and connections of a cadaver have resulted in social treatment of the cadaver as an entity worthy of special respect. The Anglo-American tradition is one of reverential treatment of the human corpse. The sanctity of human remains was not only a religious precept but also an element of law and custom. Law and custom accepted that a cadaver had been a person, still bore a strong resemblance to that person, constituted a tangible symbol of the lifetime image/identity of that person, and therefore deserved to be treated with appropriate "human" dignity even though it was no longer a person. I call the ensuing entitlement "postmortem human dignity."

This postmortem dignity required at least a modicum of protection against mistreatment of the corpse. A legal duty existed at common law—at least on the part of the next of kin or anyone in whose house a person died—to give every corpse a "decent" burial. That duty was partially impelled by public health concerns, but the requirement of a decent burial carried an element of inherent respect for the human remains. (Application of the principle of a decent burial was uneven, as later examination of potter's fields and other public indignities will show.) Another aspect of postmortem dignity was quiet repose. Even a formerly despised individual was entitled to decay in peace, and his or her corpse was protected against desecration. Any mistreatment of a cadaver "contrary to common decency" was a civil or criminal offense.

Today the impulse toward respectful treatment of human remains is still strong. "All of America's ethnic, religious, and cultural communities, regardless of class, share at least one conviction . . . respect for the dead."[57] That customary attitude of respect for the dead extends to numerous contexts. Hospital protocols for the handling of corpses customarily seek to create an atmosphere of respect and dignity for the newly dead. The mandatory nursing steps include washing, positioning, and improving the appearance of the corpse (by closing the eyes and jaw) and ensuring privacy. Mortuary workers, as they prepare a corpse for final disposition, are supposed to maintain a similar attitude of respect for the departed. Respectful predisposal rituals like a wake, a memorial service, and a disposal ceremony are customarily conducted around the newly dead. Even without ritual, anyone participating in the disposal of human remains is expected to maintain a respectful stance. As at common law, abuse of a corpse continues to be both a civil and a criminal offense under state law. In short, American public policy still treats a human corpse as a special entity entitled to be treated with a basic level of respect and dignity.

Postmortem human dignity is not identical to the human dignity applicable to living persons. For example, it is legally permissible (though very bad form) to libel a corpse with false accusations. The bottom line, though, is that the quasi-human nature of a corpse gives it enforceable legal protections. On to the legal status of human remains.

The postliving have too long been accorded casual treatment. . . . Their names are dropped from voting lists, they are no longer able to apply for or receive credit, and their pension and social security checks are ruthlessly cut off. . . . This treatment is clearly unjust. Why should a change of life status render individuals who had recognized rights into a class of those whose rights now go unprotected?

> Cynthia Kirchoff-Charles and Susan Feldman "On the Long Neglected Status of the Post Living"

The law throws around bodies of deceased human beings a protection even in their graves.

> *In re Ackermann*, 109 N.Y.S.2d 228 (N.Y. App. Div. 1908)

*Chapter 3*

# The Legal Status of the Postliving

*Do Corpses Have Rights?*

## On Resolving the Corpse's Fate

Multiple decisions have to be made about the disposition of a corpse. Most immediately, will the body or body parts be made available for use before final disposal—for autopsy, for use in research or education, or for transplantation to live persons with critical needs? What method of final disposal of the corpse or its remnants will be used—burial or some more exotic disposition? Will there be a commemorative ceremony? Will there be a religious rite? Who will speak? Will the body be displayed? How will the corpse be clothed? If the method of disposition is burial, where will the corpse be buried? What kind of container or wrapping, if any, will be used? What kind of burial ceremony, if any, will be held?

Rules for prompt resolution of such issues are necessary. Without prompt disposition, the corpse will putrefy or, if embalmed, linger in limbo (the duration of which depends on the extent of embalming) awaiting disposition. Not only should the appropriate decision maker be promptly recognized but the ensuing choice of disposition should be right the first time. It is impossible to undo some dispositions (e.g., cremation or deep-sea burial), and once a corpse has been laid to rest in some permanent fashion, there is great reluctance to disturb that repose.

Disputes about disposal of a cadaver frequently arise, sometimes arousing interest in the media and sometimes prompting judicial intervention. The introduction to this book described the unceremonious fate of Ted Williams's corpse and the legal controversy in 2002 surrounding its disposition—a legal proceeding that ended (with Williams a frozen remnant) only because his sister ran out of resources to litigate. In 2006 the matter of Teresa Schiavo made headlines. It was not sad enough that Michael Schiavo (her husband) and the Schindlers (her parents) had fought and litigated in the Florida courts for six years over the medical fate of Ms. Schiavo. (She was then a permanently unconscious patient and had survived for fourteen years only because of artificial nutrition and hydration.) Even after detachment of her artificial life support, the contestants fought bitterly over where to dispose of her body. Michael buried Ms. Schiavo in Pennsylvania despite her parents' preference that she be buried in Florida. In 2007 the disposal of celebrity Anna Nicole Smith's body was resolved judicially—amid media fanfare—after her executor/lover battled for control of Ms. Smith's remains against her long-estranged mother.

Many other controversies over the disposition of human remains are resolved with less publicity. In 2005 Sergeant Jason Hendrix's body was returned to the United States after his death in Iraq. Jason's divorced parents fought over the disposition of the corpse. His mother, who lived in California, contended that Jason had asked to be buried there. His father, who lived in Oklahoma, wanted the burial to take place in that state. Jason had finished high school there and had listed Oklahoma in his army records as his place of residence. A military tribunal resolved the dispute. After a military judge disbelieved his mother's claim about Jason's express wishes, the army invoked its handy rule granting custody of a corpse in controversy to the *older* of the two competing parents. Jason's forty-eight-year-old father got custody rather than his forty-five-year-old mother.

These cases not only pose issues about legal control of a cadaver's disposition, they also raise the question of whose rights are at stake in disputes over a cadaver's fate. As shown in the *Williams, Schiavo, Smith,* and *Hendrix* cases, a variety of surviving parties may purport to represent the interests of a corpse. Are they asserting their own rights or those of the corpse?

## Is a Corpse Property?

If a corpse were deemed to be personal property, the legal framework governing its disposal would be fairly straightforward. The starting point would be the decedent's prerogative to control the disposition of his or her own remains. That is, if a corpse were deemed to be personal property like a house or a car, that status would make enforceable the disposition of the corpse via the decedent's last will and testament (pursuant to state inheritance laws governing posthumous disposition of property). A decedent's prior decisions about postmortem donation of his or her body and its parts would be binding. On the other hand, considering the corpse as property controllable by the decedent's will would create some complications. For example, it would likely mean that a person wishing to change his or her instructions about disposition of the corpse could do so only in a formal written document. And in the absence of further legislation, creditors of the decedent might seize the corpse as property for purposes of collecting the decedent's unpaid debts.

If a corpse were, as a matter of law, deemed to be property like the decedent's other belongings but the decedent left no will, legal control over disposition of the corpse would rest with the next of kin. All property (including the corpse) would pass, according to statutes governing intestacy (disposition of property in the absence of a will), to the spouse or the next of kin. Thus, deeming a corpse to be property would reinforce the customary legal right of the descendants to control the disposition of the corpse—either as inheritors pursuant to a will or as owners of the corpse by intestacy.

The English common law has never treated the corpse as property—that is, as subject to ownership. The applicable legal term was *res nullius,* meaning something owned by no one.[1] The corpse was therefore unlike the coffin, any clothes in the casket, the headstone, or the cemetery plot—all of which were items of personal or real property. This legal treatment of the corpse stemmed in part from the fact that for hundreds of years, control over corpses and burial in England was in the hands of ecclesiastical courts and clergy. With the Church in control of a corpse's disposition, the descendants clearly had no traditional property right at stake. When the secular common-law courts took over governance of cadavers from the ecclesiastical courts in the mid-1600s, they retained the principle that a corpse could not be considered property.

In the United States, which never had ecclesiastical courts, the civil courts of equity followed the British judicial model and ruled that a corpse was not, from a legal perspective, property either of the deceased or of his or her descendants. While state courts in the nineteenth and twentieth centuries sometimes remarked that the legal status of a corpse was equivalent to a property right, most still refused to consider a corpse as property. Instead the judiciary found a protected "special status" for cadavers. "The policy of the law to protect the dead and preserve the sanctity of the grave comes down to us from ancient times. . . . This salutary rule recognizes the tender sentiments uniformly found in the hearts of men, the natural desire that there be repose and reverence for the dead, and the sanctity of the sepulcher."[2] That status flowed from the special quasi-human character associated with the remains of a former human being—the tangible representation of a unique persona bearing special attachments to survivors. Just as courts and legislatures have sometimes considered human gametes and embryos as worthy of special respect because of their *potential* for human life, the corpse, with its *past* human character and attachments, has earned the law's special respect. Protection of the cadaver against mistreatment followed even though the cadaver itself was not considered property.

From a historical perspective, deeming a corpse to be property might have strengthened the legal protection of a body and its resting place. Under the common law (which did not deem a corpse to be property), the penalties for grave robbing were less severe than those for property crimes. In the early American states, it was a felony to steal a coffin or other material objects in a grave but only a misdemeanor to steal a cadaver. Some families therefore placed a piece of cloth or a handkerchief under the cadaver's tongue or in its ear in order to upgrade the penalty for grave robbing.[3] Those steps would have been superfluous if a corpse had been deemed to be property. In addition, if a corpse had been deemed to be property, the survivors in custody might have had additional legal tools to protect the corpse. If people handling a corpse (such as funeral home or cemetery personnel) were legally deemed bailees (custodians) of personal property, they might incur more legal responsibility regarding a corpse than they currently do as providers of services.

Legal consideration of a corpse as the property of the descendants would also have significance under the U.S. Constitution. The Fourteenth Amendment prohibits state government entities from denying "due process" while interfering with people's "property." Property owners can seek legal relief in the face of due process violations. In the last thirty years, survivors as litigants have sought to make a constitutionally based claim relating to control over relatives' cadavers. Next of kin have asserted (some successfully, some not) that harvesting organs or conducting an autopsy without their consent constitutes an unconstitutional deprivation of their property interest in a cadaver without due process of law. For example, one suit contended that Ohio's law permitting a cadaver's corneas to be harvested without consent of the next of kin constituted a denial of property without due process of law. (The corneas were taken during an autopsy required by law because of a suspicion of suicide.) The plaintiff survivors sought damages, including compensation for mental anguish, for the supposedly unconstitutional deprivation of their property (their relative's corneas). This kind of constitutional claim is examined further in chapter 7, which deals generally with harvesting of body parts and exploitation of whole bodies. For now, suffice it to say that neither the U.S. Supreme Court nor the majority of lower courts addressing the issue have found that a corpse is property under the Fourteenth Amendment.

## Prospective Autonomy Rights

Though a cadaver is not property disposable by will, the question remains whether live persons are free to determine their own postmortem fate by making a premortem choice of how to dispose of their cadavers. American society relishes the concept of self-determination. One illustration is the broad protection against arbitrary or unnecessary government interference with liberty under the Fifth and Fourteenth Amendments to the U.S. Constitution. Since 1965 fundamental liberty in constitutional jurisprudence has been interpreted to include individual choice regarding the use of contraceptives, family living arrangements, intimate social association with others, decisions about terminating pregnancy, child rearing, and even homosexual practices among consenting adults. Another aspect of liberty deemed to be fundamental is freedom to decide whether or not to accept life-sustaining medical intervention—a prerogative derived from important values of self-determination and bodily integrity. But does American society accord personal liberty to shape certain events occurring after the person's death?

In some contexts, American law has been willing to give binding force to people's advance choices aimed at governing future events occurring after the chooser's mental competence has been lost. American jurisprudence, for example, respects competent choices regarding postcompetence life-sustaining medical intervention. Every state makes provision for some sort of advance medical directive and/or appointment of an agent to make postcompetence medical decisions according to the prior wishes of the now-incompetent patient.

In addition, American law has chosen to respect premortem choices concerning postmortem disposal of real and personal property. As noted, every state makes provision for enforcement of a will dictating the distribution of property owned by a decedent and for a mechanism distributing property on behalf of an intestate decedent (lacking a formal will) according to a statutory hierarchy of next of kin corresponding to the *presumed* wishes of that decedent. In short, American law recognizes the concept of prospective autonomy. It allows people to make some advance binding decisions even though they cannot know in advance the precise circumstances that will exist at the moment of loss of competence or of death.

American morals and practice have similarly upheld prospective autonomy in the disposal of human remains—as an expression of social respect for the self-determination capacity and dignity of human beings and out of loyalty to decedents. During a person's lifetime, the choice of lifestyle is important in shaping and expressing the individual's character and image. The choice of death style similarly projects the inner person to the world. Self-determination has included a person's prerogative to shape his or her memory picture not only by control of postmortem disposition of property but also by control of postmortem disposition of his or her remains. The human corpse continues to reflect in some measure the persona of the decedent. If a decedent has donated body parts to critically ill recipients, his or her lifetime image gets credit for the altruistic decision.

Enforcement of prospective autonomy also reflects the presumed preference of the great majority of living persons. That is, postmortem honoring of the wishes of a decedent reassures living persons that their own provisions for bodily disposal will be respected. As has been said about prospective autonomous control over property, "The vast majority of us are greatly comforted 'now' to know that after our own deaths the law can be used to contribute to the good of the persons and causes we care about."[4] The same attitude prevails toward the disposition of corpses, at least for those persons who care enough to spell out their preferences regarding disposal of their remains. Living persons who plan their postmortem fate want their wishes to have binding posthumous legal force.

As a matter of law, a mentally competent person has the right to dictate the disposal of his or her postmortem remains. Some statutes and numerous cases establish that principle. A New York State statute declared in 1881: "A person has the right to direct the manner in which his body shall be disposed of after death."[5] Over a hundred years later, in 1998, Pennsylvania legislation explicitly recognized a decedent's right to determine the disposal of his or her remains.[6]

Courts, while reluctant to label a corpse as property, have nonetheless tended to give binding force to premortem instructions for disposal of human remains so long as such instructions remain "within the limits of reason and decency" and do not involve "extravagant waste."[7] An 1895 decision by the Iowa Supreme Court declared that "it always has been, and will ever continue to be," the duty of courts to implement, "as far as it is possible," an express wish concerning final resting place.[8] According to another court, an individual has "a sufficient proprietary interest in his own body after death to be able to make valid and binding testamentary dispositions of it."[9] The sole legal treatise on the law of cadavers confirms that "ordinarily one has a right during life to determine the disposal of his body after death."[10] Even those courts that refuse to call the decedent's wishes for body disposal binding still urge that those wishes be given "respectful consideration" and "great weight" by those charged with disposing of a particular cadaver.[11]

As a matter of practice, survivors generally respect a decedent's wishes regarding disposal of his or her remains. This is part of the respect and fidelity accorded to the dead. (Witness my stepbrother's jazzed-up funeral.) Yet sometimes the next of kin rebel, and their failure to follow a decedent's instructions may in fact prevail. Grace Metalious was an American novelist whose scandalous account of sexual escapades in a small town (*Peyton Place*) preceded *Desperate Housewives* by decades. Ms. Metalious had provided that upon her death no funeral service should be held and that her body should be delivered to Dartmouth or Harvard Medical School for use in the interests of science. Ms. Metalious's widower and children objected and withheld the corpse from donation. A New Hampshire court ruled that the decedent's wishes would ordinarily prevail over the survivors' objections, but since the two medical schools had declined the gift cadaver (in the face of the survivors' resistance), the wishes of Ms. Metalious's spouse and children should be upheld. In theory, then, the decedent's choice of postmortem disposition would have prevailed had not the two medical schools capitulated. In reality, the decedent's wishes were frustrated by the surviving family's united opposition. A court more sympathetic to the decedent's altruistic intentions could have ruled that the corpse be donated to some other medical school willing to cooperate with Ms. Metalious's intentions.

For another successful rebellion by surviving next of kin, consider the fate of Jessica Mitford's remains. Ms. Mitford was a well-known writer who in 1968 wrote a classic exposé, *The American Way of Death,* about funeral homes' financial abuse of mourning families. Ms. Mitford, entirely disenchanted with American funeral practices, had expressed her wish to be cremated without any accompanying hoopla. Upon her death, the family invited six hundred people to a memorial service that included a carriage hearse drawn by six plumed horses and a twelve-piece brass band.[12]

The lesson is that a decedent's wishes regarding cadaver disposal may, in practice if not in law, be dependent on survivors' faithfulness. If survivors unanimously favor breach of instructions, that dereliction may simply become a fait accompli. Reluctance to intervene is especially strong when the survivors' alternative decision is reasonably understandable, as in the following example. A husband's will dictated that his money be buried with him (not a good strategy for anyone who wants to rest in peace). At the funeral, his widow slipped a check into the cadaver's pocket. No one complained.[13]

Executors of wills, families, and/or courts considering instructions from the decedent for disposal arrangements are sometimes influenced by the distress or other interests of survivors who object to implementation of the instructions. While a decedent may have a theoretical right to dictate the fate of his or her property and to control or heavily influence the disposition of personal remains, the interests of a corpse tend to be less robust when they conflict with the needs and wants of living persons. The descendants are alive and pushing their interests as opposed to the silent and immobile decedent. Remember Jessica Mitford and Grace Metalious!

Many funeral directors believe that survivors should not have to do things with which they are uncomfortable or to which they are ethically opposed. This sometimes results in upholding the survivors' preferences rather than those of the decedent. Usually the deviations from the deceased's wishes are minor; for example, the children decide that the dress their mother had selected for her public wake is simply too frumpy, and they substitute another one. Sometimes, though, the survivors' distress produces more significant changes. Grace Metalious's anguished survivors prevented donation of her corpse to science and frustrated her ultimate wish to have her remains cremated. Another judge contravened a decedent's wish regarding his place of burial in order to accommodate his widow's and child's convenience in visiting the burial site. And both executors and courts have occasionally been responsive to survivors' distress over cremating their loved ones despite the decedent's stated preference for such disposal.

Survivors' distress over a decedent's perceived religious betrayals also sometimes prevails. In one case a court permitted relatives, upset by the decedent's decision to be buried in a heretical church's unconsecrated grounds, to change the burial place. The judge was willing to interpret the deceased's call for last rites from his conventional church as a revocation of the prior expressed preference for the heretical church.[14] However, in the context of religious preferences, postmortem disputes involving the wishes and putative wishes of decedents are usually resolved in favor of a decedent's religious choices even if these are upsetting to some survivors. In a 1919 case Whitney Metcalf's widow resisted implementation of Whitney's ignominious wish to be buried in the Unitarian section of the local cemetery. Whitney's daughter went to court to compel her mother to respect her father's radical wishes about his place of burial. Counsel for the widow argued strenuously that Whitney's former preferences should not be enforced as, in his new circumstances, "his predilection for Unitarian association may have become somewhat impaired."[15] The court nonetheless enforced Whitney's premortem Unitarian preferences.

In *Cohen v. Cohen* the late Hilliard Cohen had become embroiled in friction between his non-Jewish wife, Margaret, and his Orthodox Jewish brother and sister.[16] In his 1992 will Hilliard had provided for his burial in the Orthodox family plot in Queens, New York City. (Margaret could be buried in the same cemetery, but not in the section reserved for Jewish graves.) In 1998 Hilliard and Margaret moved to Florida. There, in 2001 and 2003, Hilliard stated orally that he wanted to be buried next to Margaret in Florida. Resolving the postmortem dispute between Margaret and Hilliard's siblings, a Florida court ruled in 2005 that Hilliard's wishes, as expressed orally, should be enforced. His 1992 will provision had been revoked orally—a step that was legally binding because a corpse, as we know, is not property controlled by testamentary law.

## Premortem Planning

The law's general willingness to enforce the disposal preferences of deceased persons creates an incentive for people to engage in premortem planning on behalf of their own prospective cadavers. Relatively few do so, since people are generally reluctant to face their own mortality and prefer not to provide for future traumatic events. Only about 20 percent of persons prepare advance medical directives to control their postcompetence medical care. Less than 50 percent prepare a last will and testament governing the postmortem disposition of their real and personal property. The percentage of people who spell out their wishes for body disposal is unknown, but it is probably much less than the percentage of people who spell out their wishes for property disposition.

Not everyone recommends advance planning for body disposal. Undertaker/philosopher Thomas Lynch advises: "Once you are dead, put your feet up, call it a day, and let the husband or the missus or the kids or a sibling decide whether you are to be buried or burned or blown out of a cannon or left to dry out in a ditch somewhere. It's not your day to watch it, because the dead don't care."[17]

Nonetheless, some people—like my stepbrother, as described in the introduction—do engage in premortem planning for their own cadaver's disposal. Winston Churchill, who died in 1965, left detailed funeral instructions, including the order of march of royal guard units, the music to be played, the route of the funeral cortege, and a fly-over by the Royal Air Force. President Franklin D. Roosevelt wrote a four-page document in 1937 dictating his postmortem preferences. He prescribed, inter alia, no lying in state, no embalming, a gun carriage rather than a hearse, a simple coffin of dark wood, and an unlined grave. When FDR died in 1945, he was in fact embalmed and lay in state for days, was transported to the cemetery in a Cadillac hearse, and was buried in a copper coffin within a cement-lined grave. All of this was done not because people wanted to contravene his wishes, but because his instructions were found in his personal safe three days after the funeral. Current celebrity Oprah Winfrey has planned her own funeral, including the casket, the music, and a video eulogy.[18]

People have gone to great lengths to ensure that their preferences for their own postmortem handling are well understood. Legendary actress Sarah Bernhardt bought her own coffin and kept it in her bedroom, occasionally lying in it (presumably to ensure a continued fit). Charles V, the Holy Roman emperor who died in 1558, not only prepared his tomb within a church but also rehearsed his funeral many times. He had his servants file into the church in a procession holding black candles. Charles walked behind them, wrapped in a shroud. Once in the church, Charles laid down in his preselected coffin and joined the rehearsal of prayers to be offered for his soul.

Some testators, aware of the hazard of survivors' resistance to prescribed wishes, have tried to set up a self-enforcing mechanism for having their disposal wishes honored. One testator provided in his will that if his next of kin failed to cremate his body, his assets should be diverted from the family beneficiaries to the local cremation society. Similar disqualification provisions often appear in wills to discourage any beneficiary from challenging the will. Such provisions can create a strong incentive to abide by a testator's instructions. Still, the testator is dependent on the estate executor or some other party to implement his or her instructions if the next of kin violate his or her wishes (regarding body disposal or challenge to the will).

Advance instructions for postmortem disposal of a person's remains often represent an effort to make a symbolic statement about the lifetime image that the deceased had cultivated and the concomitant memory picture sought to be left with survivors. B. T. Collins, a California state legislator, obviously wanted to extend his image as a flamboyant bon vivant whose life warranted celebration. For his wake, he dictated that a party be held in a Sacramento ballroom accommodating three thousand guests. The instructions provided for three bars, an elaborate buffet, and a seven-piece band playing pop tunes; his flag-draped coffin (Collins was a former Marine) would stand in the middle.

Beyond a joyous wake, disposal preferences can make symbolic statements about the deceased's self-perception and character. A Brazilian legislator in 2005 had insisted on being buried in a standing position because in his lifetime he had "bowed to no one." Also in 2005 James Henry Smith, a zealous lifelong fan of the Pittsburgh Steelers, had prescribed his "viewing." His corpse would be placed in a room in front of a television set, leaning backward in a recliner with his feet crossed, a remote control at his side, a pack of cigarettes nearby, and a beer in one hand.

Mr. Smith's obvious effort to perpetuate his lifetime comforts and accessories have innumerable precedents in burial instructions. In 1899 in Buffalo, New York, Reuben John Smith was buried in a mausoleum sitting in a leather and oak recliner, alongside a table with a checkerboard, candle and matches, and a box containing clippings about the burial. Queen Victoria provided a list of items to surround her in her coffin, including photographs of Prince Albert; a plaster cast of his hand; a photo and lock of hair from John Brown, her servant for thirty-four years; jewelry; and shawls. An Indiana resident who died in 1882 was also buried sitting at a table, this time with a deck of cards, a bottle of whiskey, and a pipe. In 1964 Sandra Ilene West was buried in a baby-blue Ferrari with the seat slanted at a comfortable angle.

Sometimes people who dictate their own postmortem disposal seek to utilize body parts to make symbolic statements. John Reed, a lifelong worker at the Walnut Street Theater in Philadelphia, instructed that his head be skeletonized and used in theater productions of *Hamlet*. Reed could thus perpetuate his long association with the theater without having to memorize any lines. In 1994 Donald Eugene Russell died after requesting that his skin be stripped and tanned posthumously and that the resultant "leather" be used to bind a book of his verse. While Russell's widow wanted to implement his wish, a judge sided with the mortuary's claim that the procedure would constitute abusive mistreatment of a corpse. In 1832 the British philosopher Jeremy Bentham directed that his skeleton (after a series of invitation-only dissections of his corpse) be dressed in his clothes and seated in a chair at University College in a posture as if thinking about his writing. To this day, Bentham's remains are periodically displayed in that setting. Bentham also prescribed that if his former friends and disciples met to commemorate his memory, his executor should transport a box of memorabilia to the meeting room. Many such meetings were subsequently held, with the minutes noting: "Mr. Bentham present, but not voting."

## Public Policy Limitations on Prospective Autonomy

It will come as no surprise that public policy places limitations on the postmortem operation of various forms of prospective autonomy. Some personal prerogatives expire along with the deceased because public policy requires contemporaneous awareness for their exercise. In such instances, "prospective" exercise in advance of death is inappropriate. Voting is an example. No matter how invariable a person's partisan political preferences are, and no matter how clear the wish to continue supporting candidates of that same preference, a person generally loses the voting privilege upon death. I say "generally" because this policy is not always rigorously implemented. Former governor of New Jersey Brendan Byrne was once asked where he wanted to be buried. He replied: "In Jersey City!" Why Jersey City? "Because I want to continue voting after I die." Jersey City to the contrary notwithstanding, most jurisdictions require that a voter at least be alive and aware of the competing candidates in a public election. Jury service also demands a live body.

When a person leaves property in a will, a variety of public regulations come into play. The federal government customarily took a healthy chunk in estate taxes—a practice suspended in 2010 but likely to resume in 2011 at a rate of 55 percent. Further, state law guarantees every surviving spouse a share of a decedent's estate regardless of the testator's preference to disinherit him or her. Public policy also prevents a testator from dictating the death of a beloved pet. Nor will courts enforce the destruction of valuable pieces of art or real property or a testator's instruction to bury his or her wealth along with the cadaver. Notions of waste reinforce the adage that "you can't take it with you."

Public policy constraints likewise affect persons seeking to direct postmortem disposal of their corpse. Federal and state statutes bar the sale of bodies or body parts, a constraint applicable both to a decedent and to any other party disposing of a corpse. (That limitation is examined more closely in chapter 7.) Some state laws obstruct unfettered access to cadavers by survivors. State laws commonly permit very obtrusive forensic autopsies of corpses, regardless of survivors' objections, for reasons such as unexplained death or suspicion of a communicable fatal disease. Some state laws governing autopsies also impact the disposition of certain body parts for transplant. A number of states have allowed the harvesting (at the time of autopsy) of certain body parts, such as corneas or pituitary glands, so long as no objections from either the decedent or the next of kin are known to the pathologists handling the autopsy. (The overriding policy is to restore the health or well-being of stricken citizens—the prospective transplant recipients—by relatively unobtrusive exploitation of no longer needed body parts. Such a policy is considered in chapter 7.)

Judges also tend to follow certain conceptions of public policy when asked to implement a decedent's instructions for disposal of his or her remains. That is, social mores influence the judiciary. In 1900 the married Mr. Enos died, leaving a will as well as oral instructions directing his lover, Ms. R. J. Snyder, with whom he had lived for several years, to determine his last resting place. Mr. Enos's estranged wife and his daughter went into a California court and demanded that they be allowed to supplant Ms. Snyder in controlling the fate of Mr. Enos's cadaver. The judge granted their request, noting that the next of kin are ordinarily entitled to control a corpse's disposition. However, the judge was relying on a simplistic statement of the law. Even in 1900 a decedent's wishes about cadaver disposal were supposed to be honored. The judge's moral outrage at the premortem unfaithful behavior of Mr. Enos is probably a more accurate explanation for his decision.[19]

## Whose Autonomy Rights Are They?

As previously described, the prospective autonomy rights of the late Hilliard Cohen and the late Whitney Metcalf were enforced. But both Hilliard and Whitney were corpses at the time of the legal proceedings and the subsequent burials. Could we say that the corpses had legal rights that were being enforced? Whose rights were implemented?

Enforcement of prospective autonomy clearly implements the self-determination rights and interests of the premortem decedent. This is so, for example, when estate property is distributed according to the provisions of a will. The testator's autonomous choices, subject to constraints of taxes and public policy, govern who will receive the decedent's assets. We readily talk about a decedent's right to dispose of property by will even if the implementation follows death. It might be an executor, a beneficiary of the will, a court, or the state attorney general who makes sure that the testator's choices are respected. But the right to direct disposition belongs (or belonged) to the now-deceased testator, just as the right to receive by inheritance belongs to any beneficiary of the will.

The same framework applies to premortem instructions for disposal of human remains. Postmortem implementation of a decedent's prior wishes obviously implicates the late decedent's interest in self-determination. Other rights holders may exist in the same setting—such as the designated people charged with control of a cadaver. (A court will generally uphold a decedent's specification of who should be in charge of disposal.) The designees in control are like the executors in charge of implementing financial bequests pursuant to the decedent's will. But the control prerogatives do not displace the dispositional rights of the decedent; they merely help enforce those rights. The autonomy interest at stake is the decedent's, even if the decedent no longer exists.

Often the party who implements the decedent's wishes is the next of kin, as in the case of Hilliard Cohen's widow. (A spouse is customarily treated as the closest kin even though he or she is not a blood relative.)

Sometimes, though, the next of kin resists the decedent's wishes and another interested party steps forward to assert the decedent's rights and interests. For Whitney Metcalf, his daughter asserted her father's right to select a burial place in the face of his widow's resistance. The wish of the widow, the next of kin, was overridden.

Some disputes about disposition of a cadaver take place in situations where the decedent was estranged from his next of kin and a friend rather than a relative seeks to assert control. When Michael Stewart died of acquired immune deficiency syndrome (AIDS) in a West Virginia hospital, his parents, though long estranged from Michael, sought to arrange an Orthodox Jewish burial. Michael's gay companion, Drew Stanton, tried to intervene based on Michael's previously expressed opposition to a Jewish burial. (Michael had changed his name from Sobel to Stewart.) Mr. Stanton successfully asked a court to prevent Michael's parents from carrying out the planned religious burial. For Michael Stewart, it was his gay lover who came forward to protect Stewart's prospective autonomy right when his parents, as next of kin, refused to respect their son's wishes about his funeral.

Sometimes an institution represents the decedent's interests. For example, a cemetery has on occasion resisted efforts to remove a corpse from its chosen resting place. A judge may also be the agent who upholds a decedent's wishes. For example, a judge dictated that executed mass murderer Jeffrey Dahmer's wish to be cremated be respected, contrary to Dahmer's mother's wish to donate her son's brain for scientific study. It does not matter, for purposes of identifying the rights holder, that the decedent is dependent on various other parties for implementation and enforcement of the decedent's wishes.

### Control of a Directionless Cadaver

While a decedent's instructions about disposal of remains are generally binding, most people fail to give such directions. Who then decides the fate of the remains that are nobody's property but, according to law, still have a special status demanding respect from survivors?

Law's first mark of respect for human remains was to impose a duty to dispose of a corpse with a modicum of dignity. Traditionally, in America, a cadaver was entitled to a "decent Christian burial"—defined as the right to be "returned to parent earth for dissolution, and to be carried thither in a decent and inoffensive manner."[20] The cadaver—unless it was that of a murderer, a heretic, or a suicide—had a right to prompt burial. American courts in the nineteenth century deemed this duty of decent sepulture a "sacred trust" derived from "the universal feelings of mankind."[21] The goals were to provide respectful repose for sacrosanct human remains in preparation for resurrection and to ensure an untroubled haven for any surviving spirit. Further public interests in prompt disposition of a cadaver existed—either to prevent contagion or to avoid untended spirits' possible retaliation against the living (for neglect).

The basic duty of prompt sepulture was imposed upon the next of kin who were able (physically and financially) to provide for decent disposal of the cadaver. This was so at least when death occurred at home. American law generally made it a criminal offense to fail to provide decent sepulture. But the duty of sepulture extended beyond the immediate family. For deaths that occurred away from normal surroundings, the legal responsibility for sepulture fell on the homeowner or institution under whose roof the decedent expired.[22] The expectation was still that the expenses would be borne by the family or the decedent's estate, even if a stranger had the duty of disposal.

When surviving family members could not or would not dispose properly of human remains, the burden fell on community officials. And if someone died in isolation or without survivors, it became the duty of public authorities to provide a final repose, even if that meant burial at public expense in an unmarked potter's field. When local paupers died, often in an almshouse, the community commonly assumed control of the corpse for burial in a potter's field or for cremation.

Stemming from the legal duty of the next of kin to dispose of a corpse, the common law found concomitant rights of the next of kin to determine the place and mode of a corpse's disposition. The law created a hierarchy of control according to the proximity of family bonds, starting with a spouse and extending to close relatives—similar to current statutes governing disposition of the property of a person who dies intestate and recent statutes governing the fate of transplantable cadaveric organs (see chapter 7). The control rights lodged in the next of kin included the rights to hold and protect the body, select a manner and place of disposition (in accord with the decedent's wishes if extant), provide last rites, and assure the undisturbed repose of the human remains.

These prerogatives of control lodged in the next of kin gave rise to legal protection against third-party interference with kin carrying out the tasks of cadaver disposal. When people interfered improperly with the next of kin's disposition of human remains, the resulting legal claim was not interference with property, but rather a legal wrong—a tort—giving rise to a suit for damages. A spouse or other next of kin was entitled to receive the cadaver intact and in no worse condition than at death. A health care institution or a professional who performed unauthorized procedures on a corpse was therefore subject to suit. Many courts viewed autopsies—when unauthorized either by the next of kin or by law for forensic needs—as improper interference with the next of kin's legal control of the corpse, even if the motives for the autopsy were advancement of science and education. Even an unauthorized embalming was actionable.

The specialness of a corpse and of the intimate interest of the next of kin in human remains was recognized in the scope of damages allowed to the next of kin. Consider, for example, a situation in which medical personnel performed an unauthorized autopsy on a recently deceased patient. Ordinarily, under the common law of torts, wrongdoers in this context would be liable only for modest nominal damages for breach of their legal duty (to refrain from unauthorized use or handling of a corpse). Monetary recovery for intangible mental anguish was customarily confined to tort victims who witnessed a wrongdoer's actions. A spouse or other next of kin would therefore not be able to collect damages for mental suffering associated with the mere knowledge that an unconsented procedure had been performed on a loved one. That customary approach changed in the context of cadavers. American common law established that human remains have a special status and that a deceased's kin would likely experience extreme distress in the wake of improper interference with a corpse. Mental suffering was deemed "the natural and proximate result of knowledge" that the remains of a deceased husband or wife had been altered without permission.[23] The courts therefore allowed damages for mental suffering when a next of kin proved that a defendant had interfered improperly with control or disposal of a corpse—for example, by performing an autopsy.

Not every mishap in handling a corpse gave rise to damages for emotional suffering to the next of kin. The standard for recovery was supposed to be conduct that would "outrage" common sensibilities.[24] Also, courts and juries could disagree with a claimant on whether a defendant's conduct was sufficiently outrageous to impose damages for mental suffering. In a Vermont case, the court disallowed such damages when a railway agent stepped too close to a railroad station platform while loading a casket, unceremoniously but accidentally spilling the contents onto the track.[25] By contrast, parents recovered damages against a pathologist who, after an autopsy to which they had consented, dropped the infant's body on the floor, partially crushing its head.[26]

Descendants of decedents whose remains had been mistreated could sometimes collect for breach of contract as well as for tortious interference with a corpse. In one little-known case, a widow contracted with a funeral home to have her husband buried in his prized black Stetson cowboy hat. A few months after the funeral, she observed a relative wearing the hat. The widow collected $101,000 in a breach of contract suit against the funeral home's director.

The common assumption underlying allocation of legal control and responsibility was that the next of kin would be closely connected to the deceased and therefore inspired by reverence for the deceased and fidelity to the deceased's wishes. Of course, not every scenario matched this expectation of family benevolence. Not every decedent enjoyed affection and respect. Control of a corpse by the next of kin could be displaced when the closest survivor had exhibited hostility toward the deceased. This meant that courts were sometimes willing to overturn the efforts of estranged spouses or alienated relatives who sought to control the disposition of a corpse, even if this meant giving control to a more distant relative.[27] People who had exhibited disinterest in or hostility toward the interests of the person while alive could not be trusted to promote the well-being of the person's remains.

## Legal Protections for the Cadaver

I argued earlier that prospective autonomy rights can be classified as rights of a decedent because the choice prerogative involved is so closely tied to the wishes of that person while alive. Certain harms, though, impact primarily on the physical entity known as a cadaver. I suggest that the underlying (so to speak) legal protections can properly be considered rights of the cadaver.

Percival Jackson's legal treatise confirms that "The dead themselves have rights committed to the living to protect."[28] The first recognized posthumous right was that of decent sepulture—the previously described right "to be returned to parent earth for dissolution."[29] But a cadaver's rights extend well beyond the point of decent disposal. For example, once a corpse is given appropriate sepulture, it enjoys (so to speak) a right to undisturbed or "quiet repose." Unauthorized disinterment of a corpse is both an actionable civil trespass and a criminal offense. "The normal treatment of a corpse, once it is decently buried, is to let it lie. This idea is so deeply woven into our legal and cultural fabric that it is commonplace to hear it spoken of as a 'right' of the dead."[30] This right of undisturbed repose goes beyond the corpse's interest in protection against malevolent desecration or profanation of a resting place. Courts commonly deem it to be part of a "universal sentiment of humanity" to protect a corpse's repose even against *respectful* removal from a resting place.[31] After interment, courts of equity deem human remains to be "in the custody of the law" and judges maintain a "marked reluctance" to "disturb the sanctity of the grave."[32]

A recent incident illustrates how the concept of quiet repose survives in American culture. In 2007 exhumation of Notre Dame football legend George Gipp sparked furor and outrage in his hometown burial place in Michigan.[33] Gipp's grandnephew secured an exhumation permit by manufacturing a need related to inherited diseases in the family. The real motive was to help a sports writer who was investigating whether Gipp was in fact the father of an out-of-wedlock child whose claimed descendant had recently come forward. An ESPN crew used a backhoe that disturbed adjacent graves as well as Gipp's. The townsfolk were outraged that Gipp's resting place and remains had been disturbed.

Even when a well-meaning next of kin seeks to disturb a resting place, a court of equity may well block it in the absence of a strong justification.[34] "Disinterment of a body is not favored in the law. . . . It is the policy of the law except in cases of necessity or for laudable purposes that the sanctity of the grave should be maintained and that a body once suitably buried should remain undisturbed."[35] Cases identify "necessity" or some other strong justification as a prerequisite for disturbing a resting place.[36] Convenience to a mourning family that has moved from the burial area may not be a sufficient justification. Transfer of remains to a newly dead spouse's resting place might not be a "good cause" justification, especially if the newly dead spouse had deviated from the religious path of the deceased.[37] A report to a widow that her buried husband had been "seen alive" months after burial was not considered enough justification to dig up the estranged husband's grave.

All of this is not to say that a corpse's right to undisturbed repose is absolute. In the first place, when surviving family members agree on moving a corpse, they often do so without any judicial involvement. Second, numerous acceptable justifications exist for disturbing or moving human remains. For example, a family is allowed to move remains in a way that fulfills the wishes or presumed wishes of the deceased. In one case, transfer to a family's new cemetery plot conformed with the deceased's express wishes.[38] Transfer to a resting place adjacent to the remains of a deceased's only child was also deemed consistent with the deceased parent's presumed wishes. Restoration or reconstruction of a burial vault obviously warrants temporary disturbance of the remains therein.

Disinterment and transfer of human remains is often done to accommodate public needs for growth and development. The power of eminent domain exercised to expand roads or buildings has often served as a justification for disturbing resting places. In the 1930s, San Francisco disinterred and relocated ninety thousand human remains in order to accomplish city expansion. Of course, any family representatives of human remains affected by eminent domain are entitled to compensation for the costs of removing and reinterring disturbed remains. Long-buried remains are somehow more susceptible to disturbance, in part because representatives of the dead might not remain to enforce their ancestors' corpses' right of repose. Without some descendant to intervene, the fate of long-buried remains depends on the sensitivity (or lack thereof) of the acting government agencies. That often bodes ill for the buried corpses. New York City moved its potter's field from what is now Washington Square to Bryant Park, then to the corner of Third Avenue and Fiftieth Street, then to Ward's Island, and then to Hart's Island, all between 1794 and 1870. The buried human remains were seldom moved, as the city simply built over the former cemeteries. In 1991, a Manhattan building project unearthed a burial ground where thousands of people of African descent had been laid to rest in the seventeenth and eighteenth centuries.[39] In this instance, part of the site was set aside for a crypt to contain the gathered remains and a national monument was built to those largely unidentified ancestors.

A transfer of human remains can sometimes be justified as a mark of respect and honor. Abraham Lincoln's remains were transferred from a grave to a more secure memorial tomb. Martin Luther King's body was moved from a grave to a memorial center. Dante Gabriel Rossetti's disturbance of his wife's grave probably does not qualify as a mark of "respect and honor." When his wife died in 1862, the Italian poet buried with her the only manuscript of several love poems. The act was a gesture of eternal love. Seven years later Rossetti, perhaps then in the throes of writer's block, retrieved the poems from the grave. He disinfected and dried the manuscript and a year later published the poems. The question remains whether the poems' artistic value warranted their salvaging and the temporary disturbance of the grave.

Disinterment is also undertaken on occasion in order to solve some mystery about a celebrity's death. In the 1990s the body of President Zachary Taylor was exhumed to test whether his death had been caused by poisoning. (Taylor died in 1850, early in his presidency, after an unexplained bout of gastroenteritis had felled him for several days. An historian speculated that poisoning had been responsible. Taylor's descendants consented, and an exhumation was conducted to test for arsenic traces in hair and bone remnants. No arsenic was found.[40]) The body of Lee Harvey Oswald, who murdered President John F. Kennedy, was exhumed to show that Oswald, and not a Soviet agent, was the corpse. However, requests to exhume President Kennedy's remains in order to reexplore the cause of his death have regularly been denied in light of the Warren Commission's prior investigation.

In various periods in Anglo-American history, lack of physical space for additional cadavers has served as a necessary reason to transfer human remains. For example, burial space was at a premium in England's churchyards during the eighteenth century. At first, coffins were stacked in single burial spaces. Ultimately bodies were disinterred and the exhumed bones collected in ossuaries. Similar practices date back to the thirteenth and fourteenth centuries in England. Apparently corpses were only entitled to a single generation of "mingling human remains with the earth."[41] Other necessary reasons for disturbing graves include identification of victims of mass disasters, investigation of claimed human rights violations, and resolution of liability claims.

That corpses have rights to sepulture and undisturbed repose does not mean that all the interests of corpses are legally protected. The corpse, or at least its abiding memory picture, certainly has an interest in the preservation of the decedent's reputation, but there is no tort cause of action for libel published after the death of the defamed person, no matter how distorted, malevolent, or widespread the posthumously published claims may be.[42] This legal approach seems strange, given the corpse's continued interest in dignity as recognized in other posthumous rights of the corpse just described. Perhaps the explanation lies in the supreme importance of free speech and the difficulty of establishing truth after the subject of dispute has passed away.

A corpse also has a continuing interest in informational privacy or confidentiality, even if breaches can no longer be a source of actual embarrassment or economic harm. Legal protection of that interest is limited. In 2001 citizens tried to use the Freedom of Information Act to obtain photos of the corpse of Vince Foster, a White House counsel who had committed suicide. The photos were held in the National Archives and that institution, along with Foster's family, asserted privacy concerns as warranting the withholding of the photos. The U.S. Supreme Court upheld the nondisclosure of the photos, citing the family's interests (rather than the corpse's interests) in privacy, peace of mind, and tranquility. The Court recognized a mourning family's stake in preventing unwarranted public exposure undermining respect for the deceased person and causing anguish to the surviving family.[43] The Court did not foreclose legal recognition of a corpse's own interests in privacy, but it attributed to Congress only an intention to protect a surviving family's interests under the Freedom of Information Act.

These loopholes in the protection of postmortem interests do not vitiate the basic point that some cadaveric rights—such as decent sepulture and quiet repose—do exist. A corpse still has a special legal status entailing a certain solicitude and assurance of postmortem human dignity. The rules surrounding the treatment of corpses in American culture are appropriately "driven by a desire to treat the dead with dignity."[44] Cadavers' legal entitlement to dignified treatment is recognized and reinforced by universal criminal prohibitions of desecration of human remains—a topic explored in chapter 11.

### Can a Cadaver Really Have Rights?

Some people question whether a cadaver, a now-dead person, can have legal rights. A number of philosophers contend that because the former person has vanished permanently from the earth, "he cannot be in any true sense a subject of legal right or duty."[45] For these commentators, only a live person has the authority to assert a legal claim. A dead person, they would say, may have continuing interests such as having his or her wishes carried out or being treated with dignity, but the dead person cannot be a holder of legal rights. Ernest Partridge goes further and questions whether the dead can have interests. "Nothing happens to the dead," Partridge contends, not even harm to their legal interests.[46] To the extent that a court might consider and even protect a dead person's purported interests, it would, according to Partridge, be enforcing the rights of living persons, such as descendants or beneficiaries of the deceased.

Skeptical philosophers like Partridge concede that a decedent's survivors can exercise their own legal rights in ways that incidentally benefit the dead person's interests. But, those philosophers contend, a descendant who seeks to prevent mistreatment of a corpse is really asserting the descendant's own right to protect his or her own sensibilities against potential outrage or offense. From that perspective, a living person who seeks to enforce the decedent's instructions for property disposal is protecting the interests of survivors and beneficiaries of the decedent. A descendant who seeks to carry out the decedent's wishes for disposal of the corpse is really protecting either the peace of mind of the descendants or the general interest of all living persons in a legal system that carries out the previously expressed wishes of a corpse. (Living persons who bother to plan for their postmortem fate presumably want those plans to be carried out.)

Some juridical support exists for the proposition that the rights violated by mistreatment of a corpse are those of the next of kin or other survivors charged with decent disposal of the human remains. As noted, survivors do indeed have an established legal right to protect the dignity of a corpse and to collect damages for injury to their own feelings and emotions flowing from cadaver abuse. Some authorities have seen the survivors' rights as the only ones in the legal picture. In 1852 a legal commentator argued that damages for abusive treatment of a corpse derived not from invading "the imaginary rights of the dead, but in outraging the Christian sensibilities of the living."[47] A Colorado court commented in 1932: "Insult and indignity can, of course, inflict no injury on the dead, but they can visit agony akin to torture on the living."[48] In 1986 a Georgia court found that a pregnant woman, dead by total brain-death criteria, no longer had any personal rights that might interfere with the state's effort to preserve the fetus by continuing to use her body as an incubator.[49] Such courts share skepticism that the wronged party in a case of desecration of a grave could be a corpse mouldering in the ground.

These doubters notwithstanding, I contend that mistreatment of a corpse is a legally cognizable wrong against the corpse even though the corpse's rights might be asserted by other interested parties and even though the main monetary recovery might be for harm to survivors' feelings. Even when the party in court is a relative of the decedent whose own interests and rights may be promoted by a result benefiting the cadaver, I submit that the rights being enforced are often those of the cadaver as well. The mistreated corpse has no agonized feelings to compensate, but it does have legally cognizable interests in dignity and quiet repose.

A bearer of legal rights does not, I submit, have to be a living person. Years ago, an academic argued that trees should be recognized as having legal rights in order to protect the environmental interests of both people and trees. That suggestion never prevailed, but there is no intrinsic obstacle to legal recognition of standing for nonhumans. Animal rights advocates have long asserted that the moral stature of certain animals warrants strong legal protection. American law does recognize the interests of endangered animal species in being protected against further destruction as well as the interests of domestic animals in not being abused. Some day American law may acknowledge the independent quasi-human rights of primates. The point is that law can establish rights in beings and entities that have sufficient moral stature in the eyes of lawmakers even in the absence of moral equivalence to persons. Fetal interests provide another example. Even though a nonviable fetus does not have equivalent status to its pregnant mother, a legislature can accord significant legal recognition to that fetus, including independent protection against fatal harm. Indeed, in the third trimester, the *potential* life of a fetus gives it significant protection even against the preferences of a pregnant woman. Human corpses, with their status as former living humans and their present status as respected human remains, have enough moral stature to be accorded legal rights—hence the rights of decent sepulture, quiet repose, and freedom from desecration.

Does it make sense to talk about a cadaver as a rights holder—as a legally protected entity in its own right? I think so. The explanation lies in the durability of the human nature attributed to a cadaver and the jurisprudential willingness to accord moral stature to that nature. Going beyond the tendency to attribute feelings and emotions to the cadaver, we consider the aftermath of a human life—corpsehood—as continuing to shape a life image and possibly harboring some intangible presence. American society recognizes, respects, and legally protects an enduring presence in the aftermath of a person's life. At least certain elements of cadaveric dignity are legally protected and may be deemed to be rights of the corpse.

You may rightfully ask whether it really matters if postmortem protections are deemed to be rights of the corpse or of a current living litigant acting to protect the interests of the corpse. My response is that usually the precise locus of the rights does not make a great deal of difference, but sometimes it does. Ordinarily the interests of the corpse overlap with interests of living parties asserting their own legal claims. For example, a wife seeking to prevent disturbance of her late husband's resting place is protecting both her own interest in peace of mind and the corpse's right of repose. However, as noted above, sometimes a living party in court is not acting consistently with the corpse's instructions or interests. At that point, it is useful and important that the independent rights of the corpse be acknowledged as limiting the prerogatives of the living claimant.

Examples abound of protected cadaveric rights independent of injury to survivors. Note that desecration of a grave or abuse of a corpse is a criminal offense whether or not there are survivors whose feelings might be injured. Similarly, when a cemetery seeks to prevent wrongful removal of a body from its burial place, the main underlying harm is to the repose of the body rather than to the economic interests of the cemetery. Some states have allowed harvesting of corneas in the course of autopsies. If this is a constitutional wrong (an issue considered in chapter 7), the principal interest at stake is the integrity of the human cadaver and not the survivors' feelings. To the survivors, the corneal corpse, for all practical purposes, looks the same as any other autopsied body. The defacement (pardon the expression) occurs to the corpse. Given all the legal protections afforded to cadavers independent of their survivors or caretakers, we should have no more trouble thinking about a cadaver's rights grounded in postmortem human dignity than thinking about an animal's right to humane treatment or a human fetus's protected status.

Of course, a cadaver faces considerable natural threats without reference to abuses from human sources. I turn next to the decomposition processes that affect the human cadaver. Understanding the prospect of inexorable disintegration is a fitting prelude to the ensuing discussion of available ways to dispose of a corpse.

# Part II

# Disposition of Human Remains

Soon ripe
Soon rotten
Soon gone
But not forgotten

> Epitaph on a Massachusetts tombstone

Did you ever think when the hearse goes by,
That some fine day you are going to die?
They'll put you in a wooden shirt
And cover you over with gravel and dirt.
The worms crawl in, the worms crawl out,
They're in your ears and out your snout.
The worms crawl in, the worms crawl out,
Eating your guts and spitting them out.

> A rhyme of unknown origin

*Chapter 4*

# Decomposition of the Body and Efforts to Slow Its Disintegration

The first clue that the human body is highly degradable comes from terminology. The word "cadaver" is, at least according to court opinions, derived from the Latin words *caro data vermibus*, meaning flesh (or carrion) given to worms. That derivation is sometimes contested. Some commentators connect the word "cadaver" to the Latin *cadere*, meaning to fall. Certainly, a cadaver has, in some sense, fallen. I still prefer the first derivation, *caro data vermibus*, not because I think it is the real source of the word "cadaver," but because it contains an important truth. Depending on its mode of disposal, a cadaver will sooner or later decompose. Cremation acts quickly to disintegrate the corpse. Burial preserves the corpse longer, depending on the conditions preceding and accompanying interment. Yet the "soon rotten" inscription on the quoted Massachusetts tombstone is basically accurate as applied to burial. The questions become: How soon is soon? What, if anything, can be done to delay the rotting process? How long can the decomposition process be delayed?

**Natural Deterioration**

Left on its own, a corpse will unfailingly putrefy and disintegrate. The process begins within minutes of death. The most immediate and obvious transformation is in flesh color. A corpse promptly takes on the pallor of death. To quote Sherwin Nuland, "A man's corpse looks as though his essence has left him, and it has."[1] Blood drains from the surface capillaries and enters the deeper veins, leaving the skin paler than in life. However, not all of the skin surface remains pale. Within a couple of hours, gravity and deoxygenation come into play. Blood accumulates in the lower body parts, creating there a purple discoloration known as "livor mortis." That lower flesh darkens to red "before progressing through shades of purple and blue" as oxygen disappears from the blood.[2] By ten hours after death, that purple stain becomes fixed until the discoloration disappears in the embalming process when blood is drained from the corpse. (Livor mortis is discussed more fully in chapter 8 in the context of forensic analysis of the corpse.) Another color change occurs in an uncleansed corpse. Within forty-eight hours a greenish-black palette of bacteria growth appears on patches of skin.

The consistency or rigidity of the body mass also changes upon death. Immediately upon death, most muscles become flaccid, as is often demonstrated by the lower jaw of the corpse falling open. The body then has the consistency of a cut of meat in a butcher's display case. That status changes quickly. Within one to six hours after death the process of "rigor mortis," that is, stiffening of the muscles, begins. The stiffening is caused by the disappearance of a chemical in the muscles that assisted muscle contraction. Over a period of four to ten hours after onset, rigor mortis spreads from the face downward to the legs. Full rigor occurs within twelve hours of onset and the body is then stiff (the obvious origin of the nickname "stiff").[3] The temporary stiffness can be overcome with force, that is, massage and manipulation of extremities, but the muscles shortly begin to relax anyway.[4] Within several more hours rigor mortis ends. The muscle relaxation rate depends on many variables, including temperature, but is often complete within twenty-four to thirty-six hours after death.[5]

The physiological change that compels artificial intervention and/or prompt disposal of a corpse is putrefaction. The precise rate of decay depends on variables such as weight, temperature, moisture, and oxygen. Putrefaction—the dissolution of the corpse into liquids and gases—generally begins within minutes of death and becomes noticeable within two to three days.[6] Cells within the body begin to break down and to disperse in liquid form proteins, carbohydrates, acids, and enzymes, among other things. Bacteria colonies present in the body, especially in the large intestine, multiply, break through internal walls into the abdomen, and spread through the now passive circulatory system. "Blood is a fertile sea in which bacteria swarm and multiply."[7] The bacteria feast on the cells' by-products. The microbial action of the bacteria, together with the destructive enzymes flowing from cell breakdown, gradually liquefies soft tissue.[8] Organs are the first parts to liquefy, starting with the eyes and proceeding to the brain, stomach, and liver. Bacteria and enzymes continue to devour fatty tissue, muscle tissue, and connective tissue. The conversion of tissue to liquid starts by the seventh day after death and extends over weeks, months, or years, depending on the surrounding conditions. Temperature is an important variable. Higher temperatures speed up the decay process, while lower temperatures retard it. Artificial interventions such as chilling, freezing, or embalming delay decay.

The bacteria that spread in the body have additional noticeable effects. Within days, the bacteria-caused decay in tissue produces foul-smelling gases and liquids. The gases, including hydrogen sulfide, sulfur dioxide, methane, and ammonia, not only produce a stench but also cause the corpse to bloat. By the fourth or fifth day, gases have begun to inflate the trunk, tongue, eyes, breasts, and genitals.[9] The foul odor of death has by now permeated surrounding rooms. In the second week, the gas pressure can make the abdomen, scrotum, breasts, and tongue swell and the eyes bulge.[10] The gas pressure can also cause liquid to ooze from the nose, mouth, and other orifices and can make intestines protrude from the anus and vagina. Organs swollen by gases may begin to rupture and liquefy. Eventually gas pressure is capable of bursting the thoracic or abdominal cavities. Before embalming was common, sealed coffins sometimes exploded because of gas pressure.

Decomposition of the corpse's internal organs is paralleled by surface deterioration. By seven days after death, large blisters appear on a deteriorating corpse's skin. These patches eventually loosen, and the top layer of skin detaches. After three or four weeks, hair and nails loosen as soft tissue decays and is converted to a semiliquid state.[11]

Because an unattended cadaver becomes repulsive within four or five days of death, steps are commonly taken to retard the putrefaction process and to make the body presentable to observers during the period between death and ultimate disposal of the cadaver. Those steps usually begin immediately upon discovery of death. At the outset, they include cleaning and possibly chilling the cadaver.

Consider a hospital nurse's duties after medical certification of death. The nurse must notify both hospital personnel and the patient's family. The nurse draws the curtains, closes the corpse's eyes and mouth, washes the body, withdraws invasive devices (unless an autopsy is likely), labels the body and lays it out, as if asleep, for viewing (when that is likely) or places the body in a mortuary bag and seals it. The corpse will be transported either to the hospital morgue to await pickup (or, in limited circumstances, autopsy) or directly to a funeral home. The morgue is chilled to between 35 and 46 degrees Fahrenheit.

If death occurs in a private dwelling, a representative of a hired funeral parlor customarily arrives within hours to bag the body and transport it to the funeral home. At the funeral home, the funeral director—formerly known as the "undertaker"—prepares the cadaver for ultimate disposal. As in the hospital, early tasks are cleaning and disinfecting the surface; chilling will also occur if the body is to be preserved for disposition without embalming.

At the funeral parlor, a common next step is embalming. The primary object of embalming is to delay the putrefaction process long enough to facilitate the coming disposal steps by warding off odors, leakage, and other unpleasantness.[12] Embalming involves infusing a liquid preservative into the corpse to inhibit decay. Competent embalming will provide enough stability to permit the disposition of a body that neither looks nor smells bad.

Embalming also usually entails a cosmetic process. When viewing the body will be part of the disposal process—via either an open-casket wake or a private family viewing prior to a funeral—an undertaker uses tools and makeup to make the cadaver more aesthetically pleasing. The object of the funeral home's ministrations is to create "the sculptured image of a living human being who is resting in sleep."[13] I will shortly describe in detail both the preservative and cosmetic aspects of embalming.

There is dispute about whether embalming also serves as a public health measure by disinfecting the remains pending ultimate disposition. The funeral industry persistently claims that embalming helps protect the people working with corpses in a funeral home. However, some scientists contend that the vast majority of deaths stem from noncommunicable causes and that corpses pose no health threat to the living.[14] For those scientists, rubber gloves and disinfectants suffice to dispel any health danger.

## Without Embalming, How Soon Is a Cadaver Rotten?

The process of decomposition—putrefaction, decay, and dissolution—can continue for weeks, months, or years, depending on the surrounding conditions, especially temperature and moisture. Certain disposals, such as cremation or cryonic freezing, promptly arrest the natural decomposition. What is the effect of the more common mode of disposition—burial?

The answer is that burial can delay but ordinarily cannot prevent the bodily deterioration process. Of course, the rate of postburial decay is affected by numerous variables—including the degree of embalming or disinfecting before burial, the depth of the grave, the type of soil, the type of casket or container (if any), the temperature, and the moisture. If burial is one foot deep or less, carnivorous insects or mammals may have access to the corpse and deterioration will be rapid. The customary depth of six feet precludes that action, but putrefaction still occurs because of bacteria, cell breakdown, and degeneration of flesh. An unembalmed adult body without a coffin normally takes five to twelve years to decompose to a skeleton.[15] (The disintegration process is four times faster in water.)

Placement of a cadaver in a closed container before burial inhibits somewhat the messy decomposition process that would otherwise occur. That is, a strong, well-insulated coffin extends the time before total decomposition. The original hope and expectation might have been that a coffin would shelter a corpse and entirely prevent bodily deterioration. In early America, burial receptacles could not accomplish that objective.

The first coffins were wooden and inevitably rotted and collapsed over time. Many insects, including maggot-producing phorid flies, found their way into rotting coffins.

From the 1860s on, coffin materials included metal and stone. The object was to use durable, air- and watertight containers to preclude or retard a cadaver's decomposition and assure the undisturbed repose to which the cadaver was entitled under the common law. The metal caskets were advertised as "airtight, indestructible, and free from encroachment of vermin or water."[16]

In the late 1800s, undertakers sold porcelain-lined cast iron coffins that were welded shut.[17] These coffins sometimes achieved a significant degree of bodily preservation, though they were quite expensive. Yet the sealing of coffins never succeeded in precluding ultimate decomposition. First, it was virtually impossible to secure an airtight coffin. Second, anaerobic bacteria were still present within the cadaver and ensured the ultimate putrefaction of remains. Coffins of that era slowed but did not preclude decomposition.

Efforts have since continued to manufacture metal caskets hermetically sealed against water, insects, and bacteria. A corpse's enzymes need water for their chemical reactions; without water, bodily decomposition is inhibited.[18] During the twentieth century, metal coffins made from bronze, copper, and steel became more common than wooden ones.[19] These included some "sealer" models in which a rubber gasket was placed between the lid and the base of the coffin. (John F. Kennedy was buried in a hermetically sealed, double-walled bronze coffin.[20])

All of these sealing efforts do not succeed in preventing eventual bodily deterioration.[21] Metal caskets can have pinholes at the corners.[22] The rubber gaskets under the casket lid break down over time under the influence of percolating water, ground weight, freezing, and thawing. And even before the casket breaks down, the bodily contents begin to decompose. Anaerobic bacteria within the corpse thrive. Indeed, they create gas that can build up and even cause coffins to burst. To relieve the anticipated buildup of gas, mausoleum and cemetery personnel purposely left caskets unsealed. The bottom line is plain: "No matter how it's sealed inside the coffin, a corpse, even an embalmed one, will eventually decompose."[23] That conclusion still applies. Corpses still decompose even in metal sealer caskets.

Since the middle of the twentieth century, it has become common to lower coffins into concrete vaults preset in a grave. The concrete vault lines the bottom portion of a grave and generally is eight feet long, three feet wide at its base, and three feet high on all sides.[24] A vault may contain a ton of reinforced concrete coated inside with a waterproof polymer, plus a 1,200-pound lid with a rubber gasket seeking to seal the vault. Nonetheless, vaults are not fully watertight, and moisture eventually reaches the coffin and its contents. Even a more sophisticated vault—comprised of a steel dome lowered onto a steel plate underlying a coffin—will not prevent disintegration of a corpse. Some cemeteries require vaults, not to keep water out of coffins but rather to keep the gravesite from caving in when the casket degrades.[25]

How quickly does the inevitable disintegration of a buried corpse take place? One estimate is that a corpse buried in a metal coffin will, after forty years, be reduced to "a blackened skeleton."[26] By then, all flesh has disintegrated and a black mold covers everything, including the skeleton and the inside of the casket. Well before the forty-year mark, the corpse has become rather unpalatable. According to numerous sources, a body exhumed after years of underground repose is not a pretty sight. Jessica Mitford has described such a body as "a repugnant, moldy, foul-looking object."[27] In other words, even if the corpse is not yet skeletonized and retains its contours, the remains are still decomposed, covered with mold, and smelly. The modern coffin's primary function, then, is to help create a pleasing memory picture at the time of burial.

All the time lines on decomposition discussed up to now assume that the corpse is recovered soon after death. That is not always the case. A corpse left exposed to the elements in warm weather will, thanks to insects, be reduced to a skeleton within weeks. Such exposed bodies become quick prey to a variety of insects, especially maggots and beetles. In areas where animals have previously died, as in the woods, blowflies begin to land on a corpse within seconds. These flies can detect molecules of decaying flesh for miles around. The flies promptly lay thousands of eggs within body orifices such as the mouth, nose, and ears, as well as in any exposed wound. Within days those eggs hatch into maggots that then contribute to the stripping of the exposed corpse. Maggots can eat tissue, exude enzymes, and thus supplement the microbial dissolution taking place. In addition, other carnivorous insects such as carrion beetles can appear, depending on the corpse's location, and further hasten the decomposition process. Ultimately the insects disappear, the liquids evaporate, and bones and dry remains are left. Eventually even the bones dissolve.[28] Dust to dust.

In short, initial exposure of a corpse to flies or continued exposure to insects can considerably hasten the decomposition process. Again, a corpse exposed to the elements and hence to insects can be stripped to the bones within weeks. An unembalmed corpse in a well-insulated casket will take up to twelve years to disintegrate fully. Most corpses are embalmed. What happens in that process, and how long does it maintain the integrity of human remains?

### Embalming as a Means of Preservation

Though funeral homes urge embalming of a corpse as a matter of course, that step is not mandatory. No American state requires embalming if a corpse is to be disposed of expeditiously. Jews and Muslims neither embalm corpses nor expose them to public viewing. They bury their dead quickly (Muslims within twenty-four hours) consistent with rules restricting Sabbath activity. A secular "green" burial also eschews embalming in order to avoid toxic damage from embalming fluids.

There just are not a lot of palatable ways to preserve human remains in their lifelike form. Ancient societies used a variety of immersions, such as in honey, in an unsuccessful effort to preserve bodily integrity. By the end of the eighteenth century, anatomists had discovered that body parts immersed in alcohol would not decompose. In 1805 Admiral Horatio Nelson's corpse was transported home from the sea immersed in a barrel of spirits. In the nineteenth century physicians and others used immersion in various chemical solutions to preserve body parts as teaching specimens, displays, or curios.[29] That preservation system was fine for body parts, but it was not appealing for entire corpses.

Modern embalming entails circulating a liquid chemical preservative throughout the corpse in order to arrest the corpse's cellular decay and tissue decomposition.[30] This process is called "arterial embalming." It dates to the 1600s, when anatomists sought to preserve certain corpses for public dissection. The primary utility of embalming then was to reduce the stench during the dissections aimed at teaching prospective healers, artists, and sculptors about human anatomy.

In seventeenth- and early-eighteenth-century America, embalming was seldom used. Bodies were buried quickly or, if burial was delayed, kept on ice. Even into the mid-1800s artificial preservation of human remains was uncommon. A corpse was typically laid out at home for one to three days. If available, ice was placed under the coffin. Burial took place without administration of any artificial preservative.

In the middle to late eighteenth century, arterial embalming emerged in America as a potential means of retarding putrefaction of a corpse. Surgeon/anatomist brothers John and William Hunter were among the first to promote embalming of cadavers. They injected various chemicals into corpses and sometimes put embalmed cadavers on display in an effort to show the public how well human remains could be preserved. In 1775 William Hunter embalmed a Mrs. Martin Van Butchell.[31] The Van Butchells had an agreement (perhaps a very early prenuptial agreement) saying that Mr. Van Butchell would control his wife's fortune "as long as she remained above ground."[32] Upon Mrs. Van Butchell's death, Dr. Hunter injected turpentine and vermilion into her blood vessels, removed organs from her chest and abdominal cavities, packed the cavities with a mixture of camphor and resin, and added more chemicals to the blood vessels. Mr. Van Butchell then kept his wife's remains above ground for an indefinite period, first in a glass-covered case in his drawing room and later on display at the Royal College of Physicians. In 1857 Mrs. Van Butchell was still on public display, but her cadaver had shrunk, assumed a mahogany color, and become an unpalatable exhibit.

In the early nineteenth century, American arterial embalmers continued experimenting with various substances, including turpentine, nitrate solutions, spirits such as rum, and liquid metals such as mercury, zinc, and arsenic. (Arsenic was eventually banned because of its interference with forensic investigations and autopsies.) Not only arterial embalming but also crude cavity embalming was used. All in all, arterial embalming was not widespread. Early American embalming techniques had not yielded satisfactory enough results to draw widespread public attention. While the embalming process was embraced by some

practitioners in the mid-nineteenth century, it was used primarily to preserve cadavers for dissection in medical schools.[33]

Arterial embalming got its real impetus during the Civil War. The
prevailing custom then was to bury the war dead close to the battlefield.
Yet it had been discovered that arterial embalming with bichloride of
mercury could preserve soldiers' corpses long enough to permit their
transport home for a funeral and a more fitting burial. At first, the embalming technique was utilized for officers or soldiers from wealthy
families.[34] Over the course of the war, more and more soldiers and their
families became embalmers' customers. Bereaved families dispatched
relatives or undertakers to battlefields and grave sites in order to arrange
embalming and shipment home.[35]

During the Civil War, embalmers accompanied troops and competed for business out of tents near field hospitals. They even sought to advertise their embalming services with fliers nailed to trees near army
campsites, but Union officers did not appreciate the demoralizing influence and banned the practice. One doctor, Thomas Holmes, claimed
to have embalmed 4,028 Union cadavers over a four-year period. He
charged $100 per cadaver, so if he secured payment from all families, he
would have taken in approximately $400,000.

In the 1870s independent traveling instructors circulated throughout
the United States teaching embalming in courses lasting for a few days.
In the 1880s formal schools for embalming were established. Some embalmers took their former clients' corpses (perhaps those whose bills
were unpaid) on tours of barbershops or county fairs to exhibit their
products and promote their businesses.[36] In the same period, the American funeral industry developed because of improvements both in embalming and in cosmetic restoration. By the 1883 meeting of the funeral
directors' national organization, arterial embalming to retard bodily decay and decomposition was an article of industry faith.[37] In 1893 the
hardening capacity of formaldehyde was discovered, and formaldehyde became the preferred substance for embalming. Today formalin, a
40 percent formaldehyde solution, is still a prime ingredient of embalming fluid. By 1900 embalming was still the exception, but its appeal—
including winter wakes in the comfort of a warm room—was spreading.
Today embalming is a regular part of the funeral process, especially
when a viewing is anticipated.

## Process and Results of Embalming

Contemporary embalming has three objectives—disinfecting, temporary preservation against putrefaction, and restoration of lifelike features (at least when public viewing is in store).[38] The first task is cleansing the body. Thorough washing with a germicidal soap and disinfectant kills insects and viruses on the cadaver's surface. A disinfectant spray then reaches the nostrils, mouth, and throat. Orifices are then packed with cotton wads to prevent leakage of various bodily fluids or "purge" seeping from the interior of the cadaver.[39]

The next step, an arterial embalming process to reduce disintegration, involves significant bodily intrusions. Embalming fluid is pumped mechanically into the corpse via a tube placed in the carotid artery in the neck or the femoral artery in the thigh.[40] A drainage tube is inserted into a large nearby vein such as the jugular vein (near the carotid artery). Approximately three gallons of formaldehyde and methyl alcohol solution are circulated within the body.[41] The body is simultaneously drained of blood as embalming fluid entering the blood vessels pushes the blood ahead in major arteries and veins to drain through the drainage tube. That drained fluid then flows into the local sewerage system.

The diffusion of gallons of chemical preservatives throughout the body has several effects. The chemicals reduce the presence and growth of microorganisms in order to retard cellular decomposition. Embalming fluid temporarily hardens the body's protein to preserve tissue from enzymes and bacteria; its smell deters insects. In short, embalming fluid kills bacteria and fortifies tissue against decomposition.[42]

Cavity embalming supplements arterial embalming.[43] A long, hollow instrument called a "trocar" is inserted into the abdominal and chest cavities. Attached to an aspirator, the trocar sucks up the contents of those cavities—including blood, bodily fluids, fecal matter, semidigested food, and masses of bacteria. A trocar is also used to puncture and remove gases and liquids from each hollow organ in the cavities.[44] After the vacuuming is accomplished, a trocar infuses chemical preservatives into the abdominal and chest cavities.

In situations in which survivors may gaze upon the cadaver, part of the funeral parlor's task is to make the body presentable for viewing. An embalmer's chemical treatment of a corpse's viscera will then be accompanied by cosmetic steps to restore the integrity and appearance of the cadaver. For public viewing, the undertaker seeks to create a memory picture of the deceased laid out and looking as if he or she is engaged in normal, restful sleep.[45] The hope is to cultivate a palatable last image conducive to a mourning process.

The typical funeral home treatment enhances a corpse's appearance in numerous ways. A shave is performed where needed. Embalming fluid may include dye to add a warm tinge of life to the skin. Special attention is devoted to the exposed face and hands. A hanging lower jaw is closed and the mouth is stitched shut. An ice pack is used to reduce swelling. Plastic lens-shaped domes may be placed under the eyelids to prevent the appearance of eyeballs sinking into the skull. Discolorations can be bleached out or covered by tinted cosmetic creams or powders. Any unsightly protrusions of tissue can be cut away by scalpel incisions and covered by restorative waxes or makeup. Sags or depressions are fixable with mortuary putty or plastic forms placed underneath the depressions. Even gravity helps to remove wrinkles. Lips are colored and glued shut. A mortuary makeup kit includes, inter alia, sandpaper, mascara, lip waxes, and tinted hair sprays. Tinted cream is rubbed into the face and hands to try to restore a healthy glow. A manicure is customary along with hair styling.

Then the corpse is dressed in finery (or not) selected by the family. A tie and jacket for a man are customary but not mandatory. A semiformal dress is common for a woman. Clothes are typically split down the back both for ease in dressing an uncooperative wearer and for arranging a better fit on what is often an emaciated figure. Work uniforms or outfits are also appropriate, depending on the wearer's vocation. Commonly the displayed cadaver is "nattily attired and posed as if sleeping in a bed-like box designed to look attractive and comfortable."[46] (Given the viewing's partial objective of convincing the viewers about death, it is somewhat ironic that morticians strive to maximize the *live* appearance of the deceased both in their cosmetic ministrations and in dressing the corpse.)

The last step before a viewing is to position the corpse inside the open coffin. Props under the body stabilize the head, arms, and legs. Customarily hands are joined over the lower abdomen. The head is tilted at a 15 degree angle to ensure that mourners can easily view the face.

A central thesis of this book is that a corpse is entitled to be treated with basic dignity—what I call postmortem human dignity. How degrading are the multiple bodily intrusions accompanying embalming? Jessica Mitford disdainfully described embalming as having a corpse "sprayed, sliced, pierced, pickled, trussed, trimmed, creamed, waxed, painted, rouged, and neatly dressed."[47] She considered cosmetic efforts to deny or hide death to be grotesque.

The embalming process does indeed entail puncturing, draining, injecting chemicals, resurfacing, sewing, and smearing with cosmetics. Does that process violate a corpse's dignity? Despite those bodily intrusions, the embalming process does preserve the corpse until burial, eliminates smells, prevents leakage, and generally gives the corpse a presentable appearance for public viewing. Embalming therefore seems thoroughly justifiable despite its multiple bodily intrusions. Just as a surgeon mutilates a person during open-heart surgery in order to restore health, an embalmer's intervention aimed at making a corpse fit for viewing seems acceptable and consistent with a corpse's dignity. What is so bad about restoring an image of the deceased at peace or reminding mourners of a previously more vital persona? Perhaps a more palatable last image is emotionally conducive to mourning.

## Duration of Preservation

Duration of the preservative effects of embalming varies according to the intensity of the chemical intervention. Typical embalming for a funeral seeks to protect the corpse from putrefaction only for a matter of days or weeks. The object is to buy time for visitation and disposal during the several days following death.[48] Thereafter the formaldehyde solution breaks down and bacteria begin to do their work.

For special circumstances, such as protracted public display of a cadaver or use in medical school education, more intensive embalming can preserve a corpse much longer. A cadaver slated for dissection by medical students gets seven gallons of a more highly concentrated embalming fluid.[49] In addition, the preservative fluid is pumped into a closed vein system under pressure so that more saturation takes place in the circulatory system. After saturation, the vein system is opened and excess fluid drains. Such a cadaver will last at least for the several months of an anatomy course and for years longer if not dissected.[50]

Reinforced embalming can produce much longer-lasting preservation than customary embalming. More thorough embalming uses stronger chemicals and multiple injections of those chemicals. Vladimir Lenin's corpse is still on display in the Kremlin almost ninety years after his death. (However, his initial embalming has been reinforced many times during that period.) Eva Peron's embalmed corpse lasted for more than twenty years. After an initial embalming process lasting for three years, her body was buried in Italy. When an exiled Juan Peron returned to Argentina, he exhumed Eva's body and kept it in his Argentine attic for two years before having it entombed in a family mausoleum.[51] Civil rights activist Medgar Evers was so thoroughly embalmed that his corpse was still suitable for an autopsy decades after his murder.

You might wonder why embalming today seeks to postpone putrefaction only for days or weeks. Why don't more people insist on the Peron/Evers treatment? One answer is that larger doses of preservative fluids make it harder to produce a lifelike appearance in the corpse. Heavy chemical embalming produces an unnatural appearance in both the texture and tinge of the skin.[52] That fact, along with the perceived need for only temporary inhibition of decomposition, probably accounts for the modest preservation period typically achieved via embalming.

Mummification and plastination are possible methods for long-term preservation of a corpse. But while those processes preserve the human contours of the remains, they do not preserve a lifelike appearance. A mummification procedure might last a thousand years or more. A plastination process to preserve human remains would probably guarantee preservation of a corpse's basic contours for at least hundreds of years. For reasons to be discussed in chapter 6, which deals with modern disposal techniques for maximizing preservation of remains, neither mummification nor plastination, despite their long-lasting effects, is likely to be your chosen means of bodily disposal.

Some people consider the aboveground mausoleum to be a preferred resting place because it seems more sanitary and less claustrophobic than a coffin covered with several feet of earth.[53] Ironically a mausoleum or any other aboveground sepulcher does not typically affect the nature or pace of bodily decomposition. Corpses are embalmed before entombment in order to delay putrefaction, but not to any greater extent than for regular burial.[54] Because heat can become quite intense in a mausoleum, the locale may actually accelerate decomposition. Funeral directors may suggest either a thick plastic bag or a plastic tray underneath a mausoleum casket to hold leakage of embalming fluid or other bodily fluids over time. Occasionally a body interred in a mausoleum will explode because of trapped gases.[55]

Better long-term results from embalming seem to have been achieved with discrete body parts, particularly the heart. Separate preservation of the heart has been used at different times by different cultures. The ancient Egyptians left an embalmed heart within the mummified chest cavity or in an adjacent urn. At one stage, European Catholics buried the corpses of distinguished clergy outside the church but preserved their hearts in urns within the church structure. Apparently the hearts still tended to shrivel up. European royalty also sometimes kept the remains of forebearers' hearts in separate urns. Richard the Lionheart was buried in Fontevrault, France, but his heart was presented to the people of Rouen in gratitude for their prior assistance. It eventually withered like a leaf.

The best results—in terms of pristine preservation over a very long term—have been achieved with the bodies of saints. Saint Teresa Margaret of the Sacred Heart died of gangrene in 1770. Fifteen days postmortem her remains showed no signs of putrefaction, retained a pink hue, and had a sweet fragrance. When viewed in 1805, her corpse still had a healthy flesh color. Note, though, that when Teresa Margaret was canonized in 1934, her preserved body was dark and dry (though still uncorrupted). Saint Bernadette Soubirous died in 1879. When disinterred (once in 1909 and once in 1919), she appeared to be almost perfectly preserved.[56] So sainthood seems to be a possible antidote to bodily decomposition. However, that route to eternal preservation is generally arduous and attainable by only a tiny percentage of the population.

Interestingly, the premortem diet has the potential to retard postmortem decomposition. In one instance, a person who followed a strict, ascetic diet for several years before death produced a corpse that was resistant to decomposition. The diet consisted mostly of the nuts and bark of pine trees. It caused mental dullness and cravings for food while building up resistance to decomposition.[57] Each individual can make a personal decision on whether to follow this ascetic regimen.

To conclude, a cadaver is very likely to decompose completely over time whether treated or untreated, whether interred below or above ground, and whether placed in a sealed container or not. Embalming can delay that decomposition, but under current practices it preserves the cadaver only for days, weeks, or months. Alternatives like mummification or plastination prevent complete deterioration but leave the cadaver disfigured and perhaps grotesque. Given these facts, we can examine the multiple ways in which Americans choose to dispose of human remains.

Assume that we are confronted with the dead body of a man. What disposition shall we make of it? Shall we lay it in a boat that is set adrift? Shall we take the heart from it and bury it in one place and the rest of the body in another? Shall we expose it to wild animals? Burn it on a pyre? Push it into a pit to rot with other bodies? Boil it until the flesh falls off the bones, and throw the flesh away and treasure the bones?

> Kenneth Iserson, *Death to Dust*

The physicality of a human corpse is undeniable. It is a carcass, with a predisposition to decay, to become noisome, obnoxious to the senses, and harrowing to the emotions. Disposal of such perishable remains is imperative.

> Ruth Richardson, *Death, Dissection and the Destitute*

*Chapter 5*

# Final Disposal of Human Remains

Without proper disposal, a corpse not only gives sensory offense, it poses some danger of contagion to the living. Decent disposal also signifies respect and fidelity to the deceased, consistent with the hope and expectation of the vast majority of people that their remains will be afforded a dignified final disposition. And proper disposal of remains can give comfort and perhaps closure to survivors, often fulfilling a sense of responsibility toward the cadaver on both the natural and supernatural planes.[1]

Cultural traditions shape the appropriate mode of cadaver disposal and provide a paradigm for its safe management.[2] Rituals for the dead have been performed since time immemorial and are among "the most enduring of all cultural traditions."[3] Those rituals often aim to protect the soul or spirit of the fallen.[4] Human remains have traditionally been associated with a lingering spiritual presence—whether the lingering presence is considered to be housed within physical remains, a hovering spirit, or just part of collective memories. Survivors therefore feel a duty to "ensure the speedy release and future wellbeing of the departed spirit."[5] Few survivors ever want to offend the spirit of the departed, especially if they believe that spiritual retaliation for neglect is a possibility. The notion that the postmortem conduct of survivors could affect the soul's fate was widespread as the pattern of American funerary rituals evolved.

While assuring undisturbed rest has been the overriding object of American methods of disposal of human remains, a variety of other rites partially aimed at spiritual reinforcement commonly form part of final disposal.[6] After a corpse is transported to a funeral parlor, cleaned, and embalmed, a series of ritualized events typically occurs. A wake is held (with or without an open casket); a funeral service is held (whether at a religious institution, a funeral home, or the place of ultimate disposal); and finally, the corpse is sent to its ultimate disposition, most often lowered into the ground.[7] The last step, final disposal of the corpse, may or may not be accompanied by a brief committal ceremony.

**Burial**

Underground burial has been a principal means of securing eternal repose for tens of thousands of years.[8] Perhaps the original impetus for burial was to promptly remove the smell of rotting flesh and simultaneously prevent access to the corpse by scavengers or cannibals. Custom and religion have supplemented the original motivations for decent burial.

Ancient Romans and Greeks believed that souls could not enter the lands of the dead if their bodies had not been buried.[9] Jews adopted burial as a fulfillment of the biblical statement "for dust thou art, and unto dust shalt thou return."[10] Early Christians supplanted cremation of human remains with burial as an adaptation of Jesus Christ's entombment and resurrection. Christ himself resurrected Lazarus from his tomb. And Christ preached that "The hour cometh wherein all that are in graves shall hear the voice of the Son of God. And they that have done good things shall come forth unto the resurrection of life; but they that have done evil, unto the resurrection of Judgment."[11]

The United States was and is a largely Christian country, so burial early became "the disposal of choice" here.[12] Christian cadavers were typically laid to rest underground to await resurrection; the coffin supposedly protected against external disturbance in the meantime.[13] In colonial and early republican times, cadavers were buried without a great deal of preparation or fanfare. Puritans believed that new bodies would accompany resurrection, so earthly remains were "a meaningless husk" to be unceremoniously buried.[14] Over time, however, Americans more and more came to mark death and burial as moments for ceremony.

## Locus of Burial

> Why do cemeteries all have walls?
> It's silly beyond a doubt;
> The people outside don't want to get in
> And the people inside can't get out!
> > Robert Hatch, *What Happens When You Die*,
> > quoting British comedian Benny Hill

A cemetery is an area set apart largely for underground burial of the dead or their ashes (though some cemeteries also offer options for aboveground entombment). In colonial and early republican periods, the churchyard or the yard outside the meeting house served as the primary burial place. Gravestones in such locations date back to the mid-1600s.[15] By the late eighteenth century churchyard cemeteries had become crowded, even though their burial chambers or vaults handled several layers of coffins and/or side compartments. By 1800 the yard of Trinity Church in lower Manhattan, New York City, contained one hundred thousand remains; multiple layers of burial had actually raised the surface level.[16] As urban land became more valuable, many church burial grounds were sold and their occupants reinterred elsewhere.

Other sorts of cemeteries appeared in early America. Private family plots served as one option. In 1799 George Washington was laid to rest in a vault on the grounds of his Mount Vernon home. In the early 1800s some families with land similarly devoted a small portion to a family burial plot. Rhode Island is dotted with thousands of such family cemeteries. (Families can still choose homestead burial, though local law generally prescribes a minimum depth and requires a certain distance from any water supply.[17])

In the same period, privately owned cemetery corporations came into being. These enterprises sold a perpetual right of burial and visitation but did not convey outright title to the plot.[18] One early example of the private cemetery is the Congressional Cemetery in Washington, D.C. Despite its deceptive name, it started as a four-and-a-half-acre private cemetery in 1807. Though deeded at one point to Christ Church, it returned to private, nonprofit ownership and reached thirty-two and one-half acres by 1875. Its current sixty thousand graves include veterans from the Revolutionary War, the War of 1812, and the Civil War (both sides), as well as numerous public figures. Such cemetery grounds became resting places not only for burial of cadavers but also for aboveground entombment in mausoleums, table vaults (aboveground vaults on legs), or sarcophagi. (In other words, some well-off individuals preferred to decompose in aboveground sepulchers rather than in underground graves.)[19]

The college graveyard also developed in the early 1800s. In that period, when embalming was both rudimentary and uncommon, a college student's corpse could not be transported a long distance for a home burial. Numerous colleges set aside space for burials within the campus. For example, in 1808 Mount St. Mary's University in Maryland created a graveyard that accommodated students, priests, professors, and even a few slaves.[20] The University of Virginia's campus graveyard dates to 1828. (Interestingly, college resting places are today enjoying somewhat of a comeback, as will shortly be explained.)

Another form of cemetery, publicly owned, also developed in the nineteenth century. As churchyard cemeteries became overcrowded, towns set aside land for cemeteries with plots available at a modest fee to town residents. In addition, as municipalities took responsibility for poorhouses for the indigent, they created burial grounds known as "potter's fields" for people who died without means for a cemetery plot. For reasons to be explained, these potter's fields were a poor substitute for a paid burial in a regular cemetery.

As early as the time of the Roman Empire, public authorities had sought to confine burials to areas outside of cities. A similar push to locate cemeteries in more rural areas occurred in the United States during the nineteenth century. By the 1830s cemeteries in urban settings had become crowded and, according to some critics, were sources of pollution and health dangers.[21] Among the critics were the Sanitarians. The Sanitarian movement sought to move American cemeteries from urban to suburban locations. The Sanitarians, as their name implies, generally sought to improve public health—usually by promoting cleaner streets and more efficient garbage disposal. They also believed that corpses in urban cemeteries emitted toxic miasmas that polluted nearby air and water. They therefore pushed for more isolated burial sites as well as deeper burial (ten feet deep rather than the customary six feet) or complete embedding in cement.[22]

From approximately 1831 on, privately owned cemeteries tended to be established away from densely populated areas. Some of these cemeteries sought to attract customers by locating in rural settings that also served as parks for strolling or picnicking.[23] These rural or garden cemeteries, including woods and landscaped areas, appeared in an era when public parks were relatively scarce.[24] The first well-known garden cemetery was Mount Auburn Cemetery in Boston, established in 1831. Mount Auburn covered 70 acres and included meadows, woods, and walking paths.[25] Laurel Hill Cemetery was established in Philadelphia in 1836 and Green-Wood Cemetery in Brooklyn, New York, in 1838. Green-Wood Cemetery covered 478 acres, including four lakes and thousands of trees. For a time, this cemetery competed with Niagara Falls as New York State's most popular site for recreational visitors.[26] In 1866 the *New York Times* touted Green-Wood Cemetery as being equally "associated with the fame of our city as the Fifth Avenue or the Central Park."[27] Between 1831 and 1890 scores of parklike cemeteries featuring trees, ponds, and trails were created.[28] The garden cemetery fashion reached St. Louis in 1849 (Bellefontaine) and Chicago in 1860 (Graceland).[29] Savannah's Bonaventure featured paths along a river through cedars, magnolias, azaleas, and Spanish moss. It was described by an 1867 traveler as "so beautiful that almost any sensible person would choose to dwell there with the dead rather than [with the] lazy, disorderly living."[30]

## The Social Hierarchy of Disposal

In a sense, death is a great equalizing force.[31] The naked corpse of a rich person in a hospital morgue looks, acts, and is temporarily treated much the same way as a neighboring corpse of a person of modest means. The two corpses are likely to undergo a similar succession of events—cleaning, transport to a funeral home, embalming, a wake, a funeral, and burial. People, including those of lesser means, strive to give their loved ones respectful and decent final disposition in line with American customs. The ultimate fate of a corpse—decomposition—also transpires without much regard for wealth.

This does not mean that all corpses are treated equally. Over the course of American history, the social hierarchy has found stark expression even in the world of cadavers. All the accessories of final disposition via burial or entombment—burial location, coffins, funerary rites, and commemoration markers—tend to vary according to wealth and social status. Marilyn Yalom remarks: "Differences in wealth and status are as striking among the dead as among the living."[32]

Consider the burial of slaves in the eighteenth and nineteenth centuries.[33] On some plantations, dead slaves were simply buried, without coffins or lasting markers, in the fields or woods. On other plantations, a separate slave cemetery was created and slaves' corpses were placed in burlap sacks and dumped into shallow graves marked with a small wooden cross. Wooden markers quickly weathered and disintegrated. At best, a slave might be buried in a separate section of a local cemetery. Free blacks could aspire to coffins and gravestones, but seldom in the same cemetery or the same part of a cemetery as their white compatriots. Excavators in Manhattan in the 1990s uncovered remnants of an African American burial ground in which, it is estimated, twenty thousand people were buried between 1653 and 1796.[34] An 1810 Boston regulation stated that cadavers of "undesirables" such as African Americans and criminals should be confined to a delineated space away from more respectable cemetery sections.[35]

In most American locales, racially separate burial grounds were long the norm, either by custom or by law.[36] Southerners believed that "peace and good order" required racially separate burial grounds as well as separate means of transportation and schools. Beyond the South as well, cemeteries were allowed to discriminate on racial grounds.[37] Most states did not consider private cemeteries as places of public accommodation required to be open to all races. Forest Lawn, a famous California cemetery, was restricted to whites until 1958. Up to that time, waves of

Japanese and Chinese immigrants were excluded from West Coast cemeteries.

Wealth distinctions have always affected the locus of burial. Only the well off could afford the rural garden cemeteries that appeared in the mid-nineteenth century. Even today, costs within each cemetery vary according to the desirability or status of the burial area. In Forest Lawn Cemetery in California, burial in the Terrace of Brilliant Stars section costs twice as much as burial in the Vale of Faith.[38] Location, location, location! When the *Titanic* sank in 1912, the victims' cadavers did not receive equal treatment. Rescue boats recovered 328 cadavers. The 209 cadavers of first-class travelers were embalmed and placed in coffins for return to their homes. Second- and third-class cadavers were placed in canvas bags and recommitted to the ocean.[39]

Corpses of paupers, regardless of color, have always received inferior treatment. A pauper might be a resident of a poorhouse, a prisoner, a hospital patient, or a homeless person without relatives willing to dispose of the body. Or the decedent's family or friends might simply be too poor to afford the customary disposition. The untended potter's fields set aside for paupers' burials were a far cry from the cemeteries catering to the more affluent. A potter's field grave might be a wide, deep pit left open until it was filled with pine coffins. In New York City's potter's field, each grave received three permanent occupants before being filled in. Elsewhere, as many as twenty coffins, separated by little or no earth, might be piled into a pit until the hole was filled and covered over.[40] On the taxpayers' tab, an unclaimed cadaver was relegated without funeral rites to a shabby resting place with makeshift markers that would disappear over time. In New York City alone, over 750,000 people have been buried in its shifting potter's field.[41]

Corpses in potter's fields were also fair game for the grave robbers who supplied anatomists and surgeons with bodies for practice or teaching material in the eighteenth and nineteenth centuries. (Chapter 10 describes the body-snatching phenomenon.) The personnel in charge of poorhouses and potter's fields were notoriously corrupt. A small bribe might suffice to allow suddenly appearing "relatives" easy access to otherwise unclaimed corpses. The indigents whose corpses reached burial were still vulnerable, both because the coffins were flimsy and because the potter's field was not well guarded. In short, the corpses of the very poor, prostitutes, criminals, and immigrants provided a disproportionate percentage of the cadavers exploited by medical schools and surgeons.[42]

Wealth and class distinctions are reflected in other aspects of funerary practice beyond the burial locus. Funerary display has often served as "a powerful articulation of social aspiration and attainment."[43] As early as the mid-eighteenth century, affluent families in New York and New England tended to arrange upscale funerals featuring gifts (such as gloves, rings, scarves, or spoons) to the invited mourners and a postfuneral feast. In Puritan New England, bereaved families sent gloves as a form of funeral invitation.[44] One Boston cleric accumulated three thousand pairs of "invitations" over a thirty-two-year career. In the mid-nineteenth century and later, funerals for the wealthy were distinguished from other funerals by more invited guests, more carriages in the procession, and special gifts for mourners.

Other accoutrements of funerals traditionally reflected and continue to reflect economic status. The opulence of coffins and related disposal containers frequently distinguish the well off.[45] Funeral directors commonly urge the family to provide "the best" for their deceased loved one. This generally means an expensive coffin made with choice wood or metal, high polish, and even an inscription. In the twenty-first century a bronze casket generally costs $5,000 to $9,000, though a gold-plated version will run to $34,000.[46] Coffin interiors can be upgraded with expensive fabrics, special tailoring, and pictorial panels celebrating some passion of the deceased, such as fishing or gardening.[47] In the case of cremation, urns for ashes cover a vast price range, depending on their composition, from plain cardboard or plastic to ornate works of art made from ceramic or metal.

A hierarchy of cadaver disposal according to economic status is nowhere more evident than in the permanent markers erected to memorialize the departed. A tombstone or other grave marker has long served as a means of permanently commemorating an extinguished existence. The practice goes back thousands of years. Stonehenge in England is now considered a cemetery for cremated remains dating back thousands of years. Its majestic stones are thought to be monuments to a ruling local dynasty from about 4,500 years ago.[48]

In prerevolutionary America, only a small percentage of the population could afford permanent grave markers. Those markers were generally flat, upright stones with a rounded tympanum; the inscription often included just the deceased's name and the dates of birth and death. People who could afford to pay stone cutters could embellish gravestones with carved motifs, generally symbols of death such as death heads (a skull with wings), hourglasses, or skeletons.[49] Religious symbolism also appeared, generally cherubs or angelic faces with wings offering some hope of a benign eternity or a heavenly reward.[50]

During the late eighteenth and early nineteenth centuries permanent markers became more elaborate, with marble slabs (ledgers), marble pedestal tables, and marble boxes sometimes marking burial spots rather than flat, upright stones.[51] The early nineteenth century featured a Greek revival movement in grave markers using pedestals and columns, sometimes topped with stone urns. Egyptian motifs, especially obelisks, also became popular.

During the nineteenth and twentieth centuries the wealthy opted for more and more elaborate and ostentatious grave markers. Recall the garden cemetery movement of the mid-1800s. While those sylvan settings aspired to natural beauty, they also came to house grandiose markers of the departed wealthy. Tombstones became monuments, sometimes taking elaborate forms such as obelisks, Gothic spires, stone crosses, or columns. Cemetery statuary also became more elaborate, featuring weeping or soaring angels, cherubs, pietàs, weeping maidens, and even a bust of the deceased.[52]

Another way to display wealth during cadaver disposal was and is entombment in a mausoleum. A mausoleum is an aboveground structure, usually made of granite, with niches or vaults housing one to four coffined cadavers. It might also contain a small seating area or a chapel. A grand mausoleum has long been a symbol of stature. The original mausoleum was a giant tomb erected in the third century BC in part of the Persian Empire by the widow of King Mausolus. That structure was one 140 feet high—one of the seven wonders of the ancient world before it was destroyed by an earthquake. Pre-Christian Romans built mausoleums along the sides of roads. The larger the mausoleum and the nearer it was to Rome, the more attention and prestige it garnered.[53]

Wealthy Americans, starting in the mid-nineteenth century, adopted the granite mausoleum as a status symbol—a more visible and impressive reminder of their existence than a mere gravestone, even one that was elaborately inscribed. Many mausoleums were elaborate columned structures featuring carved friezes. These ostentatious templelike tombs "ensured that the rich and powerful would be neighbors for eternity, sharing the same exclusive community they had enjoyed when alive."[54] The peak years for these structural statements of achievement and stature were the 1870s and 1880s.[55] Philadelphia's Laurel Hill Cemetery developed a millionaire's row of spectacular mausoleums in a variety of architectural styles. In 1880 the Bowman family mausoleum was constructed in Cuttingsville, Vermont. It was described by its architect/designer as being "as imperishable as any structure ever built by human hands," a monument "to perpetuate the well rounded, honorable, successful life and name of its most noble founder."[56] Mr. Bowman's life-size statue was portrayed ascending the outside granite steps. The Bowman mausoleum also featured marble busts of the husband and wife, a massive granite door, and six bronze candelabras. When Ulysses Grant died in 1885, private contributors constructed a massive mausoleum in Riverside Park in New York City. The structure features a domed lobby decorated with murals and sculpture overlooking a sanctuary where Grant and his wife are entombed in twin granite sarcophagi. (Comedian Groucho Marx used to ask, as a consolation-prize question for losers on his television quiz show, "Who's buried in Grant's tomb?")

In the early twentieth century wealthy families like the Rockefellers and the Vanderbilts erected large, ostentatious mausoleums as final resting places.[57] Banker/financier J. P. Morgan's mausoleum in Hartford, Connecticut, was shaped like a safe-deposit box. In St. Louis the brewery barons Adolphus Busch and Lilly Anheuser Busch erected an elaborate neo-Gothic mausoleum. It stood on mausoleum row—a stretch where no money was spared and no style was too ostentatious.[58] When movie producer Irving Thalberg was interred in Forest Lawn Cemetery in 1937, his marble tomb cost $800,000.

In the twenty-first century there has been a resurgence of mausoleums built by wealthy persons aspiring to conspicuous commemoration. The Cold Spring Granite Company, a major supplier of private mausoleums, sold two thousand in 2005 compared to sixty-five in a typical year in the 1980s.[59] In 2007 the average base price for a family mausoleum was $250,000. Two recent family mausoleums—granite structures in the neoclassical pillared style—in a Daytona Beach, Florida, cemetery cost $400,000 and $650,000, respectively. The latter featured red granite, two date palm trees, a balustrade around the structure, and a view of a tree-lined lake.[60] When Leona Helmsley died, her mausoleum in Sleepy Hollow Cemetery in Westchester County, New York, cost $1.4 million. It was a 1,300-square-foot granite structure with Doric columns reminiscent of the Parthenon. One newspaper observed: "The Queen of Mean's last property is fit for a king."[61]

Apropos of wealth, Donald Trump recently wanted to build a family mausoleum and commissioned a design for a mausoleum with an altar, six vaults, and four nineteen-foot obelisks on the outside corners.[62] Mr. Trump then set his heart on a somewhat problematic location for this final resting place. He wanted to place the mausoleum next to the first tee on his beloved Trump National Golf Course in Bedminster, New Jersey. When lawyers pointed out that the local zoning regulations did not permit mausoleums, Mr. Trump initially claimed that the plans were really for a wedding chapel rather than a mausoleum. (After all, the structure did contain an altar.) When the wedding chapel idea was ridiculed he withdrew his plan, but not before an enterprising journalist, Kevin K. Manahan, investigated what the consequences would have been for any golfer whose ball landed against a mausoleum. A helpful Professional Golfers Association official explained that a mausoleum adjacent to the first tee would have been considered "an immovable obstruction," so the errant player would get a free drop without penalty. The official added, "To get in there [the mausoleum], the Donald might have suffered a stroke, but you [the player] don't have to."

Aboveground entombment had historically been an option for the wealthy.[63] However, in the mid-twentieth century the idea of aboveground entombment was adapted to accommodate people who could not afford structures for individual or family crypts. Cemeteries erected buildings containing tier upon tier of contiguous crypts (niches or slots for coffins or urns) with a veneer of marble or granite covering the end of the crypt facing observers. Jessica Mitford derisively called these structures "tenement mausoleums."[64] Massive structures housing hundreds or thousands of crypts attracted less wealthy customers to mausoleums.

The Cathedral of Memories in Hartsdale, New York, contained 8,800 vaults as well as 250 larger family rooms. The Melrose Abbey Mausoleum in Anaheim, California, contained 1,800 vaults. Woodlawn Mausoleum in Nashville, Tennessee, was twenty stories high and was built to accommodate up to 129,000 bodies.[65]

The idea of a crypt within an aboveground multitiered building is also enjoying a comeback in the twenty-first century for people of more modest means. Cemeteries are again, as they did in the mid-twentieth century, erecting massive multicrypt mausoleums. Such structures house tiered crypts for coffins and for urns containing ashes. The higher up the particular tier—that is, the farther it is from view—the less expensive the vault. A spokesperson for the funeral industry recently said, "Six feet up and not six feet under is increasingly the direction in which people want their remains stored."[66] Green-Wood Cemetery in Brooklyn recently completed a five-story mausoleum with 2,500 vaults and a common area featuring skylights and indoor waterfalls.

## Green Burials

As environmentalism has blossomed in recent decades, so have a few ideas about the disposal of cadavers in an environmentally friendly way. Advocates of green burials start with the claim that traditional funeral practices are harmful to the environment.[67] Specifically, millions of gallons of toxic fluids (primarily embalming fluid) are put into the ground each year and are eventually fated to leach into the soil. Millions of tons of reinforced concrete are buried annually, along with millions of feet of hardwood and thousands of tons of steel.[68]

Environmentalists therefore promote the notion of green burial. The basic idea—similar to that of the garden cemeteries of the mid-nineteenth century—is to bury corpses among trees and grass within an idyllic memorial preserve in which the public can hike and picnic. At the same time, special steps are taken to minimize the destructive effects of earth burial. Refrigeration replaces embalming for purposes of preburial storage, diminishing the use of toxic fluids. Burial is at a depth of three feet in a simple biodegradable coffin or in a shroud without a coffin. The hope is that the decomposing body will eventually serve as fertilizer.[69] At the grave site the prior greenery and vegetation are restored after a burial.[70] Flat ground-level grave markers preserve the natural vistas within the preserve. (Such a green burial is substantially cheaper than regular burial because there is no embalming, no expensive coffin, and no ostentatious grave marker.)

The first such green cemetery, Ramsey Creek Preserve, was set up in Westminster, South Carolina, in 1996. It covers thirty acres of forest containing a two-mile network of trails. Grave sites are located off the trails and are marked only with flat field stones adjacent to the replanted vegetation.[71] Similar memorial preserves exist in California, Florida, and Texas.

Another ecology-oriented idea for body disposal is to convert the cadaver into some sort of fertilizer used to grow plants and trees. Mary Roach, in her book *Stiff,* describes multiple methods of recycling a corpse back to the earth as compost. One way is to grind the corpse up, combine the remnants with manure and wood shavings, and spread it as compost to cultivate shrubs or trees.[72] Another method uses freeze drying to reduce the corpse to material suitable for use as part of a compost mixture.[73] None of these techniques for creating fertilizer precludes honoring the deceased via a memorial service. As is often done for people who have opted for cremation, a ceremony can precede or follow destruction of the corpse.

A third method for creating fertilizer from human remains is to dissolve the corpse's flesh in a solution of lye and water. The process is known as "alkaline hydrolysis"; its environmental utility is dubious.[74] It uses ninety-two gallons of water and four gallons of lye mixed in with the cadaver in a stainless steel cylinder. After a six-hour reduction process the dissolved remains are washed down the drain as "a brownish, syrupy" liquid.[75] A bone residue remains, similar in volume and appearance to ashes from cremation. Those remaining bone pieces are pulverized and can be used in compost or scattered.[76] At first blush, it seems somewhat undignified to be washed down the drain, but is the technique any more unseemly than being burned and going up in smoke?

## The Seawater Solution

Sea burial seems like a quick, simple, and inexpensive disposal method. Not much body preparation is required, and no charge is incurred for a cemetery plot or for perpetual maintenance. In *The Tempest*, Shakespeare seems to speak favorably about burial at five fathoms:

Of his bones are coral made;
Those are pearls that were his eyes;
Nothing of him that doth fade,
But doth suffer a sea change
Into something rich and strange.

That sea change, however, makes the reality of underwater burial less enticing. After being in water for a few hours, an exposed corpse's skin becomes white and soft and is unpleasant to sight and smell.[77] The body initially sinks, but as putrefaction occurs the body bloats with gas and buoyantly rises to the surface, sinking again only after further decomposition. This means that only a heavily weighted corpse will stay submerged permanently. Recall the *Godfather* movie in which the mob hit man Luca Brasi, after being garroted to death, slept "with the fishes." His corpse was tied to a weight, but he was not given cement slippers by his gangland murderers. We cannot know whether the weight was sufficient to assure Mr. Brasi undisturbed rest underwater. If a cadaver is exposed in seawater, fish, crabs, and small marine animals will feed on it, starting with parts of the face.[78] And the rate of decomposition is much quicker underwater than in the ground.

In the nineteenth century sea burial was common in both the American and British navies. Navy people have traditionally been careful to ensure that a sea burial is secure and permanent. Dead sailors were sewn into hammocks along with heavy cannon shot to prevent them from rising again to the surface.[79] In the nineteenth century, keeping a corpse on board was believed to bring bad luck as well as to pose health hazards because of putrefaction. Therefore, there were strong incentives for nineteenth-century sailors to dispose of human remains by tossing them overboard.

By and large, undersea burial would seem to be attractive only for a decedent who in life has been strongly connected with the sea—someone with a symbolic or sentimental reason for sea burial. Some seafarers still request a committal service and burial at sea.[80] The American military offers sea burial for active duty and honorably discharged veterans and their families.[81]

Some people arrange sea burial for strange reasons. In the 1730s New Hampshire resident Samuel Baldwin arranged to be buried at sea. He did so not because of the appeal of sea burial, but rather to frustrate his wife, who had sworn to dance on his grave.[82] Many people have ended up buried underwater as victims of circumstance. Victims of water mishaps can meet that fate, as did some of the *Titanic*'s passengers. Before the Brooklyn Bridge was built in 1883, unintentional water burial occurred when horse-drawn coffins slipped off barges into the East River on their way from Manhattan funerals to cemeteries in Brooklyn.[83] For the average person with a strong attachment to the sea—to the point of seeking permanent association with water—cremation and sea disposal of the ashes might be more attractive.

## Cremation

> It's kind of like covering up a crime—burn the body, scatter the ashes around. As far as anyone is concerned, the whole thing never happened.
> Lisa Takeuchi Cullen, *Remember Me*,
> quoting Jerry Seinfeld

> Joan Rivers: "I had to take my mother-in-law to the crematory today."
> Interlocutor: "Oh? Rough day I guess."
> Joan Rivers: "Yeah, she didn't want to go!"
> Tim Matson, *Round Trip to Deadsville*

Cremation as a formal mode of cadaver disposal originated in Greece in about 1000 BC.[84] The Greeks saw fire as a way to free the pure soul from the impure body. The ashes or cremains (in modern terminology) were placed in urns and then entombed. The Romans, toward the end of their Republic, also adopted cremation as a common form of cadaver disposal. They stored the remains in elaborate urns sometimes entombed in multiniche columbarium-like buildings. Julius Caesar, Augustus, and Caligula all ended up as cremains. By contrast, Christians came to view cremation as a pagan custom opposed to Jesus's teachings about burial and resurrection of the body.[85] Charlemagne in 789 decreed that cremation should be punished by death (of the cremator).[86] Jews also were averse to cremation, though Saul and his sons were burned on the battlefield to prevent mutilation of their corpses by the Philistines. The Jewish aversion to cremation has been strengthened by the much later experience with Nazi crematoria.

In the United States, cremation was rare during the first half of the nineteenth century.[87] In the 1820s Henry Laurens, a South Carolina merchant, chose cremation as a sure way to verify his own death after one of his children was mistakenly pronounced dead of smallpox. By the 1860s, however, cremationism emerged as a movement offering an alternative to burial. Sanitarianism had by then become a national craze, and Sanitarians believed that decaying corpses emitted noxious gases or miasmas that could pollute nearby water and air.[88] The budding cremationist movement adopted the hygienic rationale, arguing: "No human body can pass through the cheering glow of the cinerary furnace and come out in the purified and utterly inoffensive form of white ashes without contributing substantially to the liberation of earth, water, and air from this dreaded pollution [of buried bodies]."[89] Cremationists calculated that if the twenty-five thousand corpses buried in New York City each year averaged one hundred pounds in weight, those buried corpses constituted two and a half million pounds of contamination that could be avoided by cremation. They also portrayed burial as entailing vile effluvia oozing from a coffin as well as worms ravenously destroying flesh and organs, reducing the brain and heart to stinking masses. And they reminded Americans of the hazard of body snatching and dissection of corpses then plaguing the United States.

By 1874 countless pamphlets, lectures, and articles promoted burning as a hygienic alternative to burial. The cremationists argued vigorously against the Christian concern that fire might obstruct or frustrate a potential resurrection. They called it "blasphemy to state that an omnipotent God could not resurrect a cremated corpse."[90] Their own spiritual vision, like that of the ancient Greeks, saw cremation as burning the corrupt body and releasing the pure soul.

The first well-publicized cremation in the United States was held on December 6, 1876, in Washington, Pennsylvania.[91] The host was Dr. Francis Julius LeMoyne, a cremationist physician who had built a small crematory on his estate in a rural college town. The corpse was that of Baron Joseph Henry Louis Charles De Palm, an Austrian-born nobleman who had a horror of earth burial. De Palm had died six months earlier in Washington, D.C., and had been embalmed there. By the time the corpse reached Pennsylvania in December 1876, De Palm had shrunk from 175 to 92 pounds. The cremation attracted journalists from as far away as France and Germany. On the morning of December 6, De Palm's shrunken corpse was placed in LeMoyne's oven.

The fiery specter of a burning corpse repelled some of the witnesses. The cremation of Baron De Palm's corpse was reported in the U.S. press as a national scandal.[92] Journalists branded the event as an objectionable pagan farce showing no more respect for the corpse than would be accorded to a roast pig.[93] For them the event was woefully devoid of sentiment. (Although flowers had been placed on the corpse in transport, no ceremony or service accompanied the cremation.) Journalists also abhorred the "violence" of the roasting, steaming, and bubbling flesh until it was finally reduced to ashes. And they disliked the smell of burning flesh.

Cremationists still promoted incineration as a clean, efficient, and economical method of cadaver disposal. In an 1885 article Francis King Carey argued that earth burial produced loathsome material "symbolizing uncleanliness in all its forms, polluting the soil and hazarding the health of the community and, finally, offering a premium to the grave robber."[94] Carey ridiculed the "superstition" that a corpse was necessary to resurrection. He argued that buried remains ended up as dust mingled with dust, just as ashes did. If the inevitable conflation of dust with dust precluded resurrection, Carey argued, the day of judgment would "witness an extraordinary conflict of ownership."[95] Carey had no doubt that cremation would eventually become the preferred American way of body disposition.

The funeral industry of the late nineteenth and early twentieth centuries (comprised largely of funeral directors and cemetery owners) also did its best to discourage and deride cremation. It branded cremation as a heathen practice contravening the Christian vision of resurrection. The morticians saw cemetery visitation and upkeep as an integral part of a positive religious tradition. They called cremation a "bake and shake" operation or a "miniature hell," and the industry sought to associate burning with punishment of the wicked.[96]

The American public of the late nineteenth century by and large reacted to cremation with aversion similar to that of the journalists following De Palm's cremation. Though twenty-four crematories had been established by 1900, some of them were used primarily to dispose of victims of infectious diseases. The rate of cremation never exceeded 1 percent in America in the nineteenth century; it reached that level only in the 1920s.[97] The cremationist cause probably was not advanced when, in 1880, a writer suggested that mass burning of corpses could be used as an energy source. He calculated that at the contemporary mortality rate of New York City, such burning could produce one hundred ninety thousand cubic feet of illuminating gas.[98]

During the first three-quarters of the twentieth century, cremation grew modestly in popularity. The Cremation Association of North America (CANA), composed primarily of cemetery operators, was founded in 1913.[99] The funeral industry gradually sought to accommodate cremation, but also to cultivate earnings from the enterprise. That could be done by making a funeral or committal ceremony part of the cremation process, by selling coffins and/or urns for the cremains, and by providing locations for permanent disposition of cremains. In the 1970s some crematories (especially those associated with funeral homes) insisted that a corpse be placed in a coffin before being burned.[100] Some cemeteries built columbaria—buildings with niches where large numbers of urns could be placed and visited. Others adapted mausoleum vaults to serve as permanent resting places for cremains.

The rate of cremation increased slowly during the twentieth century. By 1963, when the Roman Catholic Church relaxed its opposition to cremation, only 4 percent of bodies were disposed of in that manner. In 1968, when Jessica Mitford first published her exposé of the mercenary practices of the funeral industry, *The American Way of Death*, she also suggested cremation as "a simple, tidy solution to the disposal of the dead."[101] Just as in the late nineteenth century, advocates promoted cremation as a way to save time, space, and money in final disposition.

Americans have, over the last thirty-five years, come to embrace cremation as a major alternative to burial. By 2000, 25 percent of all final dispositions were by cremation. In Oregon and Washington, cremation in that year accounted for more than 50 percent of final disposals (while remaining at around 10 percent in the Deep South).[102] By 2003, 28 percent of cadavers overall were cremated, with Washington, Nevada, and Hawaii reaching rates of just over 60 percent.[103] California and Arizona achieved rates of 50 percent. A 2005 survey supposedly indicated that 46 percent of Americans would elect to be cremated. The current website of the National Funeral Directors Association (NFDA) reports a "rising interest" in cremation. In 2007 the Catholic diocese in Metuchen, New Jersey, opened its own crematory, calling cremation "the wave of the future."[104]

The reasons for the recent upsurge in cremation are similar to the traditional reasons supporting cremation. Saving money and land are the primary rationales, but there are others. More and more people have come to understand that modern embalming does not keep a corpse intact for long, so decomposition is the inevitable fate of a buried corpse. Some of those people are averse to what they perceive as the slow and repulsive disintegration of the body within the grave. One mortician has promoted incineration as a 4-hour alternative to burial's "20 years to turn you into a puddle of ooze."[105] Funeral directors' aversion to AIDS served as an impetus to recommend cremation in the 1980s.[106] Modern transient Americans, with fewer long-term ties to their communities, may see less reason to leave behind permanent burial places.[107] And, as will shortly be described, cremation offers multiple flexible ways to dispose of the cremains. Ashes can be divided for disposal among multiple people and locations—whether the place of final disposition is burial in a cemetery, placement in an urn in a columbarium, placement of an urn on a mantel, scattering of ashes as fertilizer in the garden, or scattering over some spot dear to the departed.[108]

The funeral industry sees no contradiction between cremation and traditional funerals. Though prompt, unceremonious burning of a corpse is possible, funeral directors customarily encourage some kind of rite surrounding cremation. Ideally, from the funeral industry's economic perspective, cremation would be preceded by a traditional wake. The NFDA points out that a rented casket can be used at any viewing of an embalmed corpse slated for cremation. A traditional funeral service can be held before cremation (in a church or funeral home), at cremation (as many crematories have an attached chapel), or after cremation (at a columbarium, at the graveside before the ashes are buried, or at any place appropriate for a memorial service).[109] Most people anticipating cremation seem to favor some form of commemoration ceremony, whether a funeral or another memorial service. The funeral industry encourages not only funeral rites as an adjunct of cremation but also disposition of cremains in a final resting place associated with a ceme-tery such as an urn in a columbarium, mausoleum, or grave. Allegedly, some crematories purposely left cremains unpulverized in order to make scattering of ashes (as opposed to preservation in a container) more problematic and burial more appealing.[110] Before turning to the logistics of scattering ashes, I will describe both the cremation process and the abuses of the process that have sometimes occurred.

While any corpse is a candidate for cremation, some precautions have to be taken before consigning a corpse to incineration. For example, pacemakers should be removed to avoid the hazard of a small explosion. Some tooth fillings contain toxic mercury. In May 2006, a bill requiring precremation removal of mercury fillings was introduced in the Maine legislature. Funeral home owners protested, and the bill was buried in a rectangular metal file cabinet. Some states require a forty-eight-hour waiting period before cremation in order to permit a coroner's or medi-cal examiner's investigation of the cause of death, where appropriate.[111]

Before placement in a crematory oven, a corpse is generally placed in a combustible cardboard container. Funeral directors have sometimes urged that, as a mark of respect, the loved one's body be placed in a wooden coffin for incineration. The waste of good wood is obvious, and common sense has prevailed. Special rented caskets have a cardboard bottom that permits the corpse to be slid out after any ceremony has ended, then covered by a cardboard lid and transported to the cremato-ry. The great majority of crematees are not burned in wooden coffins.[112]

The incineration process starts with the corpse and its cardboard container being slid into the furnace. A low-intensity burner first inciner-ates the cardboard, and then the furnace heats to between 1600 and 1800 degrees Fahrenheit. (For obese corpses the temperature may be raised to as high as 3000 degrees Fahrenheit.[113]) The burning process takes be-tween one and four hours.[114] The corpse quickly chars, and the skin and hair burn first. Other soft tissue then burns, the limbs and head first.[115] As the body disintegrates, all organic material burns and all traces of DNA go up in smoke. Metal remnants may be left among the ashes. These include gold or silver tooth fillings and steel or titanium dental posts, as well as hip prostheses and orthopedic plates.[116] In the last stage of cremation, bones glow white and fall apart.[117] The ashes that are left (cremains) are mainly skeletal remains, including chunks of large bones such as vertebrae and pelvis. Because of these remaining bone fragments, the cremains must be pulverized to a grainy powder before any scattering of ashes. A mechanical processor performs the pulverization task, though a kitchen blender could do the job. Male cremains average 7.6 pounds and female cremains average 6.1 pounds.[118]

While a fresh corpse is usually readily identifiable, cremation leaves only a grainy powder indistinguishable from other powders or other cremains. This fact has, over the years, led to some outrageous practices by funeral homes or crematories. Corpses are supposed to be cremated separately and the remains collected separately and dispensed to mourning kin. Yet there are many instances in which crematories incinerated multiple or successive corpses and distributed the commingled remains to loved ones in containers labeled with only one decedent's name.[119] A 1991 class action suit (later settled) accused one crematory of treating thousands of corpses in that manner.[120] In other, more isolated cases, dentures showed up in the ashes of a nondenture wearer and a refrigerated body was discovered in a mortuary four months after its supposed cremains had been distributed.[121]

In still other instances, a proper cremation took place but the cremains were never disposed of as promised. In 1988 containerized ashes of 5,342 corpses were discovered stored on land when they were supposed to have been scattered in air.[122] In 1997 5,200 boxes of cremains entrusted to a pilot for scattering over the sea were discovered dry in an airplane hangar and a storage locker. Another pilot who promised to scatter remains over distant mountains ended up dumping them on nearby land.[123] In 2006 California suspended the license of a Glendale cemetery after finding the unburied cremains of 4,000 people (probably unclaimed remains of poor people) crammed into storage rooms and trash containers.

The worst cremation atrocity was committed by Ray Brent Marsh in Noble, Georgia, between 1997 and 2002. Marsh ran Tri-State Crematory during that period. In February 2002 Georgia authorities discovered 339 unburned, decomposing corpses on the Tri-State property—buried in shallow pits; crammed into vaults, vehicles, and storage buildings; and piled in nearby woods.[124] The cremains that Tri-State had previously returned to families turned out to be cement dust. Marsh was sentenced to a twelve-year prison term.

## Disposing of the Ashes

The growing popularity of cremation raises the question of how to dispose of the cremains. Unsentimental types may view cremains as just another form of human waste and may be happy to deposit them in the trash. The vast majority of people see cremains as an embodiment of the decedent and as deserving of respect and dignified treatment. For them a wide variety of respectful disposal methods are available. Indeed, there is no limit to the creative ways in which ashes can be inurned or scattered. Cremains also can be divided among multiple parties for disposition. This division of remains is reminiscent of the European practice of making multiple relics out of body parts of kings and saints. Many churches or towns then shared the honor of housing part of a revered dignitary's corpse. Cremains can likewise go to multiple honored recipients.

A 2005 survey of people contemplating cremation showed that a majority (56 percent) wanted their cremains to be placed in an urn. If survivors want to use an urn, a funeral home or crematory will sell a wide range of keepsake urns from cheap plastic to expensive gold-plated models. Also, more and more professional artists are designing and selling decorative urns suitable for permanent display in a home or an office.[125] These artistic urns can come in untraditional shapes and materials, such as a silver piece in the shape of a hand or a glazed porcelain container with guardian angels sitting back to back on the lid. One grieving daughter placed her mother's cremains in a ceramic prayer wheel etched with leaves. She commented that once in a while "I'll walk by and give Mom a spin." An art gallery for "personal memorial art" opened in 2007 in Northern California with forty artists contributing urns to "a new aesthetic of death."[126] Keep in mind, though, that only a small portion (10 percent) of people desiring their ashes to be inurned want the urn to be retained at home.

Before spending a lot of money on an artwork funeral urn for the home, consider the following story. Two couples (call them the As and the Bs) lived in adjoining houses in suburban New Jersey. The Bs customarily traveled to Florida for a month each winter, asking the As to keep an eye on their house. One winter, after the Bs had been in Florida for a few weeks, the As noticed a break-in at the Bs. They immediately notified both the police and the Bs, who promptly flew home to assess the damage. After inspection, the Bs reported to the As that the burglars "didn't take much, but we lost Uncle Max." In shock, the As responded: "Why on earth didn't you tell us he was in there? We would have been glad to check on him." The Bs then had to explain that the burglars had taken an ornate urn (containing Uncle Max's cremains) from their living room coffee table. One lesson of the story is that even if a valuable artistic urn is insured, the emotional value of lost remains is irreplaceable.

Another "work of art" disposal method is to have the ashes blended into paint to be used and preserved in paintings. One artist mixed her mother's ashes into paintings that she then gave to relatives as decorative mementoes.[127] Another artist prescribed a similar fate for his own ashes. He dictated that his ashes should be mixed with oil paint to be used in a posthumous portrait of himself.[128] (Such a painting is bound to "capture" the subject, but it might seem too self-absorbed for most people.)

Besides the home, many other options exist for final placement of urns. One-quarter of the people surveyed indicated that they wanted a cemetery to be the final resting place of their urn. A cemetery, in turn, can supply several options for disposition of an urn, burial perhaps being the most common. Among those people who indicated a preference for cemetery disposal of their urns, two-thirds anticipated burial. Cemeteries are happy to bury an urn either within an existing grave site or in a separate grave. Grave markers can be installed as in any other burial. A committal service can be held at the grave.

Cemeteries often offer an aboveground location for an urn. One trade association recommends inurnment in a "niche, a vault, or urn garden" as possible final resting places.[129] The references are to a niche within a columbarium where many urns are stored, a vault within a mausoleum containing coffins and/or urns, or a cultivated garden or section of the grounds set aside for urns. Not every cemetery has all of these facilities, but many local cemeteries have more than one option for urns.

A cemetery "garden of remembrance" may be used either for urns or for scattering of cremains. The NFDA, however, comments on its website that mourners may find it "hard to simply pour the mortal remains" on the ground, implying that keeping the ashes in an urn is preferable. Note that Catholic ashes are supposed to be kept in one place, such as an urn within a mausoleum, rather than scattered (coherence presumably facilitates resurrection).[130] Hillside Memorial Park in Los Angeles recently built a stream and waterfall system in which urns are placed on an island surrounded by floating candles.[131]

It is common to choose a final location for cremains consistent with the decedent's sentimental attachments. For example, there has been a recent surge in the use of college or university campuses as final resting places for cremains.[132] It has been speculated that people in a mobile society may decide that their sentimental ties to a college are as strong as those to any other place. Those college years might have been the best years of their lives. One journalist has labeled the phenomenon "the ultimate college reunion."[133] The University of Virginia in 1991 built a columbarium wall with 180 vaults for urns and has recently formulated plans for 200 more multiurn vaults. Chapman University in California and The Citadel in South Carolina have also created on-campus columbaria, the latter in a carillon tower. Colleges, in turn, see the provision of final resting places as a way to raise money. Duke University charges $25,000 for burial of alumni cremains in Duke's memorial garden. The price for a college resting place seems to correlate with academic prestige in the outside world. In contrast to Duke's $25,000 figure, Chapman University charges only $2,500 for placing an urn in its columbarium.[134]

Approximately 40 percent of people anticipating cremation want their ashes scattered in some emotionally significant place. The idea is to scatter the ashes in a place beloved by the decedent as a result of prolonged work or play. Recall Ted Williams and the Florida Keys where he had fished. Recall Donald Trump and the first hole at Trump National. A widow sought to scatter her golfer husband's ashes in a sixth-hole sand trap where her late husband had often stood. When the golf club denied permission, the widow stowed the cremains in her golf bag and covertly raked them into the sand trap.[135] Another widow wanted to scatter her husband's ashes around a favored blackjack table. The casino convinced her to place the remains in an urn decorated with a poker symbol.[136] Think also of comedian Steve Allen's idea of an appropriate placement for a gum manufacturer's ashes. Allen announced on a 1981 television show: "Morden W. Chicklett, the chewing gum heir, died today. In accordance with his wishes, he will be cremated and his ashes will be stuck to a chair in a nearby restaurant." Others have sought to prolong an association with their work. The legendary labor radical Joe Hill, before his death in 1915, dictated that his ashes should be distributed among various chapters of his beloved Industrial Workers of the World.

Scattering of ashes in nature is common. Jessica Mitford spoke of cremation's appeal "to the nature lover and the poet who visualize their mortal remains scattered over sunny hillside or remote strand."[137] For forest and field lovers, the National Park Service regularly grants permits to scatter cremains in national parks. The park rangers ban urns or memorial markers of any kind and forbid scattering within one hundred yards of streams. While some rangers apparently adopt a "don't ask, don't tell" policy for sentimental scatterers of a private citizen's remains, they will not allow a business to exploit federal lands. Fran Coover recently sought to operate a cremains disposal business, "Ladies in White," on federal lands in western Montana.[138] She planned to charge $390 for a ceremony, a scattering, and a GPS fix. The Park Service denied her a permit. Ms Coover turned to a nearby private rancher for an alternative scattering site.

Ted Williams was not the only decedent who wanted his cremains to commemorate a personal bond with the sea. The Neptune Society arranges low-cost committal services in conjunction with the scattering of ashes at sea.[139] The cost is even less if the memorial service is skipped and the ashes are scattered unceremoniously at sea. Celebrities whose ashes have been scattered at sea include John F. Kennedy Jr., actress Ingrid Bergman, and actor Robert Mitchum.[140] (If you've never heard of Bergman or Mitchum, you're probably too young to be reading this book.) When Kennedy's ashes were scattered from a naval ship at sea, the wind blew the remains back on board the vessel.[141] A better technique is to scatter the ashes from a stationary or slowly moving boat. Other solutions exist for the disposal of ashes at sea. Cremains can be placed in biodegradable urns that dissolve shortly after being placed in seawater.[142] The urns are "shaped like giant seashells the size of toilet lids."[143] Alternatively, cremains can be mixed with other materials, such as concrete, and made part of nature-friendly "eternal reefs." The artificial reef, composed of large concrete balls containing the cremains of many people, becomes a habitat for coral, sponges, fish, and other sea life. The crematee's family receives a record of the map coordinates where their loved one's cremains are permanently entombed on the ocean floor.[144]

Wind is sometimes useful in scattering ashes, but not always. Consider this story along with the previously mentioned saga of John F. Kennedy Jr. A New Jersey legislator died after requesting that his cremains be scattered over his beloved Cape Cod Bay. The late legislator's son, an amateur pilot, decided to fulfill his father's wish. The son rented a small plane and flew over Cape Cod Bay. At an appropriate moment, he slid open the cockpit cover and turned over the urn—only to have the roaring wind plaster all the cremains against his face and the back of the cockpit. This was not exactly what the decedent had in mind when requesting "scattering" over the bay. (Apparently the pilot son had either never heard the expression "don't piss into the wind" or had failed to absorb its message.)

Other examples of bad judgment in scattering cremains over beloved places have surfaced in recent years. In May 2002 a widow's effort to have her husband's ashes scattered over his favorite team's baseball park ended badly. The cruising plane caused a terrorism scare and prompted evacuation of the entire stadium.[145] In November 2005 Christopher Noteboom ran onto the playing field during a football game between the Philadelphia Eagles and the Green Bay Packers. Noteboom was attempting to dispose of the cremains of his mother, an avid Eagles fan, in a way that would make her "always a part of Lincoln Field and of the Eagles." As Noteboom ran, a fine powder trailed from a plastic bag until he dropped to his knees at the thirty-yard line and crossed himself. He was promptly arrested. The arresting officers expressed zero tolerance for someone who runs onto the playing field and dumps an unknown substance in a crowded stadium. (Couldn't Noteboom have accomplished his goal discreetly on an Eagles' practice day or during the off-season?)

Officials of the Hamburg Soccer Club (HSC) in Germany have found a way to satisfy, constructively and profitably, their fanatical fans who seek to have their ashes scattered on the club's stadium field or buried at the penalty spot in front of the goal. The soccer club recently made an arrangement with the cemetery adjacent to the stadium. Under this arrangement, a sector of the cemetery has been set aside exclusively for Hamburg soccer fans' remains. The sector accommodates up to five hundred graves, and its entrance gate is shaped like a soccer goal. The cemetery sod is taken from the stadium. The HSC cemetery sector was dedicated on September 9, 2008. Twenty-five HSC fans have already made their reservations, expressing hope that surviving soccer fan/ friends will ultimately take "time out" to visit the cemetery adjacent to the stadium.

Now that I have covered the sea, land, and air as potential locales for scattering cremains, the last medium is outer space. At the turn of the twentieth century, James O'Kelly of New York proposed that corpses be launched permanently into the stratosphere in elliptical metal cylinders that would be jet propelled by igniting gases produced from acid infused into the corpse.[146] That method, to the best of my knowledge, has never been mastered. Survivors of crematees have, however, successfully launched fireworks containing cremains into the sky, spewing the ashes over a wide area.[147] A more ambitious method, and perhaps a more environmentally benign one, is to launch a symbolic portion of cremains into space orbit within a closed container. One company had a plan to orbit a columbarium containing the cremated remains of ten thousand people. Another company currently offers to send one gram of cremains within a lipstick-sized container into Earth orbit. The company notes that launches are subject to delays and that the orbit is for less than eternity.[148] The charge is $5,300, not including a prelaunch memorial service. In April 2007 the cremains of *Star Trek* engineer Scotty (actor James Doohan) and of Mercury astronaut Gordon Cooper, as well as those of two hundred other persons, were fired into suborbital space in a joint venture of Spaceport America and U.S. Aerospace under contract with Celestis of Houston.[149]

Forget exotic space disposal that helps no one! For people who want to be useful in death as well as in life, disposition of cremains can be done in a semiutilitarian way. Funeral director/philosopher Thomas Lynch calls for the deceased "to get off their dead ashes and be good for something beyond the simple act of remembrance."[150] As constructive ways to use ashes, Lynch suggests plastic worms for fishermen, bowling balls for sportsmen, and poker chips for gamblers. Fertilizer has already been mentioned as a constructive use of ashes. One application of this theory consists of mixing wildflower seeds and ashes in a biodegradable paper urn so that cremains can help cultivate flowers.[151] Another semiutilitarian function of cremains is in jewelry. Tiny bits of ashes can be placed in charms for bracelets or necklaces.[152] It is also possible to extract carbon from cremains and press and shape it at high temperatures to create diamonds. This service is commercially available.[153]

Human cremains are not always treated with respect.[154] Cremains can be reviled and mistreated just like disfavored corpses. One widow completed her divorce only days before her former husband expired. She nonetheless presided at a brief memorial church service for his cremated remains. At the conclusion of the service, she asked the pastor about the nearest restroom. Taking the urn holding her former husband's ashes with her, she entered the nearby restroom; mourners then heard the toilet flush several times. When she emerged, the widow announced: "You can have this urn back. I just flushed that sorry SOB down the toilet where he should have been all along."[155] Along the same lines, consider ingestion of cremains. This technique was used occasionally in remote cultures as an honorific gesture intended to absorb the positive characteristics of the deceased. But considering the terminus of the digestive tract, the fate of swallowed cremains seems more insulting than complimentary.

Chapter 6

# Eternal Preservation of the Deceased

*Literally and Figuratively*

The common forms of cadaver disposal leave few remains in the end. Cremation reduces a corpse to about seven pounds of nonorganic dust. A buried corpse gradually decomposes into a dark, moldy, undifferentiated mass. Contrary to popular belief, typical modern embalming postpones decomposition of the human corpse only for days or weeks. Within twelve years the buried cadaver will deteriorate to a moldy mass and, over an additional span of years, will become skeletonized. Increased amounts of embalming fluid can extend the period before decomposition, but would leave a corpse distorted in initial facial configuration, body shape, and skin tone.

Can human flesh be prevented from decaying and dissolving? Are there ways to preserve all or a substantial portion of a cadaver in an aesthetically acceptable condition for an indefinite period? The whole idea of eternal preservation may seem to be a vainglorious conceit (and perhaps it is for those rich and famous persons who seek eternal preservation of their remains). It seems presumptuous to think that the world needs or wants a cadaver—a desiccated and highly debilitated version of a previous self—preserved for the indefinite future. There are, however, reasons besides conceit explaining why some people seek permanent preservation of their cadaver.

Some religious believers think that a future resurrection of their corpse or a reunification of their body and soul will occur and that the event would be facilitated by preservation of their bodily form. Even without religious grounding, some people consider their lasting remains as a testimonial or a reminder to survivors of their existence. For them, eternal preservation "holds out hope that death will not be the end of us, that there is some salvation from the final annihilation that we fear awaits us all."[1] Other people think that science will eventually succeed in re-vivifying the essence of a person and that their bodily form will be useful in that process. That is a central object of the cryonics (freezing a cadaver) movement. Some people want to live forever, and they think that preservation of their corpse might ultimately promote that goal. Still others simply feel a strong revulsion at the prospect of postmortem bodily disintegration and therefore wish to avoid that fate.

Sometimes people other than the decedent have reasons to seek indefinite preservation of human remains. In nineteenth-century medical schools, specimens of diseased organs, limbs, and tissue were kept in preservative-filled, sealed jars or cases and were used for medical education, for research, or as curiosities.[2] Preserved corporeal specimens are still on display, usually in formaldehyde-filled jars but sometimes embedded in clear plastic, in medical museums like the Mutter Museum of the College of Physicians in Philadelphia. Northwestern University's medical school museum displays 170 jars containing anomalous fetuses and newborns, including one newborn with a huge cyclops eye and another with a nose like a penis.[3] Cornell's psychology department still stores seventy brains remaining from an original collection of six hundred brains once studied to try to find correlations between certain human characteristics and brain size or structure.[4]

Surgeons and pathologists in the nineteenth and twentieth centuries also kept preserved specimens of pathological or anomalous body parts on display in their medical offices or laboratories as educational tools, symbols of medical expertise, or curiosities. Some of these preserved body parts derived from surgery and others from autopsies. Into the 1970s, pathologists sometimes retained (for display, teaching, or research) organs or tissue extracted during autopsies.[5]

Financial gain provided another motive for keeping and displaying cadavers or anatomical specimens. In the mid-eighteenth century "Egyptologists" unrolled mummies in front of curious paying customers. In the late nineteenth and early twentieth centuries, entrepreneurs created nonmedical "museums" that displayed exotic skeletal remains or deformed body parts in an effort to attract and titillate a paying public.[6] What was purported to be Napoleon's penis—which by then looked like a maltreated shoelace or a shriveled eel—was once displayed in the Museum of French Art in New York.[7] Today traveling expositions of plasticized human remains purport to educate the public about human anatomy; they have attracted huge paying audiences. (Chapter 12 considers the ethics of using preserved corpses as items of display for educational or other purposes.)

Political motives sometimes account for extraordinary efforts to preserve the bodily remains of public figures. For example, when Vladimir Lenin died in 1924, Russian authorities sought to embalm his body and keep it on perpetual display (eventually in a mausoleum built for that purpose). After five weeks the corpse showed signs of change and decay—such as retracting facial muscles that altered Lenin's appearance—while the lines of mourning viewers had not diminished.[8] Russian morticians came to the rescue by devising a special preservative process for Lenin's corpse.[9] After eviscerating the corpse, they injected it with formalin and soaked it in a formalin bath. They then immersed it in a secret chemical concoction (containing glycerine) before restoring Lenin to his mausoleum in Red Square. Thereafter, every eighteen months they immersed Lenin's corpse in a glass tub filled with the secret concoction of preservative chemicals. They then wrapped most of the body in rubber bandages before dressing it and storing it at 61 degrees Fahrenheit. Every two weeks they wiped embalming fluid on the corpse's face and hands.[10] Lenin's corpse has survived to this day and is on display in his Kremlin mausoleum.

Communist leaders apparently liked the idea of a preserved corpse as a permanent symbol. Ho Chi Minh of Vietnam and Kim Il Sung of North Korea sought and received postmortem treatment similar to Lenin's. When Chinese leader Mao Tse Tung died in 1976, Chinese authorities wanted to preserve his body for veneration, as with Lenin. The Chinese, however, refused to use experienced Russian morticians and embalmed Chairman Mao themselves. They initially botched the job by using too much formaldehyde. "Mao's face became as swollen and distended as a soccer ball . . . [and] his bloated ears stood out like inflated flippers."[11] Emergency surgical intervention restored Mao's corpse's appearance to a semblance of its former self.

Some corpses have been preserved as political symbols and later have been moved or disposed of according to the political fate of their causes. Katherine Verdery has written about and documented the "political symbolism" of celebrity corpses during the twentieth century.[12] For example, after Joseph Stalin died in 1953, the Kremlin gave his corpse a Lenin-style embalming and exhibited his remains in a glass-topped coffin next to Lenin. In a clear reflection of political fortune, Stalin's remains were expelled from the Lenin mausoleum in 1961 and buried unceremoniously nearby.[13] When first lady of Argentina Eva ("Evita") Peron died in 1952, her widower, Juan Peron, had her cadaver injected with chemicals, submerged in baths of acetate and potassium nitrate, and coated with plastic. Evita's body was so well preserved that Peron took it into exile with him and sometimes displayed it in his house in Madrid.[14] A subsequent Argentine junta repatriated Evita's body.

Religious influences have come into play in the long-term preservation of bodies and body parts, especially in Europe. Relics (body parts) of former religious, royal, or civilian notables have been stored and sometimes displayed in cathedrals and churches throughout Europe. Remains of approximately one hundred saints, martyrs, and other religious figures, known as "the incorruptibles," have shown extraordinary endurance over time. Some of these corpses have retained a suppleness and a lifelike appearance for centuries.[15] (Note, however, that plastination has recently been used to reinforce the resilience of some of these relics, including those of Saint Hildegard from the twelfth century.[16])

The long endurance of these religious and/or royal remains might be attributable to divine intervention, to secret embalming, or to natural mummification (to be discussed below). In the supernatural realm, saints' corpses have, in a few instances, miraculously remained intact without any signs of human intervention. Saint Zita has lain in a basilica in Lucca, Italy, for more than seven hundred years; her body has shown neither decay nor traces of human preservation. (Moreover, Saint Zita's cadaver has demonstrated other miraculous traits; some pilgrims seeking her intercession have experienced restoration of sight or speech following prayer at the site of her remains.)

In some instances, though, survivors took covert steps to ensure a notable corpse's durability. Church authorities or royal courtiers called in people to secretly embalm or mummify dignitaries for long-term public viewing. That meant removing the cadaver's internal organs and packing the cavities with resinous substances. Saint Margaret of Cortona's body resisted decay for centuries but was ultimately discovered to have undergone embalming by evisceration and drenching in preservative lotions. The motive for such preservation may have been to give the local church or cathedral a miraculous aura that was helpful in attracting visitors. The relevant morticians therefore hid the incisions or other signs of artificial preservation.

In the case of royal figures, embalming was necessary to preserve the corpse until loyal subjects and dignitaries could arrive from remote places to view the corpse and pay respects. Again, the technique was evisceration of internal organs, packing of cavities, and immersion of the body in resinous substances. From these corpses, relics were sometimes cut and distributed to multiple localities. In most instances, the relics ended up as shriveled and darkened remains.

There are only a few known methods for truly long-term preservation of cadavers. The three described here are mummification, plastination, and cryonics.

## Mummification

The very first mummifications were performed seven thousand years ago by the Chinchorro people of coastal Chile.[17] They eviscerated organs and filled the cavities with vegetation before wrapping the corpse and covering it with clay. Because the Chinchorros removed skin, organs, and some soft tissue, the remains look like a stiff bundle of bones shaped like a human form.

The ancient Egyptians are known for their process of mummification that preserved much of a corpse's bodily tissue, including skin, muscle, and bone, for thousands of years. Egyptians believed that the spirit (Ka) and personality (Ba) left the body at death but could return and reoccupy the body, leading to an eternal life in a netherworld.[18] It was obviously important that the returning spirit be able to recognize and reoccupy the body, thus creating for Egyptians an incentive for maximal corporeal preservation. A mummified corpse might become dry and shriveled, but it was apparently still useful to the returning spirit.

The first Egyptian mummies were created about 3000 BC using a simplified process in which the dried corpse was covered with baking soda and then wrapped in bandages soaked with resin. Only the wealthy and/or royal corpses got the treatment.[19] By 1550 BC, mummification was widely available to commoners as well as dignitaries, but at varying prices and qualities of work. By the seventh century AD, when mummification ended in Egypt, hundreds of thousands of mummies had been created.

Only a wealthy ancient Egyptian could afford the deluxe mummification process. King Tutankhamen (King Tut) got the full treatment in 1343 BC, leaving an elaborately prepared mummy and a tomb filled with stunning treasures that amaze modern viewers. Deluxe mummification was a long process. The first step was evisceration of the cadaver's chest and stomach cavities—except for the heart—as well as extraction of the brain. (The Egyptians believed that the heart contained the essence of a being, including feelings and intelligence, which were critical to the mummy in the next world.[20] After 1500 BC, though, the brain was also left in the mummy.[21])

The extracted internal organs were washed, dried, and sealed in jars to be placed in the mummy's tomb. The Egyptian morticians then filled the cadaver's empty skull with resin and stuffed the body cavities with sawdust and bundles of cloth soaked in resin. The mouth and cheeks were padded to adjust the facial features. The eviscerated and repacked corpse was then dried for forty days with a strong desiccant, natron, resulting in a dry, hardened body. The mummy was shriveled not just because viscera were gone, but also because body fat turns to soluble fatty acids that can evaporate or be wicked into the surrounding sand along with the body's water.[22] After washing the dried cadaver with alcohol, morticians massaged oils into the mummy in order to soften the hardened remains.[23] The final steps consisted of wrapping the mummy in up to three hundred yards of linen cloth, smearing the wrapped mummy with a black liquid resin that would eventually fuse with the cloth, and placing it in a form-fitting mummiform (resembling a coffin).[24] Given the full Tut treatment, a mummy could probably last forever. The dry Egyptian climate and the absence of bacteria in the sand and air facilitated the long-term preservation of mummies. Tomb robbers long ago and archaeologists more recently spoiled innumerable mummies by unwrapping and exposing the remains.

In Europe, in a number of monasteries, resident monks mummified and displayed their deceased brothers' corpses.[25] In Palermo, Sicily, Capuchin monks over centuries desiccated eight thousand bodies. They initially placed each corpse in a sealed chamber for six months, then bathed it in aromatic herbs and vinegar, and finally placed it to dry under the hot Mediterranean sun.[26] The monks then stuffed the shriveled bodies with straw, dressed them, and displayed them in catacombs in niches along the walls. A similar practice took place in a Franciscan church in Toulouse, France.

Natural mummification can occur where climatic conditions permit. This can happen in regions featuring very low humidity and resting places excluding air and protecting against insects and carnivores. Shallow covering in desert sand can naturally dehydrate and mummify a cadaver.[27] For example, hundreds of naturally mummified corpses have been found in the barren Taklamakhan desert in northwest China.[28] In such environments, body tissue dries, shrinks, and becomes brittle. The natural mummy is usually quite fragile and is liable to turn to dust upon disturbance.[29] But that is not always the case. Certain bogs in Ireland, Denmark, and the Netherlands have a chemical composition that prevented full decomposition of hundreds of buried corpses. Apparently the presence of sphagnum moss in the bogs caused chemical reactions slowing bacterial growth and tanning the skin. Still, the bog mummies have shriveled over the centuries; they now look like "moldy prunes" without much facial detail.[30] In Guanajuato, Mexico, the local soil and climate naturally mummified corpses. Residents disinterred dozens of such mummified bodies and displayed them as tourist attractions.[31] Natural mummification may also account for the durability of some of the incorruptibles in Europe. One theory is that when deceased notables were interred in stone vaults beneath church floors, the cool, dry environment naturally desiccated flesh and preserved the shrunken corpses for centuries.[32]

In the United States, intentional desiccation and wrapping of a corpse by some ancient continental natives have left hundreds of mummies. They have been discovered in remote caves in many states, including caves in Texas overlooking the Rio Grande River. The most famous North American mummy was named Little Alice when found in a Kentucky cave in 1875.[33] Little Alice was renamed Little Al in 1958 when x-rays revealed male genitalia. According to the radiology findings, Little Al was ten years old when he died two thousand years earlier.

Today in the United States at least one entity offers mummification service. In 1975, Summum Bonum Amon "Corky" Ra, the mortician formerly known as Claude Nowell, founded a company called Summum Corporation. That corporation, located in Salt Lake City, offers mummification of human and animal corpses.[34] Summum Corporation's mummy-making process is long and complicated, starting with removing, cleaning, and returning internal organs to the body.[35] This is followed by immersion of the corpse for six months in a vat containing a secret preservative formula. After being removed from the vat and cleaned, the corpse is covered with a lanolin cream and wrapped in twenty-seven layers of gauze. Afterward, three more layers are added to the mummified corpse—a covering of resin, a seal of polyurethane, and a plaster cast covering. Finally, the mummy is placed in a one-quarter-inch-thick bronze mummiform, ready for shipment anywhere in the world or permanent storage in a Utah mountain sanctuary.[36]

The price of Summum Corporation mummification is $25,000 for a cat or dog and between $67,000 and $300,000 for a human. The base price may be increased by enhancements of the mummiform in material and/or decoration. Stainless steel is more expensive than bronze. Decorative add-ons include a death mask to be attached to the outside of the mummiform. Corky Ra states that the Summum process keeps the body supple and that the mummy will last for thousands of years—a claim not yet verified. As part of his business pitch, Mr. Ra suggests that cells from the mummy can ultimately be cloned and that some day science will even be able to restore memory to a revivified or cloned mummy. Summum Corporation claims that as of mid-2007, it has enrolled 1,457 paid-in-advance customers, including dozens of celebrities. Mohamed El Fayed, the former owner of Harrod's in London, had supposedly chosen Summum mummification and ultimate rest on the second floor of Harrod's, next to an existing sphinx with El Fayed's face already carved on it. Summum mummification has been performed on numerous dogs and has been tested on approximately thirty unclaimed corpses (presumably obtained from Salt Lake City welfare authorities) that were later cremated.

Corky Ra is still asking, "Why go to pot just because you've died?" The answer, if you do not believe in reanimation of corpses, is that mummification entails traumatic treatment of a corpse and ultimately leaves a figure that is not very appealing.[37] The protracted chemical bath and tight sealing steps may be distasteful to many people. Unless Summum Corporation can preserve mummies in a fashion never yet accomplished by artificial mummification, the end product will be dark, shriveled, and bearing little likeness to the decedent. Cells for cloning can be preserved in other ways.

## Plastination

Over the last thirty years, a process has been developed that turns corpses into what look like skinned plastic or fiberglass replicas of the human body. The crucial step is removal of a cadaver's water and fat and replacement with polymers. This plastination process creates an odorless, flexible, lightweight, indefinitely preservable specimen on which body components like muscle or ligaments can be lifted or folded to expose normally invisible body parts. Different colored polymers then articulate or highlight exposed focal points such as the nervous system, the circulatory system, muscles, bones, joints, or any other body component. Plastinated bodies or body parts have been used in two primary settings—in traveling educational displays for the public in which adjacent text explains the nature of the exposed body elements, and in permanent medical models useful for training in veterinary and medical schools both by display and by manipulation.

The process of replacing body liquids with polymers takes up to a year and costs approximately $60,000 for a full body job.[38] The first step is to embalm the corpse, usually via immersion in a formaldehyde solution, to halt decomposition. Next, any dissections necessary for isolating or highlighting certain body parts or portions of the body are performed. The specimen is then immersed in an acetone solution at freezing temperature; the acetone draws out cellular water and replaces it with acetone. In the next step, the specimen is placed in a bath of liquid polymers and a surrounding vacuum is created. The vacuum results in vaporization of the acetone and its replacement with liquid polymers from the bath solution. That part of the process is called "forced vacuum impregnation." The specimen can then be shaped, sometimes into lifelike poses like a football player or skateboarder, and cured by heat or ultraviolet light in order to harden the plastic. In short, plastination produces from a corpse a light, pliable replica of a person without identifying facial features.

Though plastinated remains are expected to last thousands of years, plastination and storage are not yet appealing as a mechanism for final disposition of a corpse (as opposed to long-term display as an educational tool). Perhaps this is because the skinless finished product takes on a plastic, manikin-like appearance that is difficult to identify as any particular decedent. Or perhaps no appropriate cemeteries or other final resting places have been created for final disposition of plastinates. This situation could change if appropriate final resting places are found or created, if individual identification is given, and if plastinated cadavers bear a greater resemblance to the decedent. A company called Corcoran Laboratories, located in Traverse City, Michigan, offers plastination, or "eternal preservation," as a method of preserving corpses "virtually forever" but only suggests burial as the locus of final disposal.[39] Burial of a plastinated corpse in a laid-out pose might someday have mass appeal — especially to people who want their buried corpse to retain its original shape and features and who come to realize that embalming will not achieve that goal.

Another downside of plastination is that the current process entails a great deal of corporeal alteration that will repel some people who are contemplating various means of bodily disposal. The extensive chemical dissolution of flesh, infusion of polymers, hollowing out, and carving may seem distasteful to people who value body integrity. In the meantime, the idea of dedicating one's corpse to plastination still might appeal to altruistic people who are interested in leaving their remains for purposes of education and research.

The originator of plastination, Gunther von Hagens, first documented his technique in 1977 when he applied for a patent. In 1990 he did his first full-body plastination. In 1995 his traveling exhibition of plastinated bodies and body parts, called Body Worlds, made its first appearance (in Tokyo). In 1998 Body Worlds came to Germany. In 2001 von Hagens set up a cadaver processing center in Dalian, China, employing two hundred workers, followed by a processing plant in Germany.[40] Body Worlds exhibitions have come to a number of American cities, including Los Angeles, Philadelphia, and Houston. Worldwide, Body Worlds has now attracted over twenty million visitors, each paying approximately $20.[41]

A competitor to Body Worlds, called Bodies: The Exhibition, has also surfaced in the United States. Using a format very similar to that of Body Worlds, this rival opened in Tampa in 2005 and has since reached New York.[42] Bodies: The Exhibition contains 260 plastinated body parts, including diseased lungs, livers, and arteries, as well as full body plastinates in action poses.

Body Worlds and Bodies: The Exhibition have aroused controversy during their operations. One criticism involves the origins of the cadavers that have ended up as plastinated public displays. It is universally deemed indecent to perform a chemical transformation on a corpse and put it on public display without informed consent from the decedent or an appropriate representative. In Germany in 1998, critics contended that the cadavers in Body Worlds exhibitions were those of executed Chinese prisoners whose bodies had been confiscated and sold by the Chinese government. Von Hagens insisted that he personally was only aware of cadavers obtained by informed consent, though he conceded that his representatives might have bought some executed Chinese corpses. Currently, von Hagens's exhibitions apparently possess signed consent forms relating to all the corpses on display. Allegations have arisen that Bodies: The Exhibition obtained corpses of deceased inmates in Chinese mental hospitals. Producers of that exhibition have recently conceded that they cannot demonstrate consent for their plastinated subjects, but they deny any illegal or unethical conduct.

Whatever the origins of the first corpses used in Body Worlds and Bodies: The Exhibition, the future supply of corpses for educational exhibition can be met by genuine, informed donations. As a result of written solicitation at exhibitions, over seven thousand people have already agreed to donate their bodies for plastination for educational use.[43] Body Worlds tells such potential donors to arrange to have their corpses sent to an embalming facility in Upland, California. From there the corpses will be sent for plastination either to laboratories of the Institute for Plastination in Germany (founded by von Hagens) or to the production facility in China. Over four hundred bodies have already been delivered to Body Worlds in this fashion; half of them have been used in traveling exhibitions and half for teaching in universities worldwide. Plastinated teaching models are in place in several hundred universities.[44]

A further criticism of exhibitions of plastinated bodies relates to the dignity of the displays. Some critics have labeled Body Worlds "a macabre spectacle" that violates human dignity.[45] Part of the claim of disrespect toward the plastinated remains is directed at the action poses of some full-body plastinates (a runner, a basketball player dribbling, a football player carrying the ball). The notion is that this creation of action-figure cadaver displays is "voyeuristic" and disrespectful, involving the pursuit of artistic and financial ends rather than education.[46]

Plastinates in action poses are closer in appearance to statuelike works of art than to learning tools. The question remains whether such artistic displays of corpses are intrinsically disrespectful. That issue is considered in chapter 12 in its discussion of the abuse of cadavers and the asserted indignity of cadaver displays. Suffice it to say here that the willingness of over seven thousand people to contribute their corpses tends to show that the Body Worlds displays are not intrinsically humiliating or distasteful. While some of the over twenty million visitors were undoubtedly voyeurs who had come for titillation, the vast majority of visitors learned an enormous amount about the human body and its internal systems. That assessment is based not only on my own observations at exhibitions but also on the remarks people leave in exhibition guest books after visits. The educational impact of labeled plastinates is fairly clear.

Moral issues may some day arise concerning the ultimate disposition of plastinated bodies and body parts. What becomes of plastinates after the traveling exhibitions are over? Bodies: The Exhibition has stated that the plastinates will either be given to medical schools or returned to their countries of origin for cremation.[47] Those ultimate fates seem to constitute respectful disposition of the corpses of people who have given informed consent to plastination.

## Cryonics

Extreme cold has long been known to prevent putrefaction and decomposition of cadavers. Before embalming became widespread, cold storage (over blocks of ice) was the only American method of preserving cadavers for enough time to permit long-distance transportation for burial, or for prevention of putrefaction long enough to permit distant mourners to arrive before final disposition. In 1912, after an expedition to the South Pole was caught by a blizzard and decimated, the frozen bodies were found seven months later in perfect condition by a relief party.[48] Today morgues are refrigerated.

In the 1960s the concept of cryonic suspension—freezing of a corpse and long-term preservation for future resuscitation whenever medical science becomes sufficiently advanced—surfaced in the United States. The theory was that the human brain, which is the locus of personality, memory, and identity, could be frozen and ultimately restored. Moreover, though whole bodies could be frozen, it would be enough to freeze a corpse's head and ultimately construct a body to go with the restored brain.

The first organization to promote cryonics was the Cryonics Society of New York, established in 1965. The first cryopatient (or cryonaut) to remain in cryonic suspension was James Bedford, a seventy-three-year-old psychology teacher who died in California in 1967.[49] The movement to advance cryonic preservation led numerous private, for-profit companies to offer such services in the 1970s. Many mishaps occurred within this budding industry. More than once, companies negligently failed to maintain low temperatures and corpses decomposed. Other companies went out of business without fulfilling their paid contracts, sometimes leaving unattended cryopatients and depleted stores of coolant.[50]

From this spotty history two contemporary cryonics enterprises have emerged—the Alcor Life Extension Foundation (Alcor) in Scottsdale, Arizona, and the Cryonics Institute (CI) in Clinton Township, Michigan.[51] Alcor currently houses 98 cryopatients, most of them in "neurosuspension," meaning that only the head is preserved. Ted Williams is still the most famous occupant. As of 2010, Alcor charged $150,000 for full-body treatment and preservation and $80,000 for neurosuspension. Alcor also has 921 dues-paying members (prospective cryopatients) at $398 per year.[52] Alcor's cryonics rival, CI, has 81 stored cryopatients, all of them full-body. CI offers no-frills cryosuspension at $28,000. ("No frills" means bodies encased in frozen sleeping bags as opposed to the steel tubular containers at Alcor. Families seldom visit at CI.) CI offers a life membership in its support institute for $1,250. (A third American cryonics operation, located in Nederland, Colorado, cannot be taken seriously. It keeps its cryopatients in a home freezer in a shed.[53] It exists apparently to help attract tourists to the annual "frozen dead guy" day in Nederland.)

Alcor offers the most sophisticated process for cryonic suspension.[54] A "standby team" of Alcor technicians is placed on twenty-four-hour alert, sometimes reaching the bedside by the time a prospective cryopatient dies. Upon declaration of death, the team swings into action. To prevent ischemic (oxygen-deficient) damage to the brain, the team may temporarily connect the corpse to a heart-lung machine to maintain blood circulation and an oxygen supply. To prevent damage to tissue cells from freezing, a cryopreservative, a glycerol-based solution, is pumped through the body, replacing blood in the circulatory system.[55] This solution drives water from cells and replaces it with preservative. The corpse (or the surgically removed head) is cooled to –108 degrees Centigrade and immersed in silicone oil for two days. Then the corpse is transported to Arizona and its metallic tube resting place, where it is further cooled by liquid nitrogen for long-term storage. At the Alcor facility, a five- to seven-hour perfusion process diffuses a fresh cryopreservative into the cryopatient. Since 2001, Alcor's cooling process has sought to accomplish vitrification—deep cooling resulting in solidification but avoiding freezing, crystallization, and concomitant cell damage.

The paltry number of existing cryopatients (fewer than two hundred) testifies to the failure of cryonics to attract many participants. This failure, in turn, is due in part to widespread skepticism about whether the cooling and regeneration process will ever succeed.[56] The notion of reanimating and restoring a cryonically preserved cadaver has been likened to turning a piece of hamburger back into a cow.[57] That skepticism is currently well grounded, given the enormous hurdles facing cryonics. One hazard is cellular damage caused by lack of oxygen between death and the administration of preservatives. Another hazard is cellular damage caused by the freezing (or supercooling) process. As freezing occurs, water in cells freezes into crystals that rip the walls of neighboring cells. Once significant crystallization has occurred, cryonics may amount to freezing meat, not living cells.[58] Scientists say that the freezing process used in cryonics before 2001 has caused profound and irreversible damage to brain tissue, making impossible the restoration of the memory and personality unique to those decedents.

Cryonics bolstered by vitrification might have some future. New cryopreservative substances and new cooling techniques may diminish cell damage from freezing. Future techniques of stem-cell engineering, combined with nanotechnological tissue repair, might someday overcome previous tissue damage. Even then, strong obstacles to successful resuscitation would remain. Cryopreservatives may well produce their own toxic effects. Vitrification may cause thermal stress. In order to regenerate a cadaver successfully, the damage caused by the original fatal pathology would have to be reversed. As to heads in cryosuspension, regenerating an entire body and grafting it onto a resuscitated head also poses great neurological and physical challenges. And in order to re-create the same person from the corpse, a technique must be found to maintain the decedent's unique brain contents, including memory and character.

Nonetheless, vitrification offers some hope of successful cell preservation in cadavers. Recently, the brilliant futurologist Ray Kurzweil signed on for postmortem processing at Alcor. He is convinced that within thirty years science will permit people to live forever, and he wants to be able to benefit from that development. His hope is that in the event of his expected interim death, Alcor's treatment and storage will keep his cadaver fit enough long enough for that to happen.

Putting aside the enormous technical difficulties, successful cryonic preservation and bodily regeneration would create interesting legal problems. There would be considerable pressure to alter the definition of death. Cryonicists want to be able to supercool now living but fatally ill persons in order to maximize the cellular vigor of the preserved cryopatient. In 1992 Thomas Donaldson, an Alcor member suffering from a malignant brain tumor, wanted to advance the cryopreservation process before cancer decimated his brain. He petitioned a California court to declare that premortem freezing of his head for purposes of cryonic preservation would not constitute homicide. The court correctly rejected the petition, ruling that the freezing process would precipitate Mr. Donaldson's death and must be considered a form of unlawful homicide.[59] If citizens were able to point to a substantial chance of successful postmortem regeneration, the pressure on courts and legislators to alter the current definition of death—which now uses criteria that entail total brain dysfunction—would be considerable. People like Mr. Donaldson would have a powerful incentive to demand acceleration of their dying processes.

Other thorny legal questions would surround successful revivification of dead persons. How much regained brain content would be necessary to make the regenerated being the same person as the frozen decedent—that is, how much memory and character constitute self-identity? Assuming that the reconstituted person will be the same person as his or her progenitor, what is the legal status of the cryonically preserved corpse in the interim period? What happens to the former (and perhaps continuing) spouse, children, and other survivors? Can the spouse remarry? Are the heirs free to dispose of the decedent's property while the corpse is in frozen limbo? Could they decide to thaw the corpse without revitalization? Are they responsible for paying continued maintenance to Alcor or CI?

Suppose that the memory transference during the cryonic revivification process turns out to be inadequate to make the regenerated person the same person as the decedent. Is the vivified successor entitled to any of the assets of the predecessor who, after all, was a different person? Is the successor person responsible for the social and legal obligations assumed premortem by the decedent? Does he or she have a duty to support the predecessor's children? Another issue is the successor's financial well-being. Presumably the predecessor, while alive, can set up a trust or make explicit provision to secure the financial well-being of the newly animated successor. In the absence of an explicit provision of this sort, who bears responsibility for the maintenance of the successor if the successor is not immediately self-sufficient?

The science is still relatively primitive, so most of these legal problems are not likely to arise for many years. Lawyers, judges, and scholars will have more time to ponder the legal status of a regenerated corpse. But some of the preliminary issues—such as the definition of death and the responsibility for frozen cryopatient maintenance—are already at hand.

### Commemoration of the Deceased

Many people have no pretensions to an eternal presence, either physical or spiritual. They are content to have their remains unceremoniously and expeditiously disposed of, whether by cremation, prompt burial, or conveyance to an educational or research institution.

Most humans, though, want to leave a mark on the world as part of an urge to find meaning in existence. Says undertaker/philosopher Thomas Lynch: "We need our witnesses and archivists to say we lived, we died, we made this difference. Where death means nothing, life is meaningless."[60] For many people, their important legacy is in the hearts and minds of people previously touched, and that impact, they think, is recorded before they become "a piece of meat in a box."[61] Lifetime deeds perhaps become the best means of ensuring postmortem memories. Still, a variety of postmortem means exist for perpetuation of memory in the wake of death. An elaborate monument or mausoleum, as described in chapter 5, was and is a memorial device used by some wealthy decedents. Other memorialization practices cross socioeconomic lines. Commemoration is an important element of most of the rites accompanying disposal of a corpse.

The presence of the corpse at a wake can facilitate recollection and memorialization of a former persona in accord with particular cultural traditions. Subcultures such as fraternal groups, veterans' groups, law enforcement organizations, or unions may employ their own honorific customs. In 1991 his colleagues gathered to recall and honor the fallen Inka Dink the clown. Inka Dink was laid out in full regalia, including yellow wig, immense red bow tie, red striped stockings, and giant yellow shoes.[62] Many of those who came to pay their respects also wore full clown regalia. In another subculture, Irish wakes were sometimes boisterous affairs, including storytelling, singing, dancing, and card playing (occasionally dealing the corpse in).[63] An Irish corpse might be propped up in a chair with a pipe in its mouth; on one occasion, the corpse's head (decapitated in a work accident) was placed on a chair with a pipe in its mouth.[64] A Syrian orthodox archbishop, Althanius Y. Samuel, was "laid out" seated in a thronelike chair at St. Mark's Cathedral in Teaneck, New Jersey.[65] Lifelike presentation of a corpse perhaps undermines the effort to remind survivors that death has occurred, but it can certainly trigger recollection.

Funerals or memorial ceremonies typically contain a commemorative element—an effort to remember the departed, reminisce, pay tribute to certain attributes, and celebrate a former existence. Religious ritual used to dominate funerals, but at many contemporary funerals the emphasis is on remembering and celebrating the extinguished existence. The National Funeral Directors Association (NFDA comments about contemporary funerals: "Families want the funeral ceremony to no longer focus on death, but rather a celebration of life."[66] As part of the commemorative focus, people who knew the deceased rise and reminisce in stories and tributes. People may contribute readings or poetry or music. Some sort of pictorial display—by still photos or videos—may help recreate the image of the deceased.

The modern celebration of life may succeed in elevating mourners' spirits. Funeral director Thomas Lynch talks about celebrations of life as capturing the "fun" in "funeral" and the "good" in "goodbye."[67] But an emphasis on memory and celebration does not erase the sadness of loss. Says one observer of the funeral scene: People "did not grieve any less because they chose to celebrate a life even as they mourned a death."[68] A jumble of emotions typically accompanies a sense of permanent loss—regret, sorrow, guilt, anger, fear, love, and longing.[69] The ambivalence and confusion may increase when a celebration of life includes "multiple sets of ex-spouses and children along with their attendant neuroses and baggage."[70] Usually, though, the prevalent impulse at this stark last confrontation with the deceased is to make things as right as possible through fond recollection.

A combination of clergy, family, and friends typically rises at memorial services to present eulogies. People who deliver eulogies understandably tend to glorify the departed or at least to focus on whatever positive attributes he or she had. This is consistent with the ancient inscription above a mortuary door: "De Mortuis Nil Nisi Bonum" (Speak nothing but good about the dead).[71] A degree of exaggeration or selective recall is often evident in reminiscences, at times in large measure. At some funerals I have attended, I wondered whether the person being eulogized was really the same one I had known; testimonials tend to recount fables rather than foibles. Jessica Mitford wryly commented about the exclusive focus on a decedent's virtues: "No provision seems to have been made for the burial of a Heartily Disliked One, although the necessity for such must arise in the course of human events."[72]

Glorification of the deceased is not invariable. Sometimes the truth about the deceased is so notorious that it will out. One widow, marking a forty-year marriage to her departed spouse, is quoted as saying, "This is the first night in all those years that I *know* exactly where he really is!"[73] At another funeral, an incredulous son piped up during the eulogies: "Quit telling all of these lies. My mother was a mean person and everyone here knows it!"[74]

Perhaps the focus on the decedent's positive qualities is appropriate for a being who is no more and who is unavailable to offer a defense to negative statements. The people who really knew the deceased are probably well aware of his or her foibles and need no reminders. At a memorial service, recollection of endearing rather than infuriating habits might also help to calm mourners and bond survivors in respectful remembrances. Perhaps a common awe or fear of the dead also influences survivors' testimonials at funerals. We do not really *know* what follows death. Suppose that the departed's spirit is still around, and suppose that it is capable of mischief or retaliation against any demeaning voices. Why take a risk with derogatory recollections of the deceased?

A written obituary provides an opportunity to acknowledge a death and to summarize a lifetime's accomplishments. Who among us does not aspire to have his or her obituary appear in the *New York Times*—preferably in the form of a eulogy prepared in advance by the *Times* staff and printed as a public service? In this era of newspaper distress, many papers, including the *New York Times*, will accept paid death notices. Lengthy notices cost hundreds of dollars. Even the display or reading of a name can constitute a moving form of remembrance. Consider the Vietnam War memorial in Washington, D.C. Consider the frequent readings of names of victims following the destruction of the World Trade Center—a memorial exercise that is repeated annually.

Another way of memorializing a vanished existence is by presenting visual images of the departed. During the first half of the eighteenth century carved faces sometimes appeared on gravestones, though the carvers were not skilled enough to make accurate representations of the deceased.[75] During the nineteenth century death masks of prominent individuals were made from clay molds and displayed. The Princeton University library has a large collection of such death masks, including those of the early American personages Aaron Burr, Thomas Paine, Daniel Webster, and Samuel Taylor Coleridge. Between 1830 and 1860, paintings of the cadaver, singly or surrounded by family, offered affluent survivors a form of reminiscence.[76] In the second half of the nineteenth century, photography replaced painting as the genre of remembrance for the affluent. After the advent of photography, families who could afford it often commissioned keepsake photos of the cadaver.[77] Such photos supplied "a lifelike reminder of a former presence."[78] Sometimes photos reproduced death scenes showing the dying patient or his or her cadaver on a death bed surrounded by family.

In the modern era, photos are still often used to bear witness to departed lives. A display board of photographs of the deceased is a frequent accoutrement at the funeral home. After 9/11 the photos on the "wall of the missing" at the 69th Street Armory in New York City (where unidentified bodies were collected and where relatives searched desperately for news of the missing) formed a poignant testimonial to the people lost that day.[79] Similar photo montages appeared in many public places in New York City, such as the Port Authority bus terminal (in memory of dead transit police officers). Some cultures attach photos of the departed to gravestones.[80] When Senator Edward Kennedy lay in repose in Boston in August 2009, his casket was accompanied by several large photos of the senator at different stages of his life.

A more permanent form of written commemoration is an epitaph—the inscription on a gravestone or on a plate located at a grave. Typically the inscriptions on American gravestones have been simple, often merely noting the deceased's name, dates of birth and death, and perhaps the familial role as husband, wife, son, or daughter. Simple formulaic folk epitaphs, some employing religious themes, have always been popular. These include "RIP" (*requiescat in pace* or rest in peace); "*memento mori*" (remember, you must die); "gone to rest"; "asleep in Jesus"; and "Blessed are the dead which die in the Lord." Before 1800 epitaphs sometimes focused on the inevitability of death and decay, with "As I am now so shall you be" being a common lament.[81] In 2005 a cardboard epitaph was taped above the still-exposed body of a hurricane Katrina victim, Alcede Jackson: "d. Aug. 31, 2005, Rest in Peace In the Loving Arms of Jesus."[82] Any permanent marker, even one with just a name and date, makes a statement by recording an existence that created enough impact to warrant a marker and an inscription.

Some epitaphs offer more personalized commemoration. Some record a salient fact about the deceased, a few noting death by a tragic event. In the eighteenth and nineteenth centuries, these events included Indian raids, falls from horses, hunting accidents, stagecoach mishaps, and railroad disasters. The 1884 inscription on the grave of John Heath in Boot Hill Cemetery in Tombstone, Arizona, reads: "taken from county jail and lynched by Bisbee Mob." In Albany, New York, Harry Edsel Smith's 1942 gravestone reads: "Looked up the elevator shaft to see if the car was on the way down. It was."

More frequently, epitaphs seek to highlight and honor some salient fact or characteristic about the life of the deceased. Notation of the occupation or hobby of the deceased is not unusual. When Captain Thomas Coffin died in 1842 in Rhode Island, his gravestone noted: "He's done a-catching cod, And gone to meet his God."[83] Lawyer John Strange's epitaph reads: "Here lies an honest lawyer, and that is Strange." In the late nineteenth century, placing symbols on tombstones had become a way of marking a decedent's lifework—for example, carvings of sausages on the headstone of a butcher or a baker's gravestone in the shape of a cake.[84] Such symbolic markings of a final resting place continued into the twentieth century. Monuments carved in the Lower East Side of Manhattan often included symbols signifying the lifework or passion of the deceased—a spool of thread for a seamstress, scales of justice for a lawyer, a tennis racquet, a violin, or even a slot machine.[85]

Tributes to skill, accomplishment, or character can appear in epitaphs. An 1878 epitaph for Captain Augustus Littlefield reads: "An experienced and careful master mariner who never made a call upon underwriters for any loss."[86] Early epitaphs on women's graves tended to praise their domestic virtues with words such as "faithful," "prudent," and "loving."[87] Later, female accomplishment was acknowledged. When Mary Arnet Galt died in 1854 in Williamsburgh, Virginia, her gravestone extolled her not just as a wife, friend, and neighbor, but also as the "matron of the lunatic asylum for 40 years."[88] Elizabeth Gurley Flynn is memorialized in stone as "The Rebel Girl Fighter for Working Class Emancipation."[89] (Flynn was a fiery supporter of labor struggle who served as an officer of the American Communist Party in the 1950s.) Harriet Tubman is memorialized as the "Heroine of the Underground Railroad, Nurse and Scout in the Civil War."[90]

Not all epitaphs carry benevolent messages. Anna Wallace's grave in Ribbesford, England, is inscribed:

> The children of Israel wanted bread,
> And the Lord sent them manna;
> Clark Wallace wanted a wife,
> And the Devil sent him Anna.

When Bezalel Wood died in 1837 in Winslow, Maine, the inscription read: "Here lies one Wood, Enclosed in wood; One Wood within another. The outer wood is very good; we cannot praise the other."[91] In another instance, surviving family members castigated a fellow surviving relative with this inscription: "a brother of the deceased . . . although benefited thousands of dollars from her estate . . . absolutely refused to contribute more than $10 toward the erection of this monument."[92]

People have an opportunity to leave a lasting message by formulating their own epitaphs. My favorite epitaphs are those that demonstrate the acute sense of humor of the deceased and/or their descendants. One example is "Here lies Johnny Yeast; Pardon me for not rising."[93] Another example is the notation on a grave in a Princeton, New Jersey, cemetery: "I told you I was sick."[94] A West Virginia miner left instructions for cremation and composed his epitaph: "I made an ash of myself." A locally renowned housewife and cook had a recipe carved on her gravestone along with the message "I always said the only way you would get this recipe was over my dead body."[95] A humorous epitaph seems to enhance the chances of truly perpetuating one's memory.

The point is simple: People strive to immortalize themselves in diverse ways. Some seek to preserve their bodily remnants. Some create permanent symbols or markers of their presence in the form of structures or monuments. Others leave permanent inscriptions—messages that encapsulate the life that was. Another way to perpetuate oneself is by donating cadaveric tissue to be used by a needy living person. Organ donation is the subject of the next chapter.

# Part III

# The Multiple Roles of a Cadaver

Don't take your organs to heaven;
Heaven knows we need them here

Bumper sticker, circa 2002

Every hour another person dies waiting for an organ transplant. Despite significant technological improvements and numerous publicity campaigns over the past several decades, the substantial shortage of organs, tissues, and eyes for life-saving or life-improving transplants continues. This shortage persists despite efforts by the federal government and every state legislature to improve the system.

National Conference of Commissioners on Uniform State Laws, Comments to the Uniform Anatomical Gift Act (UAGA) (2006)

*Chapter 7*

# The Cadaver as Supplier of Used Body Parts

A host of uses can be made of a human cadaver. Some of them are utilitarian, such as using ground-up human remains for crop fertilizer or for filler in artificial reefs. Other uses are more humanitarian, as in education and research for the advancement of medicine and science. Corpses or parts of corpses are used beneficially as teaching tools in medical education or as practice tools for health care providers. Preserved human remains appear in museums and exhibitions that teach about human evolution and anatomy. Corpses as subjects of scientific research contribute to therapeutic advances in medical knowledge. A basic autopsy, for example, may help identify sources of fatal afflictions—a first step in leading to a cure. Or an autopsy may determine how effective various drugs or prostheses have been within the deceased's body. Research using cadavers examines how the human body responds to various traumas and tests the effectiveness of related protective devices.

No use of a cadaver is as immediately beneficial and appealing as transplanting a needed body part to a fatally afflicted or seriously ailing person. For decades, health care organizations and government agencies have sought to encourage cadaveric organ transplantation. Successful tissue transplant techniques in the United States date to the 1940s, when orthopedic surgeons began using bone taken from one patient (a live donor) to repair fractures in another patient. Within a few years, surgeons discovered that cadavers could be a useful supply source for such bones.[1] In 1951 a naval surgeon set up a body-donation program, and his Naval Tissue Bank became a source of tissue for civilian as well as military hospitals. The first successful kidney transplant occurred in 1954, using a live donor.[2] Successful kidney transplants from cadavers started in 1962. By the late 1960s surgeons were using cadavers as a source not only of kidneys but of corneas, pituitary glands (to obtain human growth hormone), skin, and hearts as well.

The development of immunosuppressive drugs enormously increased the success and scope of organ harvesting, making human cadavers a true "potential source of life [and well-being] for others."[3] Progress in tissue transplantation extended well beyond lifesaving organs like kidneys and hearts. By the 1980s nonprofit tissue banks were regularly supplying bone, ligaments, and tendons for repair of injuries. Also in the 1980s profit-making companies founded a "tissue-processing" industry to supply certain body parts for both transplantation and teaching purposes.[4] By 2000 at least twenty-five different types of tissue or organs were transplantable, including liver, lungs, pancreas, veins, heart valves, cartilage, blood products, and collagen.[5] In theory a single corpse can now benefit as many as one hundred tissue recipients. In 2004 a million tissue transplants were performed annually in the United States; today the total is close to a million and a half.

### Authority to Retrieve Cadaveric Organs—Informed Consent

Any legal framework governing organ transplantation from cadavers must reconcile the enormous potential benefits of organ and tissue recovery for living recipients with traditional concern for the integrity and dignity of the human cadaver. American social and legal traditions have established that human remains should not be disturbed or violated except for very good reasons. A cadaver itself ordinarily has rights to be decently disposed of and to quiet repose. Removal of body parts could easily qualify as unlawful abuse. At the same time, virtually no one disputes that salvaging the lives and restoring the health of stricken humans can, upon appropriate authorization, furnish a good reason to disrupt the normal tranquility of a cadaver. The question is who weighs the competing interests and decides whether a particular cadaver's repose should be preceded by removal of one or more organs for transplant.

Decedents and their families have traditionally been accorded considerable leeway in disposing of human remains—especially with regard to the place and mode of disposition. Given such customary American emphasis on prospective self-determination and survivors' prerogatives, it is no surprise that today recovery of cadaver organs and tissue for transplant is based primarily on consent (as determined by the previously expressed wishes of the now-dead potential donor and/or the current wishes of the next of kin).[6]

In theory, at least, decedents control the availability of their own remains for transplant. All states authorize a decedent's antemortem donation of his or her cadaver or its parts for purposes of transplant, research, or education.[7] The first state statutes governing cadaveric organ transplants were adopted in the 1950s, and state legislation gathered momentum following drafting of the Uniform Anatomical Gift Act (UAGA) in 1968. (The UAGA was formulated by a national commission as a recommended statutory model for regulation of organ transplantation within each state.) The model UAGA, some version of which is now followed in all states, operates on the principle that "the right thing to do [concerning organ transplants from cadavers] is to respect the will of the deceased."[8] The 1968 UAGA gave binding force to an organ donation document previously signed by the decedent in the presence of two witnesses. A 1987 amendment required only a signed document. The 2006 revised version of the UAGA, already adopted in over forty states, makes even an oral declaration binding.[9] Health care organizations readily provide wallet-size cards for potential donors, and several states ask people to indicate on their drivers' licenses whether they wish to contribute their organs upon death. The revised UAGA explicitly validates the forms found on the back of drivers' licenses

Despite the ostensible authority given to the decedent's wishes, surviving family members have often been able, as a practical matter, to thwart those wishes. Counter to the UAGA's intention to give a decedent's wishes prevalence over survivors' preferences, health care institutions have commonly sought family members' approval of organ or tissue removal and have deferred to their opposition to such harvesting.[10] One physician described this phenomenon in a 1983 magazine article: "You could die with an organ card in every pocket, and another one pasted on your forehead, and still no one would touch you if your [family] said no."[11] Roy Reeves recounts the story of a fifty-eight-year-old male who was a card-carrying organ donor. Upon the would-be donor's death, his wife sought to honor his wishes. She was legally entitled to determine the fate of her husband's remains. Yet, because the dead donor's mother objected to the organ harvesting, the health facility violated not only the decedent's wishes but also the legally authorized spouse's wishes, by failing to salvage the usable organs.[12]

Health facilities' long-standing practice of following an objecting family member's wishes, rather than the decedent's wishes, is not hard to understand. The stunned, mourning family member's objection is based on upset at the image of a loved one's corpse being surgically invaded and its (previously) vital organs extracted. Or perhaps the mourner believes that all organs will be useful to the deceased in an anticipated afterlife. The health institution wants to respect mourners' feelings rather than provoke their anger and upset. The emotional well-being of survivors is an understandable institutional concern.

Health care personnel may try to persuade family objectors to go along with organ transplant, but they have not been prone to unilaterally override family opposition. Even if the institution is legally entitled to override survivors' objections, organ harvesting in the face of a family member's opposition might provoke emotional upset, outrage, or even litigation. Health care institutions are understandably sensitive to potential public relations nightmares. A newspaper headline trumpeting a health care institution's "plundering" of a cadaver over family members' objections is not a palatable outcome.[13] No institution relishes devoting time, money, and effort to defending a lawsuit—even if the institution would ultimately prevail. Lawyers representing health care institutions, as well those representing doctors, tend to be extremely risk averse in such situations. The less risky path is to defer to the survivors' objections.

Such nonadherence to decedents' wishes to become organ donors deprives decedents of their legal right to donate their organs or tissue for transplant. The decedent's prospective autonomy prerogative then remains a theoretical legal right without a remedy if neither the health facility nor another family member chooses to contest survivors' objections to implementing the decedent's wishes.

The newly revised UAGA makes a valiant effort to overcome health care institutions' tendency to abide by any family member's opposition to fulfilling the decedent's express wish to donate an organ. The 1987 version of the UAGA had stated that a decedent's donation is valid and "does not require" concurrence from the surrounding family. The 2006 version emphasizes that a decedent's wish should not be blocked by others. It states that a decedent's wish (either for or against donation) "is not subject to change by others."[14] Accordingly, if the decedent previously consented to organ or tissue donation, there is "no reason to seek consent from the donor's family" or even to search for the next of kin before harvesting the donated organs.[15] Only time will tell whether the new UAGA will in fact change institutional deference to the surrounding family. Hospital personnel, not the drafters of the UAGA, will have the burden of coping with distraught relatives who object to implementation of the decedent's wishes.

In the absence of prior expressions from the decedent about the fate of his or her organs, the next of kin are entitled to decide whether usable organs and tissue are to be harvested for transplant (or research or teaching). This allocation of authority is consistent with the common law's recognition of a family's right (as described in chapter 3) to determine the disposition of a cadaver. That right of disposal includes a right to receive the cadaver "as is" without tampering.[16] As stated by a North Carolina court in 1914, a next of kin's right to dispose of a cadaver includes "a right to possession of the body in the same condition in which death leaves it" (an exception for forensic autopsy notwithstanding).[17] The next of kin's prerogative to dispose of a cadaver and its parts is reinforced by an entitlement to damages—pursuant to state tort law—for emotional distress caused by any mutilation of a corpse.[18] Removal of a body part without consent, including for purposes of transplant, is a form of mutilation. In 1968 the UAGA built on that judicial foundation by giving the next of kin (in descending order) the right to decide whether a cadaver or its parts would be donated for purposes of education, research, or transplantation.[19]

The primary mechanism for obtaining cadaveric organs and tissue for transplant, then, is consent—voluntary donation by the decedent or the next of kin. That consent framework also governs postmortem, posthospital harvesting of nonvital tissue for transplant purposes. The tissue processing industry, which accounts for hundreds of thousands of annual therapeutic transplants, uses donated muscle, bone, tendons, skin, and so on.[20] Those donations come mainly from consent obtained in the context of autopsies, funeral homes, crematories, or gifts of cadavers to medical schools. (Family consent need not be obtained immediately upon death because nonvital tissue remains salvageable for transplant even days after death.)

While the applicable legal framework clearly calls for informed consent, abuses have sometimes corrupted the harvesting of nonvital organs. On occasion—in the context of funeral homes, crematories, and donated body programs in medical schools—such tissue has been retrieved without *any* consent.[21] A 2006 news report refers to "a motley collection of grim reapers who sometimes secretly and [sometimes] with dubious consent harvest skin, bones, tendons, organs, and even brains from funeral homes, burial sites, and morgues."[22] The harm is exacerbated when the reapers fail to screen adequately the donors and tissue, so that communicable disease can be transmitted to the ultimate tissue recipient.[23] That form of cadaver abuse—unconsented, reckless transfer of human tissue—is described in chapter 10 under the heading of "Modern Body Parts Snatching." But it is useful to keep this chicanery in mind in exploring means for obtaining badly needed organs or tissue for transplant.

Even without the decedent's or family's consent, an autopsy can lawfully be performed for forensic purposes (such as an inquiry following an unexplained death).[24] But a government pathologist's temporary postmortem control over a corpse's viscera for purposes of investigating the cause of death does not create a broad legal prerogative to use autopsies as a source of transplant tissue. A forensic autopsy does not permit the harvesting of organs for transplant. A significant exception to this legal framework demanding voluntary consent to organ retrieval is found in a few state statutes that authorize the taking of corneas and/or pituitary glands in the course of forensic autopsies absent known objections from the decedent or the decedent's family.[25] This statutory authorization for harvesting tissue provides a significantly different approach than the prevailing consent-based model. The utility and constitutionality of a system of government-authorized systematic retrieval of transplant tissue will be considered shortly.

## The Current Shortfall in Transplant Organs

By all accounts, the current consent-based system of obtaining organs for transplant has failed to meet social needs.[26] As of August 2007 ninety-seven thousand potential organ recipients were awaiting organs; that figure increased to 108,122 in 2010. Only a fraction of those organs become available each year. Over six thousand people die each year while awaiting a donated organ.[27] The average wait for a kidney for a dialysis patient is more than three years—time often spent bearing the burdens of dialysis in the face of advancing kidney disease. This protracted wait means not only that many people will die before receiving an organ but also that the chances for a successful transplant (once an organ is found) will have diminished. The gap between the supply of donated organs and the need for organs is widening; the total number of cadaveric organ donors has decreased since 2007.

This shortfall in supply exists despite valiant efforts by health-related organizations to increase public awareness and to distribute donor consent forms, as well as efforts within hospitals to sensitively solicit consent for transplantation from the families of qualified dying patients. The encouragement of consent to organ donation goes well beyond the bumper sticker level. The routine for in-hospital solicitation of donation at transplant centers is well established. Upon notification about a dead or imminently dying patient who is a potential source of organs, trained personnel from an organ procurement organization (OPO) investigate the suitability of the relevant organs for transplant and check whether the patient has previously given instructions about organ donation. The OPO solicitor can then approach the patient's family and raise the possibility of donation. Solicitors from OPOs can be aggressive in pushing for transplant. They have been criticized for not fully disclosing the procedures accompanying a transplant, such as administration of drugs to assist organ perfusion.[28] If family consent is given and once death is pronounced, a new team of transplant surgeons does the harvesting according to the scope of consent obtained.

In their request for donation, solicitors in hospitals focus on benevolence—the opportunity to save life (as in kidney donation), to ease suffering (as in skin donation), or to remedy disability (as in cornea donation).[29] In other words, one theme of the appeal to potential organ donors is to satisfy altruistic urges. Another appeal is the opportunity for the organ provider to "live on" after death. Something of a dead donor's self is transmitted and preserved in the surviving organ within a tissue recipient.[30] Tissue donation thus provides "a way to guarantee one's memory after death"—or at least to leave a positive mark on earth.[31] Surviving family members might find some comfort in knowing that a humanitarian benefit is being derived from the patient's death.[32] Surviving families, though, are not always so benevolently inclined. At least 40 percent of solicited families decline to authorize organ retrieval. While improved training of procurement personnel and cooperating hospital personnel can increase the rate of organ recovery, improved solicitation techniques are not likely to fill the need for cadaveric transplant organs.

Many methods have been suggested or tried to increase the number of organs available for transplantation. Proposals exist to mandate solicitation of organ donation from the next of kin in all instances when a patient with usable organs dies in an institution.[33] Another suggestion is to legally require all citizens to register their wishes about the postmortem fate of their organs, sometimes as a condition for renewal of a driver's license. Still another proposal calls for providing an incentive to agree to cadaveric organ donation by giving such "volunteers" preferred status in the event that they themselves develop a need for an organ transplant.[34] Programs already exist for "paired donations" in which a healthy person who wants to donate an organ to a loved one, but whose blood type is not a match, will donate to an appropriately matching donee in return for an organ from the donee's cooperating donor. An online registration system at MatchingDonors.com seeks to facilitate such exchanges. None of these methods or suggestions is likely to produce the number of donated organs needed.

The continuing reality is that a legal framework confined to explicit consent for transplant does not produce nearly enough organs to meet pressing public health needs. That failure raises the important question of whether the existing mechanisms for securing human tissue from cadavers should be altered and, if so, how. Reliance on human organ transplants to save dying persons may someday end. Artificial organs are being perfected, xenotransplants (such as pigs' heart valves) may become more common, and stem-cell technology may ultimately create replacement organs.[35] In the meantime, though, ways still have to be found to increase the supply of cadaver organs for transplant. As long as the next of kin still form the main portal to organ donations from cadavers, it will not be easy to secure unanimous consent from bereft families to exploit the cadaver of a loved one, even for the noble purpose of salvaging others' lives. Additional approaches will be necessary.

## Organ Removal after Pronouncement of Death by Cardiac Criteria

One method of increasing the organ supply is to expand the eligible sources of transplant organs. Until recently, the vast majority of organ providers were accident or crime victims who had sustained severe brain trauma and had been connected before death to machinery supporting their lung and heart functions. In such instances, when brain function declines to the point that whole-brain death is detected, organs can be removed while machinery continues to perfuse or keep fresh the organs to be harvested. This system of harvesting from cadavers pronounced dead by brain death criteria (DBD) maximizes the chances of successful organ transplant. Yet only 2 percent of deaths occur while people are already connected to respirators in this fashion.[36]

Many medical sources now urge an increase in organ transplants from people whose death is pronounced on the basis of cardiac stoppage (as opposed to the 2 percent of people whose whole-brain death is recorded while the potential donors are connected to respirators).[37] This approach—called transplant from non-heart-beating donors (NHBD) or donation after cardiac death (DCD)—has been successfully employed in numerous medical centers.[38] In 2007 DCD accounted for only about 5 percent of transplant tissue. But DCD has the potential to become more widespread, increasing both the number of potential donors and the actual recovery of organs.

In planned DCD cases, disconnection of life support is scheduled in advance, and organ transplant surgery can be undertaken so long as the patient dies within ninety minutes following disconnection (i.e., when solid organs are still fresh enough to be recoverable).[39] The withdrawal of life support is performed either in an intensive care unit (ICU) or in an operating room, with a transplant surgery team outside poised to act.[40] A family member can be present. Once cardiac stoppage takes place, the attending physicians wait between two and five minutes—depending on the hospital protocol—to ensure that autoresuscitation will not occur. At that point, an attending physician's pronouncement of death is deemed to be conclusive (a conclusion still disputed by some medical sources as discussed in chapter 1) and organ harvesting proceeds. The survival rate of recipients and the endurance of transplanted kidneys in DCD cases are close to those in transplants involving DBD.[41] Even when DCD results have not matched those of DBD, physicians are confident that more careful donor selection will result in making DCD an important additional source of organs for transplant.[42]

Several legal/ethical objections have been raised about NHBD transplant protocols, but all of them can and should be overcome. The most serious assertion is that the DCD technique violates the dead donor rule by pronouncing death prematurely (after two to five minutes without a heartbeat). In chapter 1 I reject the contention that a two- to five-minute wait after heart stoppage is inadequate to pronounce death. The speculation that a dying patient who has rejected (or whose representative has rejected) further resuscitation might have had a tiny chance for a fleeting glimmer of life (if the transplant team had waited a few more minutes) does not seem incompatible with the dead donor rule. This DCD methodology for pronouncing death in a moribund patient does not appear likely to undermine public confidence in the medical establishment's organ transplant practices. The specter of ending life prematurely is no greater in this context than in the context of removal of organs from a DBD corpse that is still pink, warm, and breathing (with mechanical support) immediately after being pronounced dead by whole-brain cessation criteria.

A separate issue of premature causation of death or of harm to patient well-being arises when physicians inject substances into a moribund DCD donor primarily for the purpose of promoting successful organ retrieval. The disputed substances promote successful transplants by increasing oxygen perfusion of organs that are about to be transplanted. Substances that aid perfusion include anticoagulants such as heparin and vasodilators such as regitine (for widening blood vessels).[43] The problem is that such substances are nontherapeutic for the donor and could possibly have the effect of hastening death. Some commentators contend that these substances risk causing brain hemorrhage or reduced blood pressure in the moribund patient.[44] Commentators also point out that these nontherapeutic measures are sometimes undertaken without explicit consent from the patient or the family. (Another controversial adjunct to DCD transplant is premortem installation of a femoral cannula in the moribund organ donor to be used postmortem for mechanical perfusion of a transplantable organ.[45])

For me, this criticism of nontherapeutic interventions preceding DCD or NHBD organ transplant is a tempest in a teapot. It is empirically unclear whether the nontherapeutic substances are in fact hastening death. Further, as Norm Fost has pointed out, it seems reasonable to imply assent by organ donors to the modest steps being taken to facilitate a successful transplant.[46] A donor wants the transplant to succeed and should be willing to allow the use of facilitative substances that create no real imposition on the moribund patient and that pose only a slight risk, if any, of hastening an imminent death.

It would be better practice to fully inform potential organ donors about the possibility of using nontherapeutic substances such as anticoagulants. Existing guidelines for DCD transplants do provide for including information about such nontherapeutic agents within the consent process.[47] In the meantime, the current practices surrounding consent to DCD transplants are defensible, though not ideal.

A recent incident tends to support the thesis that the use of so-called nontherapeutic substances during DCD or NHBD organ transplants need not violate legal or ethical bounds. In 2007 criminal charges were filed in California against Dr. Hootan Roozrokf for allegedly hastening a prospective donor's death while participating in a planned DCD transplant of a kidney and a liver. Sometime during the eight hours that the patient survived after withdrawal of life support machinery, Dr. Roozrokf administered three substances—morphine; an antianxiety medication called Ativan; and Betadine, an antiseptic substance.[48] Dr. Roozrokf characterized the medications as palliative—intended to relieve the suffering of the moribund patient—but the Betadine was probably intended to help prevent infection in the organ intended to be transplanted. (The anticipated organ transplants never took take place because the patient died so long after the artificial life support machinery was disconnected that the organs were no longer usable.) By the time a criminal trial took place in late 2008, the charges had been reduced to one—abuse of a dependent adult.[49] After a two-month trial, a jury acquitted Dr. Roozrokf.

The verdict upholding Dr. Roozrokf is not surprising. Prosecutions of this sort in the context of DCD are not likely to succeed. As noted, a prosecutor claiming that homicide has occurred must prove that the physician-administered substances did in fact cause death—a difficult task in the context of patients already afflicted with fatal diseases. Even if causation is somehow proved, a transplant surgeon's conduct aimed at preserving transplantable organs appears to be lawful. Both medical practice and the relevant jurisprudence give physicians certain leeway in using substances that have legitimate objectives (such as pain relief) even if they risk accelerating death.[50] Just as pain relief to a suffering patient can be a legal justification for administering a risky substance, preservation of an organ to be transplanted can serve as a justification for creating some risk of hastening death. A patient or patient's representative can consent (certainly explicitly and perhaps implicitly) to the use of such substances, and a physician can use them so long as the dosages are not known to be fatal and are not excessive for accomplishing the legitimate objectives. In other words, a physician attending a DCD patient is entitled to facilitate transplant so long as the conduct does not pose reckless dangers to the dying donor.

It does not matter that the substances given to the moribund DCD patient—such as anticoagulants and vasodepressors—are nontherapeutic in terms of the health of the dying patient. A surrogate decision maker, in deciding what course of medical intervention (or nonintervention) is in the best interests of the incompetent patient, need not extend the patient's life at all costs. A surrogate acting in good faith might determine that the now-incompetent patient would want his or her own best interests to include facilitation of a successful organ transplant. That is, a surrogate is not violating any fiduciary duty by approving salutary steps (facilitating a successful organ transplant) that pose only a tiny risk of hastening death, at least when the surrogate in good faith believes that the patient would concur. By analogy, a surrogate could also enlist a dying patient in nontherapeutic medical research that carries minimal risk. Benefit to medical science can be a legitimate justification for such nontherapeutic conduct.

Another tempest in a teapot involving DCD organ retrieval concerns maintenance of dying potential organ donors on life support machinery despite a patient's advance medical directive (AD) possibly dictating an end to life-extending medical intervention in the circumstances at hand. The controversy centers on the 2006 and 2007 amendments to the UAGA. The accusation is that the UAGA now permits physicians harvesting organs to keep potential organ donors alive in contravention of an AD indicating the patient's preference to be allowed to die.

The revised UAGA does go far in seeking to promote organ transplant donation following cardiac death. It anticipates that an OPO will investigate the suitability as an organ supplier of any hospitalized patient who is at or near death. This means investigating the medical and social history of the potential donor and examining the medical suitability of the patient's organs.[51] If the patient is a suitable donor, the officer checks the record for evidence of prior consent to organ transplant and seeks consent from the next of kin.[52]

An OPO investigation may also turn up advance patient instructions regarding end-of-life medical intervention, either via a formal AD or some other recorded means. Revised UAGA Section 21 provides that in the event of an ostensible conflict between life-extending measures (while investigating the "medical suitability" of transplantable organs) and an AD dictating removal of life-sustaining medical intervention, the investigative, life-extending measures should proceed. This provision has been decried as an intolerable interference with a patient's or patient representative's control over end-of-life medical intervention.[53]

I wrote the book on ADs, and I do not see the revised UAGA as a threat to patient autonomy.[54] The UAGA's supposed violations of an AD or other expressions of a moribund patient's preferences just don't seem very daunting in the context of maximizing successful organ transplants. My lack of alarm is attributable to several elements. First, the typical AD states in somewhat opaque terms that medical intervention should be foregone when it "only" serves to prolong the dying process.[55] That is, most AD instructions do not anticipate and are not intended to preclude temporary life extension for the purpose of successful organ transplant. Second, the disputed UAGA Sections 14 and 21 support continued medical intervention only to a limited extent. The drafters' comments to the revised UAGA suggest that any interference with normal handling of a dying patient (for example, to investigate medical suitability) will take place within "a relatively short period of time."[56] The comments also instruct an attending physician to continue mechanical intervention only if it is "not contraindicated by appropriate end-of-life care." This means that continued intervention is not authorized for a patient whose extreme suffering, discomfort, or indignity in a moribund state dictates prompt withdrawal of life support. Most importantly, revised Section 21 authorizes continued medical maintenance only long enough to allow the attending physician to confer with the patient or the patient's representative and to determine the potential donor's likely wishes in the transplant circumstances.[57] If the patient's likely wish is determined to be prompt termination of medical intervention, that choice is to be implemented even if a viable organ is sacrificed.

Revised UAGA Section 21, then, respects the wishes expressed in an AD. A typical AD contains vague language that deserves careful consideration and interpretation. To the extent that the AD is suspended temporarily pending inquiry into what the now-incompetent patient would want done in an apparently unanticipated circumstance, that temporary disruption pales in comparison to other ways in which legislatures have imposed nonvolitional, nontherapeutic limitations on ADs. Consider the numerous state statutes that dictate that a pregnant patient's AD should be overridden or those statutes that preclude removal of artificial nutrition and hydration (ANH) unless the AD explicitly mentions ANH among the medical measures to be foregone.

A different hazard to the preferences and well-being of a potential organ provider is presented in the revised UAGA. That model legislation authorizes the use of machinery to oxygenate (perfuse) salvageable organs even after the provider has died. The object is to preserve an organ pending investigation of medical suitability (and presumably to permit efforts to secure transplant consent).[58] The machinery performing artificial extracorporeal blood reoxygenation and recirculation after cardiac arrest is called ECMO.

ECMO intervention makes organ harvesting possible even after unscheduled or unanticipated cardiac arrest. This possibility is important when a moribund scheduled donor has "premature" cardiac arrest or when a recent trauma victim has died by cardiac criteria either at or on the way to a hospital. When a potential donor's death is unexpected, as in the case of a trauma victim, heart/lung machinery was not in place to keep blood flowing through the body. Without such machinery in place, the absence of oxygenated blood flow will quickly harm transplantable organs. ECMO machinery perfuses organs until donor suitability is investigated, consent to transplant obtained, and organ recovery procedures undertaken.[59]

Where ECMO interventions occur after DCD death, questions arise as to whether maintenance of corpses tethered to possibly unwanted machinery is ethically and legally sustainable. If ECMO machine maintenance following cardiac death occurs in the context of a planned and agreed-upon disconnection of life support, the relevant donor (either the patient or a representative) has either explicitly or implicitly consented to having machinery in place in order to accomplish the tasks incidental to organ transplant. In the context of cardiac death without previous consent to organ harvest, ECMO maintenance to preserve the possibility of organ transplantation is more problematic. In effect, the revised UAGA allows physicians to presume that a person would consent to having his or her cadaveric organs mechanically perfused while consent to transplant is sought from the next of kin and the transplant process is arranged (once consent is obtained). Commentators tend to favor this result, pointing out that ECMO intervention assures the family the option of donating a vital organ.[60]

Keeping a cadaver temporarily connected to obtrusive machinery does not seem to violate intrinsic postmortem human dignity. Keep in mind that these mechanical intrusions are maintained only temporarily pending resolution of consent to organ transplant and performance of the transplant when appropriate. A mechanical limbo just as intrusive as ECMO occurs regularly in the context of DBD—donation following pronouncement of death by whole-brain criteria. In that instance, the dead donor (as measured by whole-brain criteria) is kept connected to heart/lung machinery that maintains blood and oxygen flow until the transplant surgery can be set up and performed.[61]

Temporary ECMO is a mild imposition on dignity compared to state laws precluding disconnection of life support machinery in the absence of prior explicit consent from a now-incompetent patient. Such an approach to end-of-life care, which exists in a few states, offends human dignity by precluding withdrawal of life support no matter how degraded the patient's condition is. If long-term maintenance of a totally insentient human (to take one example) does not breach intrinsic human dignity, then short-term perfusion of a DCD corpse also does not.

Could a corpse be held indefinitely in a tethered ECMO limbo? Willard Gaylin once envisioned a corps of neomorts being sustained in mechanical suspension as suppliers of body parts for living persons. Current standards of postmortem dignity would not permit such exploitation of a cadaver. Even permanent unconsciousness—such as a permanent vegetative state—is alien and distasteful to the vast majority of people contemplating their own demise. An extended, indefinite period of ECMO mechanical perfusion of a corpse's salvageable organs may constitute an intolerable indignity for a dead human even though it was undertaken for the worthy purpose of aiding another human being. On the other hand, perhaps our instinctive revulsion at the concept of protracted postmortem limbo as a supplier of body parts will change if people give fully informed consent to this mode of tissue retrieval. American culture tolerates and even welcomes a variety of postmortem cadaveric mutilations grounded on informed consent. I am referring to the dissection of cadavers for medical education, an autopsy's invasive slicing and dicing of a cadaver in the interests of medical and forensic science, and the bodily mutilation of human remains via plastination for educational display. These legitimate modes of disposition of a corpse—modes not deemed to violate intrinsic human dignity—are arguably no more distasteful than prolonged mechanical perfusion of critically needed body parts.

## Buying Organs for Transplant

Another plausible approach to increasing the supply of cadaveric organs for transplant would be to provide financial incentives. As early as 1885, a Baltimore physician, Francis King Carey, recommended giving financial rewards to a deceased's estate (for having donated the deceased's corpse to be dissected in the interests of medical science).[62]

American law unequivocally prohibits the sale of organs for transplant. A federal law passed in 1984, the National Organ Transplantation Act (NOTA), makes it a crime to transfer, for transplantation purposes, any human organ (except regenerative tissues like blood and sperm) for "valuable consideration."[63] The UAGA since 1987 has also prohibited the sale of body parts for transplantation or therapy.[64] The revised 2006 UAGA continues to use the term "valuable consideration" and makes it clear that the UAGA's ban on organ sales is still "consistent and in accord with" NOTA.

The prohibition on the sale of transplant organs is based on several perceived problems. One is undignified "commodification" of the human body.[65] Making body parts marketable is supposedly a demeaning objectification of humans in a way reminiscent of the sale of slaves. Then Senator Al Gore admonished in 1983: "People [or their parts] should not be regarded as things to be bought and sold like parts of an automobile."[66] Ethicist Leon Kass also sees the sale of a body part as an intrinsic human debasement. He asserts that "if we come to think about ourselves as pork bellies, pork bellies we will become."[67]

An associated moral concern is that economic incentives to surrender organs will disproportionately exploit poor persons (in the case of live donors) and poor families (in the case of dead donors).[68] The exploitation claim is based on a vision of poor, uninformed people being impelled by economic exigency to sacrifice their body parts for the benefit of affluent others.[69] There already exists an international market (or black market) in which affluent people seeking organ transplants travel to India or China to buy kidneys from impoverished residents.[70] Most of this transplant tourism involves live organ suppliers. The trade in China, though, has extended to dead suppliers as well. Chinese law allowed procurement of organs from executed prisoners. While such organ harvesting was supposedly limited to unclaimed corpses or to situations where the next of kin had consented, thousands of executions were and are carried out in China without notification to families. The executed prisoners' organs were simply harvested and sold.[71] Chinese law was purportedly changed, as of 2004, to ban the sale of human organs, but the impact of this law on executed prisoners is still unclear.[72]

These predictions about the negative consequences of financial incentives are largely speculative, particularly as applied to organs obtained from cadavers rather than live providers.[73] The notion of intrinsic debasement of humans via commodification is particularly shaky. The commodification card can be played too often. Voluntary autopsies were once opposed on the ground that the human body was being objectified and degraded in being used as a study tool to benefit surviving humans. In addition, in the early nineteenth century, the marketing of life insurance was opposed as "merchandising in human life" and as inappropriately measuring life in financial terms.[74] In short, now-accepted practices, including some constructive arrangements involving monetary exchange, were initially greeted with an outcry of commodification or objectification.

A certain moral incoherence is reflected in the squelching of financial incentives for procurement of lifesaving organs in light of existing practices affecting human tissue. Robust markets in a few body products already exist, and some are even applicable to live suppliers. Sales of regenerative tissues such as blood, sperm, and ova are allowed. For example, graduate students receive thousands of dollars for supplying eggs to infertile women for reproduction purposes or to scientists for stem cell research.[75] While some objections are made to the ova sales based on their commodification tendency and their exploitation of economically vulnerable young women, the only convincing objection is to the inadequate information given to potential egg donors about the discomforts and hazards accompanying egg harvesting.[76] The well-grounded objection about the lack of informed consent in ova sales can be met without eliminating the market.

In the context of cadaver tissue, objections about commodification also ring hollow. Despite the ostensible bans on the sale of organs and tissue for transplant, "rapidly growing and increasingly lucrative secondary markets in human tissues" already operate.[77] There is a multibillion-dollar industry, including at least two thousand companies, involved in the procurement, processing, and delivery of transplantable body parts such as bone, ligaments, tendons, skin, and corneas.[78] In addition, there is a secondary market for whole cadavers, brains, hands, and feet to be used for research and health education purposes.[79]

How, you ask, can secondary market participants make much money if NOTA (the 1984 federal statute) and the UAGA (as adopted in state legislation) prohibit the sale of human organs and tissue for transplantation? The answer is that the bans on "valuable consideration" under NOTA and the UAGA still permit "reasonable payments" associated with transplantation support services—the processing, preservation, storage, and testing of tissue.[80] The permitted reasonable payments, in turn, include not just the return of costs, but also "normal profits."[81] Major tissue processors may well be earning inflated profits by exploiting both patents for tissue preparation techniques (e.g., cryopreservation or novel sterilization machines) and brand recognition by loyal medical customers (e.g., medical transplant centers) who are willing to pay a premium.[82] Secondary tissue market participants can also hide some profits by inflating their costs.[83] Excess profits are likely being reaped by some tissue processors and intermediaries.[84] No federal or state agency closely monitors the tissue industry in order to enforce the limits on sales contained in NOTA and the UAGA (as adopted in all states).

The opportunity to earn money by obtaining and selling cadaveric tissue has led to some unsavory and even criminal practices under the current statutory schemes. Because some cadaveric tissue is salvageable for days following death, consent for donation is sometimes obtained in funeral homes, crematories, and morgues. In those contexts, body parts have sometimes been harvested without consent and sold without appropriate safety steps to protect the ultimate recipients. (Details are provided in the section of chapter 10 called "Modern Body Parts Snatching.") Screening failures and false medical histories have resulted in serious illness and infection in some tissue recipients. Yet Food and Drug Administration (FDA) inspections of 153 tissue recovery firms in 2006–2007 found "no major deficiencies."[85]

Abuses in the secondary tissue market do not disqualify the use of financial incentives to increase the supply of cadaveric organs for transplant. Note that the secondary tissue market does not affect procurement of major organs—such as kidneys, lungs, or livers—that are harvested and transplanted immediately upon death to waiting recipients under the auspices of OPOs operating strictly on a nonprofit basis.[86] Note also that the secondary market does not involve the impact of money on the donor/suppliers (decedents and families) of cadaveric organs. Instead intermediaries such as tissue processors and brokers maneuver to reap the financial benefits of sales to ultimate transplant recipients who are willing to pay big bucks for tissue. Financial incentives to a decedent donor's estate or family for solid organs that are transplantable directly to a patient recipient would not implicate the profit-making entities that now benefit most from tissue processing services.

The growing gap between the demand for and supply of lifesaving kidneys, livers, lungs, and hearts is producing increasing calls for pilot projects using economic incentives to obtain organs.[87] The Pennsylvania legislature in 1994 offered to pay the burial or cremation expenses of organ providers but never implemented the system out of fear of violating federal law. In 2009 Senator Arlen Specter suggested the use of federal tax incentives for cadaveric suppliers. Another notion is a "futures market" in which potential organ sources prospectively agree to organ harvest from their cadavers in return for future payment to their designated beneficiaries.[88] Such proposals for economic incentives include a provision to ensure that the organs secured are distributed according to equitable criteria without reference to a recipient's wealth. They also provide for full and careful disclosure of all relevant facts to the affected parties.

There are reasons to be wary of economic incentives for providing transplant organs. An important question is whether financial incentives directly to the donors or to their families would indeed increase the availability of cadaveric organs and tissue.[89] Opponents of payment for organs fear that current rates of voluntary organ donation will drop as organ procurement becomes viewed as a matter of economic exchange rather than altruism.[90]

Pilot projects should certainly be initiated in the United States to test the consequences of economic incentives. The corrupting effects of such incentives may not materialize in the context of cadaveric organ transplant. On the other hand, economic incentives are also unlikely to eliminate organ supply shortages.

## Routine Retrieval of Cadaveric Organs

The practical need to increase the number of cadaveric organs for transplant is glaring. In terms of the certainty of increase of such organs, nothing could be better than routine posthumous recovery of medically suitable organs. By making every fresh cadaver a potential provider of organs and tissue, this system would maximize the material available for transplant and eliminate any cloud of social discrimination in sources of tissue supply. Every dying patient with salvageable organs would be eligible. Systems of routine organ recovery have been proposed.[91]

Is there a satisfactory moral justification for a legal framework employing routine retrieval despite potential mutilation and disturbance to the quiet repose of a human cadaver?[92] Current social values of autonomy and altruism provide a moral foundation for the current system's reliance on actual consent to organ retrieval. Some commentators insist that the only moral basis on which to seize a cadaver organ is explicit prior consent by the now-deceased person.[93] Yet it is by no means clear that actual consent by a donor should be the exclusive moral basis for organ harvesting.

A communitarian rationale for nonconsented organ harvesting would be that a now-dead citizen owes some return to the community that had previously benefited him or her.[94] Every living person gets some unpaid benefit from his or her community—even if it is in the form of subsidized garbage pickup, an uninterrupted water supply, or roads and bridges built by previous generations of taxpayers and now being used. Past benefit to citizens is presumably the basis for estate taxes traditionally imposed on decedents. The federal government formerly collected 55 percent of any decedent's estate, and both federal and some state governments will probably continue to extract enough estate taxes to take a healthy metaphorical bite out of cadavers. Some supporters of systematic organ retrieval likewise invoke the notion that cadaveric organs should be treated like a social resource for the community's benefit.[95] In short, a return-of-benefit rationale provides a possible moral base for utilizing human remains.

Note the extent to which states have already "expropriated" tissue from cadavers in order to benefit the health needs of living persons. Despite the pretense that American organ retrieval depends entirely on voluntary donation, some states have allowed limited forms of organ harvesting without consent. Every state has, since 1968, adopted some version of the UAGA (a recommended but not mandatory basis for state legislation). And the UAGA has, in all of its incarnations, authorized some mode of nonvoluntary organ retrieval.

In its 1968 version the UAGA contained a provision establishing, in descending order, the people authorized to donate a cadaver organ when the decedent had failed to make his or her wishes known. This statutory ladder of surrogate decision makers started with a spouse and ended with a broad provision giving authority for organ donation to "any other person authorized or under obligation to dispose of the body." That authority to make a cadaveric organ donation applied if no one higher on the statutory list was available to make a decision and so long as the now statutorily authorized person was not aware of any opposition to donation by someone higher on the decision-making ladder. The nonavailability of higher-ranked deciders could be determined with attention to the time constraints applicable in organ harvesting. This 1968 UAGA provision was apparently intended to give government medical examiners doing forensic autopsies discretion to harvest organs in the absence of known opposition and without assiduous effort to locate responsible family members. Such a provision still exists in a few states. It is not clear, though, to what extent this provision is in fact being utilized by medical examiners as a basis for organ harvesting in the absence of consent by the decedent or the next of kin.

In 1987 the UAGA was amended in its relevant part. The above sweeping provision was omitted. In its place, a new section explicitly authorized a medical examiner in lawful possession of a cadaver to release a body part for transplantation so long as need was expressed by an organ procurement agency, no known decedent opposition to transplantation existed, and the examiner had made a "reasonable effort"—taking into account the time constraints surrounding transplant of the relevant organ—to inform the next of kin of their option to object to transplantation. Twenty-eight states adopted the 1987 version of the UAGA, and approximately fifteen of those states incorporated this provision relating to medical examiners.[96] The Texas version allowed the coroner to harvest any "nonvisceral" organ after four hours of effort to contact the next of kin. Louisiana legislation ostensibly permitted the coroner to act without making any reasonable efforts to locate a family decision maker. Again, approximately fifteen states adopting the 1987 UAGA made organ harvesting possible without explicit consent when a cadaver was in the custody of a medical examiner. Approximately nine of them actually implemented that organ harvest prerogative.[97]

The 2006 version of the UAGA—adopted in some form by more than 40 states to date—purports to revoke the authority of medical examiners or coroners to remove tissue without explicit consent from an authorized source. (This unfortunate step by the UAGA drafters was based on the erroneous assumption, discussed below, that a medical examiner's unconsented retrieval of transplant tissue would constitute an unconstitutional violation of survivors' "property" interests.) Section 22(b) of the 2006 UAGA ostensibly prevents removal of any body part by a coroner "unless [the part is the] subject of an anatomical gift." Yet it is clear that this provision will not entirely preclude unconsented removal of tissue even in states adopting the 2006 UAGA.

State legislatures adopt the UAGA with various alterations. Some states may omit the Section 22 language ostensibly barring tissue harvest absent explicit consent from a decedent or next of kin. Some states may even retain language in their version of the UAGA authorizing medical examiners to retrieve transplant tissue in the context of forensic autopsies (after a reasonable effort to inform next of kin).[98] In a few states adopting the 2006 UAGA, Section 22 will have to be reconciled with existing statutory provisions explicitly authorizing medical examiners in the context of statutorily permitted forensic autopsies to harvest corneas and/or pituitary glands where the examiner, after a reasonable effort to contact next of kin, has no knowledge of objections to such tissue removal.[99] Some states may, as Georgia has done, repeal their separate statutory provisions relating to cornea retrieval; others will leave such provisions in effect.[100]

Even in states without separate provisions relating to medical examiners' jurisdiction over corneas, there is room to interpret revised UAGA Section 22 as not precluding all nonvoluntary tissue harvest for transplant. The drafters' comments on the 2006 version of the UAGA concede that even under the new Section 22(b) some unconsented tissue harvests may continue. Those comments point out that the newest hierarchy of people authorized to consent to tissue removal includes, at the end of the list in new Section 9(10), "any other person having the authority to dispose of the decedent's body."[101] Thus, the 2006 version of the UAGA leaves room for interpreting Section 9(10) as authorizing medical examiners to make "an anatomical gift," as required for an organ harvest under Section 22(b). Where a medical examiner is authorized to dispose of a corpse—as when a forensic autopsy is performed and no one claims the body—medical examiners might still permit the harvesting of tissue or organs. The drafters' comments assume that tissue (but not solid organs) will be harvested in this manner, probably on the theory that by the time the corpse is officially unclaimed, the solid organs will no longer be salvageable.[102]

All of these variables in state statutes governing organ and tissue removal indicate that some medical examiners will—in limited circumstances—continue to be authorized to remove cadaver tissue without the consent of either the decedent or the family. In other words, confiscation of tissue for transplantation will continue to occur in some states in the context of forensic autopsies. Unconsented harvesting of cadaveric tissue necessitates consideration of whether such government conduct is constitutional.

## Constitutionality of Government Expropriation of Cadaver Tissue for Transplant

Constitutional challenges to unconsented tissue harvesting can be based on the Fourteenth Amendment's restrictions on government's taking of "property" (cadaver parts supposedly belonging to the next of kin) or on government interference with "liberty" (of the next of kin normally entitled to determine a relative's postmortem disposition).[103] These challenges apply to any statutory proposal for routine retrieval of organs without prior explicit consent. The challenges also apply to state authorization of organ recovery, usually involving corneas, at forensic autopsy (especially when the relevant pathologist is not required to make a reasonable effort to notify the decedent's family about the pending surgical action). Yet even aggressive forms of unconsented retrieval of organs seem, upon analysis, to withstand constitutional challenge.

One constitutional claim by the next of kin is that their Fourteenth Amendment property interest in their loved one's cadaver and its parts has been infringed. While the issue of whether a corpse is property for constitutional purposes is still unresolved, some legal precedent already exists. A 1991 federal circuit court of appeals decision—called *Brotherton*—concluded that an Ohio coroner's statutorily authorized removal of a corpse's corneal tissue without notice to the next of kin violated the constitutional property rights of the next of kin without due process of law.[104] The drafters of the 2006 version of the UAGA were well aware of the *Brotherton* case. In explaining why the 2006 version did not continue the 1987 UAGA provision allowing organ harvesting after a reasonable effort to contact the next of kin, who might object, the drafters' comments simply cited *Brotherton*. A few cases agree with *Brotherton* that a cadaver part constitutes property for purposes of the Fourteenth Amendment, but there is significant judicial precedent in disagreement.

In my estimation as a constitutional law professor for thirty-five years, it was extremely rash of the drafters of the 2006 UAGA to rely on *Brotherton*. The arguments against deeming a cadaver part to be constitutionally protected property are strong. States have traditionally refrained from deeming cadavers to be property. (Recall the description in chapter 3 of how the ancient common law refused to label a corpse as property in light of the jurisdiction of ecclesiastical courts.) Moreover, the reasons for states' refusal to deem bodies and body parts to be property are understandable and defensible. Denying property status can have collateral benefits within a state legal system. For example, a decedent (while still alive) might more easily change an instruction for final disposition of his or her cadaver if it is not deemed property controlled by estate laws demanding a written will. Once upon a time, the legal position that a corpse is not property also helped to prevent creditors from holding debtors' corpses hostage until the survivors paid off their debts and also helped to prevent grave robbers from receiving excessively long sentences for stealing property.[105] A state can protect against abuse to the dignity and well-being of a corpse without calling it property. Under state tort law, damages for mental anguish can be obtained by next of kin offended by outrageous conduct toward a loved one's cadaver.

Federal constitutional jurisprudence looks to a state's practice and tradition for guidance in deciding what interests qualify as property interests for purposes of the Fourteenth Amendment. Given that a state has this leeway to define the bounds of property, it would be strange to overturn a state legislature's determination that a corpse's corneas are not strictly property.

Even if a corpse's body parts were deemed to be property for constitutional purposes, the typical state statute providing for unconsented harvesting of corneas (and/or other tissue) might still be upheld. The typical provision requiring a reasonable effort to locate objecting next of kin might satisfy procedural due process. Even if a constitutional violation of procedural due process were found, the legal relief for this violation might be sharply limited. The most to which the next of kin would be entitled for an unconstitutional taking of property would be monetary compensation rather than damages for emotional distress. Monetary compensation for a cornea, pituitary gland, or patch of skin might be modest indeed. A 1999 case restricted the damages available to the next of kin protesting a coroner's unconsented removal of corneas.[106] The monetary award was for "nominal" damages—that is, a token amount not worth suing for. Beyond nominal damages, the market value of a corpse's corneas (as a possible measure of damages) would still be modest. Even a corpse's foot would only bring between $200 and $400 in the secondary market for research material.[107]

A different constitutional challenge can be made to a state's harvesting of a corpse's body parts for transplant without having obtained explicit consent. The question becomes whether such government measures deprive the next of kin of their protected liberty under the Fourteenth Amendment. That is, is it constitutional for government to interfere—by unconsented confiscation of a deceased's organs—with the traditional prerogative of the next of kin to receive and dispose of a cadaver with all of its parts still in place?[108]

To resolve a Fourteenth Amendment liberty challenge, a threshold question is whether the next of kin's prerogative to determine the fate of a decedent's organs is "fundamental." Under prevailing constitutional jurisprudence, a liberty interest has a higher level of judicial protection against government interference if it is deemed to be a fundamental liberty interest. (If liberty to dispose of a corpse's parts is not fundamental, government need only have a legitimate—as opposed to a compelling—

justification for its impingement on the family's choice.) A determination about fundamentality depends on judicial assessment of a particular liberty interest's fundamentality according to the "traditions and collective conscience" of the people.

The Supreme Court's application of that fundamentality test has been rather uneven. The Court did determine in 1973 that a woman's interest in terminating a pregnancy is a fundamental liberty.[109] A woman's bodily integrity and liberty to procreate (or not) were critical elements supporting the finding of fundamentality. Yet the Supreme Court has ruled against fundamentality with regard to a person's choice of nonrelated living companions and with regard to a terminally ill person's claim for assistance in dying. Liberty interests deemed to be fundamental to date have been limited to certain intimate and personal choices relating to marriage, procreation, choice of sexual partners, family living arrangements, and child rearing.[110] None of these precedents bodes well for judicially attributing fundamental status to a family's control over a cadaver's tissue.

Family control of a corpse's body parts might not qualify as a fundamental aspect of Fourteenth Amendment liberty. True, a venerable American tradition (as codified in the UAGA) gives deference to a family's decision about the disposition of a corpse's body parts, as well as according respect to a corpse as a special entity not generally subject to exploitation even for salutary purposes.[111] Nonetheless it is quite possible, if not probable, that the Supreme Court would refuse to deem the family's interest in the disposition of a cadaver's body parts to be fundamental.

Keep in mind that family control of a cadaver has traditionally been qualified by a variety of government interferences. First is the limitation on the means of disposal of a corpse. Considerations of public health and decency customarily confine the places and ways in which the next of kin can dispose of human remains. Government agents (medical examiners) have long been allowed (for reasons of public inquiry into causes of death) to perform on cadavers the massive bodily incursion of an autopsy—even in the face of family opposition. Since the advent of organ transplantation in the 1950s, some states have authorized significant intrusions on the control of a corpse and its body parts. A number of states authorized removal of corneas or other transplant tissue during a forensic autopsy—either with or without a reasonable effort to locate next-of-kin objectors—for purposes of helping others.

The Supreme Court might ultimately conclude that the government interests behind retrieval of cadaveric tissue for transplant—saving or greatly improving lives—sufficiently justify the impingement of family liberty to withstand a Fourteenth Amendment challenge. The gains to public health from tissue transplants surely qualify as significant government interests. Several courts have already recognized that the assistance to seriously limited lives provided by transplanted corneal tissue qualifies as a strong government interest.[112] Cases upholding the confiscation of corneal tissue have found that such confiscation has restored sight to tens of thousands of blind people over the years.[113] These courts have ruled that reliance on voluntary donation of corneal tissue was inadequate both because most corneal tissue was donated by older decedents and because many families could not be contacted for purposes of consent during the limited hours when corneal tissue was still usable.[114] Those courts have also pointed out that at least in the context of an autopsy, removal of a cornea is "an infinitesimally small intrusion."[115] At least in the context of statutes related to cadavers under the jurisdiction of medical examiners, alleviating serious incapacity can constitute a strong government justification for permitting cadaveric tissue recovery without consent from the patient or a representative. That justification might even qualify as a compelling government interest (in the event that a family interest in controlling a corpse's fate is deemed to be a fundamental aspect of liberty).

What about the constitutionality of "routine retrieval"—harvesting of salvageable organs from every healthy cadaver whether in the jurisdiction of a medical examiner or not? As to solid organs for transplant, a government interest in preserving human lives—those of the thousands who die each year waiting for organ donation—offers a strong justification for systematic government recovery of cadaver organs. Preservation of life has been deemed to be a strong public interest in many medico/legal settings. For example, in 1990 the U.S. Supreme Court upheld Missouri's insistence that a permanently unconscious patient had to be maintained on life support absent some prior expression by the patient rejecting such life support.[116] That case upheld state interference with the traditional prerogative of the next of kin to determine the end-of-life medical handling of relatives, even though this state interference would leave the permanently insensate patient in a highly undignified status and impose continued burdens on the next of kin. This interference with customary family control over end-of-life decisions was upheld in the interest of preserving human life. The interest in preserving human life also prevailed in the 1987 Supreme Court cases rejecting challenges to state statutes prohibiting assistance with suicide. In short, any organ recovery program aimed at salvaging lifesaving cadaver organs is at least supported by a compelling government interest.

My conclusion, then, is that statutory programs permitting recovery of transplant tissue during the course of an autopsy—so long as the pathologist is not aware of contrary wishes from the patient or family— are easily sustainable on constitutional grounds. (I am not referring to whether these programs are politically viable.) A further statutory program for systematic retrieval of organs would be supported by a compelling government interest, but it would ride roughshod over the customary prerogative of decedents and/or their families to maintain the integrity of a human cadaver. The constitutional fate of systematic organ retrieval is therefore uncertain (and its political fate dismal). However, there is no need to adopt such an extreme measure when a better solution to organ shortages is readily at hand.

## A No-Brainer: Presumed Consent to Be a Tissue Supplier

The severe shortage of cadaveric transplant organs must be corrected. If you think that financial incentives would be too crass or corrupting or insufficient by themselves to end the shortfall, and if you recoil from systematically retrieving transplant tissue from all neomorts, how about a system that allows organ harvesting from the corpse of every citizen unless that citizen or an agent has previously recorded opposition? The basic proposition is that every adult citizen should be deemed to be a willing cadaveric tissue supplier unless, prior to death, the citizen or an authorized representative has given notice of a contrary preference. A presumed consent regime (hereinafter ironically called PC even though it is anything but politically correct) has been endorsed by some quite respectable sources, such as the AMA's Council on Educational and Judicial Affairs.[117] PC is the existing system in several European countries and is credited by some commentators with significantly increasing there the supply of organs for transplant.[118] (Other commentators dispute whether the European experience is really successful.[119])

The attractions of a PC system of organ retrieval are considerable. A main one is that the system allows autonomy—personal choice over the fate of human organs—to continue to prevail. Any reasonable PC system would provide wide publicity to educate the public about the possible removal and transplant of cadaver tissue and would create an easy and efficient system for people to opt out.[120] Among the well-publicized, easy means for people to record objections would be a check mark on a driver's license, or on a tax return, or on any application for government benefits.[121] As long as a PC framework provides such ample means for a person or his or her representative to opt out of providing cadaveric transplant tissue, the approach does not constitute forced government confiscation of organs. That fact undermines any constitutional claim about government expropriation of property or deprivation of liberty to control a cadaver's fate. Envision a government scheme in which your home will become government property upon your death unless, before you die, you register an objection. In other words, your home will remain your home so long as you opt out of an imposed future change in ownership by following a well-publicized, easily accessible, unburdensome objection route. Not so daunting! You want your tissue to remain in your cadaver despite the existence of a PC system? Just opt out. In the meantime, the public interest warrants retrieval of salvageable organs to benefit the multitude of needy organ recipients.

True, PC in application would not always reflect the decedent's actual preference. Some people who don't really want to become organ donors would procrastinate, fail to register their opposition, and thus have organs taken in contravention of what would have been their wishes, if articulated. This price for dereliction in failing to revoke the presumed consent—retrieval of cadaveric tissue—does not seem to be too high. The adverse impact of inertia under a presumed consent system is like the current consequence when people fail to prepare a will governing the distribution of their assets upon death. State law universally distributes the assets of people who die intestate to the next of kin in a statutorily fixed order. Some people, who are neglectful in failing to write a will, end up with their hard-earned assets distributed to despised relatives whom they had no actual wish to benefit. They could easily have avoided that consequence.

A default presumption in favor of organ availability makes sense. The fate of a corpse is often determined by what the uncommunicative decedent, if only asked, probably would have wished to be done. This rationale is similar to a "substituted judgment" approach employed by the next of kin or guardians making medical decisions on behalf of now-incompetent patients. In the context of organ retrieval, a presumption of cadaveric organ availability arguably reflects the wishes, albeit not always explicitly expressed, of a large majority of decedents. Surveys show that a distinct majority of competent adults are, in the abstract, willing to donate organs upon death to medical patients with acute needs. Even if many of these same prospective donors are averse to facing their own mortality and ultimately refrain from effectively communicating their donative wishes, the distinct majority still favor cadaveric organ donation to needy recipients. This assumption is strengthened when the decedent did not utilize a widely publicized and easily accessible opt-out option. In short, it is logical to treat a corpse's imputed preference as mirroring the preference of a distinct majority of people, especially if the decedent refrained from opting out of that majority preference.

Note, as we consider PC for organ harvesting, that for approximately a century the United States relied on a variation of presumed consent to supply medical schools with cadavers to be dissected in the course of medical education. Roughly between 1829 and 1929, states allowed access to unclaimed corpses as dissection material for medical students of anatomy. (Some of those laws are still on the books; medical schools just don't need that cadaver source as much as they previously did.) That nineteenth-century system for procuring corpses for dissection focused on the poor, the homeless, and the socially detached as cadaveric sources. A contemporary PC system would have the distinct advantage of applying to every cadaver. And the system's benefits would be immediate and material—the saving and/or improvement of innumerable human lives.

Suppose that I'm right in thinking that a PC system for harvesting cadaver organs would be efficient and constitutional. What would be the limit of any state effort to facilitate removal of cadaver tissue? Would every corpse be subject to exploitation regarding the multiplicity of body parts potentially useful to live recipients? Imagine the surviving family collecting the remains of a corpse that has been plundered of eyes, teeth, hair, patches of skin, and vital organs, as well as some bone, ligaments, veins, and arteries. How much violation of the integrity of their loved one's remains must the family tolerate? (Not everyone accepts the vision of a human cadaver as nothing more than disposable, inanimate matter destined to undergo earthly decomposition and decay.) And how long could any PC program keep cadavers on ice, so to speak? Could neo-morts be maintained indefinitely on ECMO oxygenating machinery until relieved of their supply of needed organs and tissue?

Political constraints operate in defining the palatable bounds of organ harvesting under a PC regime. Legislators must inevitably be sensitive to "the dignity of the human body in its final disposition."[122] The human cadaver, while not equivalent in status to a live human, still embodies elements of human identity cognizable by both legislatures and their constituencies.[123] Both their constituencies and the courts would remind legislators that every cadaver is entitled to intrinsic postmortem human dignity. The question becomes how intrinsic postmortem human dignity applies limits in the context of organ and tissue harvesting pursuant to a PC regime.

One element of postmortem dignity involves aesthetics: the physical appearance of a corpse. Though respect for the dead is a universal precept, the physical sanctity of a corpse is not absolute. A corpse may be subjected to a variety of physical alterations without breaching its intrinsic human dignity. Embalming, cremation, dissection, and autopsy are all potentially compatible with corporeal dignity. Nonetheless, any legislative body contemplating adoption of PC will be influenced by concerns about aesthetics and postmortem dignity. One golden rule in both autopsy and embalming is that the external appearance of a corpse should not be negatively impacted by postmortem procedures. This is not a difficult standard to meet. Even victims of extreme trauma (including an autopsy) can be stitched and patched and padded to present a reasonable appearance to mourners. Vital internal organs and tissue can be removed without disturbing the outward final appearance. Still, the aesthetics of disturbance to a cadaver's appearance are likely to curb legislators' exuberance in increasing organ availability via PC.

A further element of dignity is the association between certain parts of a corpse and the personal identity attributed to a corpse. People commonly associate certain body parts—such as the heart, brain, and face—with the soul or essence of the deceased person.[124] Legislators are well aware of these associations, which serve as political checks on public exploitation of body parts. When I called PC a "no-brainer" in the title of this section, I meant that the system was obviously desirable and worthy of trial. In application, though, PC might become a no-brainer in a more literal sense. As a practical matter, the smaller and more unobtrusive the body part, the greater the chance that it would be made salvageable under a PC statutory regime. In other words, the less importance people commonly ascribe to the postmortem integrity of certain body parts, the more likely those parts can be exploited. Corneas are an illustration. Tendons might be another.

People's religious beliefs also have a political impact on legislators. Some people believe, on religious or philosophical grounds, that physical remains can be restored and be useful in an afterlife. Perhaps a legislature would, as a political matter, build in a conscientious objection exemption from a PC system. That is, a PC regime would likely exempt any decedent whose religious or philosophical beliefs encompassed the critical nature of postmortem bodily integrity.

An interesting and important boundary question for a PC regime is whether postmortem family objections might, as a practical matter, prevent even statutorily authorized organ retrieval. In countries that have embraced PC, medical staffs tend to be unwilling to rely on PC in the face of objections by the surrounding family.[125] Imagine a PC arrangement in place in an American state. And imagine a scenario in which surviving family members seeking to block organ removal are claiming that the beloved decedent was decidedly opposed to being an organ provider and had simply neglected to register his objections. Or imagine that the family's recently shaped (but widely shared) religious principles oppose organ removal. It is at least possible that medical institutions' reluctance to override an objecting family would carry over to this context. In other words, the practical application of PC to organ donation might end up working the way explicit consent currently works in the United States: Objections to organ transplant by the surrounding family generally prevail even if the family is improperly violating the decedent's express (or implied) wish to donate.

What is the point of PC if the next of kin are able to veto the statutorily authorized retrieval of an organ? There would still be a couple of important benefits. One would be a psychological impact on families who would be encouraged by the statutorily expressed default position to be more receptive to organ donation. By acquiescing in organ retrieval, they would be doing "the right thing" as defined in public health legislation. The PC framework would also help inform families who are uncertain about what their deceased loved one would have wanted. A decedent's failure to opt out of PC despite an easily accessible notification system could help reassure the surrounding survivors that organ retrieval does not violate the decedent's likely preferences.

To conclude, a PC framework—at least on a pilot project level— deserves a chance to provide a solution to the current shortage of cadaveric organs. One expert opposing PC opines that it "would probably be ineffective and counterproductive in the United States."[126] He speculates that people opting out of the statutory presumption might preclude what would otherwise have been family organ donations. Maybe, maybe not. Let's find out!

All of this discussion relates to the harvesting of cadaver parts for purposes of transplantation in order to help tissue recipients. The next chapter considers the fate of a cadaver and its parts that are potentially useful for educational or experimental purposes.

> Who would not prefer . . . to be useful, even after death, to his
> survivors, rather than to fester and decay—to feed the numerous
> worms and to undergo the slow and disgusting process of
> chemical decomposition?
>
> > Report of an 1830 Massachusetts Legislative Committee,
> > as quoted in Gary Laderman, *The Sacred Remains*
>
> *Taceant colloquia. Effugiat risus.*
> *Hic Locus Est Ubi Mors Gaudet Succurrere Vitae*
> (Let talk be silenced. Let laughter be banished.
> This is the place where death delights to come to the aid of life.)
>
> > Inscription above the entrance to the New York City
> > Medical Examiner's Office

*Chapter 8*

# The Cadaver as Teacher, Research Subject, or Forensic Witness

Most people assume that death ends their period of service to fellow human beings and seek to implement their historic entitlement to quiet repose. They contemplate a final disposition that allows their remains to rest in peace. They worry only about the comparative dignity of various means of disposal, the associated costs, and the toll on surviving loved ones.

A different paradigm of final disposition abjures quiet repose in favor of postmortem service to humanity. The previous chapter notes a cadaver's opportunities to save or improve human lives by supplying critical body parts for transplantation. Further opportunities to benefit humanity exist in teaching, research, and investigation of deaths.

## Teaching Medicine by Dissection of Cadavers

The human cadaver has long been recognized as an important source of learning about human beings and their afflictions. Dissection of cadavers provided knowledge about the functioning of the human body and the causes of dysfunction. The Roman physician Galen (c. AD 250) was renowned for his work in correlating events that affected the live body with internal consequences disclosed in postmortem examination.[1] (Galen was well situated for analytic dissection due to his post as medical supervisor of the gladiatorial amphitheater.)

In Europe, medical figures in the early Renaissance continued to dissect cadavers in order to increase their knowledge about human anatomy, and they began to make dissection a part of formal education. As early as 1405 dissection was introduced into the academic curriculum at the intellectual center in Bologna.[2] In 1482 Pope Sixtus IV approved human dissection for educational purposes.[3] By the sixteenth century, dissections regularly took place in public in order to educate a variety of people about human anatomy—people aspiring to medical practice, curious citizens, and artists. Observing artists wished to sharpen their creative skills in depicting the human form. Some fairly good artists benefited from witnessing and/or performing dissections. Michelangelo Buonarroti, Leonardo da Vinci, and Tiziano Vecelli (Titian) all performed dissections—with da Vinci producing a set of thirty drawings based on such dissections.[4] Rembrandt depicted the performance of a dissection in his famous 1632 painting "Dr. Tulp's Anatomy Lesson."[5]

Public dissection permitted efficient use of the small number of cadavers available for purposes of dissection. At a public dissection, the crowd could see, hear, and smell the proceedings. The procedure took place on a raised platform where a cadaver, a learned anatomist, and one or two barbers or surgeons shared the stage. The anatomist served as director and commentator, while the surgeon(s) did the actual slicing and dicing.[6] The dissection equipment included saws, knives, scissors, drills, pipes, tubes, wires, and buckets.[7] In Italy three people participated in the dissection. A lector read the medical text, an anatomist commented on the relation between the text and the ongoing disassembly of the cadaver, and a barber or surgeon performed the manual labor on the cadaver.[8] Dissected body parts were deposited in basins or buckets for later disposition as waste.

Dissection as an educational tool also existed in the American colonies. The earliest example was a public dissection performed on a Native American executed for murder in Boston in 1734.[9] As in Europe, dissection of cadavers in America became a part of both formal and informal medical education. In the mid-eighteenth century aspiring American physicians traveled to England or elsewhere in Europe to enhance their medical knowledge. There they were exposed to the strong European belief in the importance of anatomy and dissection to any mastery of medicine or surgery. When they returned to America, these same respected physicians emphasized dissection as an integral part of the training of apprentices and of the sharpening of their own surgical skills. Personal dissecting experience became an important part of any medical career. In 1762 William Shippen Jr. began teaching anatomy classes in Philadelphia using both anatomical models and cadavers.[10] In 1767 Samuel Clossy introduced anatomy courses, including some dissections of dead slaves, at King's College (later Columbia University) in New York City.[11]

In nineteenth-century America, dissection of cadavers continued to be a useful way for people involved in medicine to learn anatomy. Though the overall standard of medical education was poor in the early nineteenth century, anatomical knowledge was viewed as a cornerstone of a sound medical education.[12] Performing and/or witnessing dissections helped students and apprentices to memorize body parts and their arrangement. Increasingly dissection became a technique for learning not just about bodily arrangement, but also about anatomical changes caused by various disease processes, about the correlations between symptoms and anatomical changes, and about surgical or medicinal correction of derangements. During the second half of the nineteenth century, numerous medical schools opened and they all deemed performance of an anatomony (dissection) to be an essential part of medical education, a prerequisite for graduation.[13] In the same period, practicing physicians and surgeons also relied on cadaver exploration to improve their skills. Knowledge of the interior structure of the human body was deemed to be integral to surgical practice.[14] The Civil War and its battlefield experiences underlined the need for enhanced surgical training and skill.

The twentieth century did not diminish the role of cadavers and dissection as a key to advancing medical knowledge and skills. Learning anatomy via dissection became (and remains in the twenty-first century) "a powerful initiation ritual that signals entry into the medical profession."[15] On the first day of medical school, medical students are assigned to their teaching material—the cadaver through which they will learn the ins and outs of human anatomy.[16] The number of students per cadaver depends on the number of available cadavers. A typical arrangement is two working pairs of students per cadaver—that is, two students to dissect either side of the cadaver.

Over the course of a semester or more, medical students probe the cadaver, beginning with the trunk and internal organs and ending with the neck, face, and head. The exercise not only teaches anatomy but also helps students to gain enough clinical detachment to overcome their initial revulsion to the dead and to the mutilation of cadavers. Students need to develop detachment because the dissection process has plenty of violent aspects. Cracking open the chest cavity and extracting and minutely examining the viscera is just the beginning. In succeeding weeks a pelvic hemisection is performed, involving splitting the genital parts, sawing through the pelvis, and pulling the legs apart from the trunk.[17] One former participant in a first-year dissection describes the disarticulation of the pelvis as "about as close to 'rending a person asunder' as we are ever likely to get."[18] As the legs are manipulated and pulled apart from the sacral vertebrae, a tearing noise is heard like that produced by the wrenching of a turkey leg from a holiday turkey. In later weeks, when the dissection process reaches the cadaver's head, the scalp must be peeled back over the face; ultimately, the brain has to be freed from the skull and severed from the connective tissue in the neck. The dismantled cadaver ultimately looks like "a shambles of muscle and bone, cut away and divided."[19] During the course of the educational exercise, dissected body parts are collected in metal pails for later disposal (usually by cremation).

Is the dissection of cadavers still a necessary way to learn anatomy?[20] Alternative ways to study anatomy include cutting into computer-controlled mannequins and "virtual" dissection on computer models. For the most part, though, these alternatives are considered inadequate substitutes for hands-on dissection and the actual confrontation with human death.[21] Systematic exposure of muscles, blood vessels, and nerves maximizes students' understanding of the human body. Also, cadavers or their parts are still necessary for the continuing education of numerous medical professionals outside of medical schools—surgeons who seek to learn new techniques, researchers, mortuary technicians, and forensic pathologists, among others. For example, any surgeon who is learning a new procedure, such as laser surgery, needs a corpse for practice. At the annual meeting of the American Academy of Orthopedic Surgeons, some seminars about new techniques feature hands-on training using parts of cadavers. Annie Cheney describes a 2003 seminar at which thirteen urological surgeons used six men's torsos to learn laparascopic nephrectomy.[22] A fledgling plastic surgeon usually starts on a cadaver's face by practicing nose jobs and face lifts before doing any makeovers on live patients.[23]

Serving as a dissection subject has never had mass appeal—even for altruistic people interested in advancing medical science. People contemplating the fate of their own cadaver did not relish the thought of having their remains publicly picked apart and unceremoniously discarded as trash. For many centuries, only the cadavers of the most socially marginalized served as the source of dissection material. During the Renaissance, the corpses of executed criminals, vagrants, or other undesirables served as the major source of dissection subjects. Vesalius, the fifteenth-century physician who wrote the first important anatomy textbook, stole the corpses of hanged criminals as one source of material.[24] Executed criminals and deceased vagrants continued to serve as major sources of dissection subjects in England for centuries.[25] In 1540 in the reign of Henry VIII, a statute permitted the barber-surgeons of London to exploit the bodies of executed felons for the betterment of "knowledge, instruction, insight, learning, and experience" in medical science.[26] In 1752 the British Parliament mandated that every executed criminal be either gibbeted or dissected.[27] However, there were too few bodies of executed criminals to meet the demands of British anatomists. By the end of the eighteenth century in Great Britain, body snatching and grave robbing by so-called resurrectionists constituted a significant source of cadavers for dissection.

American anatomists also had to cope with an acute shortage of cadavers. During the Revolutionary War, the battlefields had been strewn with unidentified and unclaimed bodies that supplied plentiful material for dissection.[28] Thereafter, American medical education's increasing emphasis on anatomy and dissection resulted in a chronic shortage of cadavers until the late nineteenth century. When the supply of cadavers of executed criminals and social castoffs did not meet American medical educational and practice demands, American physicians did just as their British counterparts had done: They turned to resurrectionists to supply cadavers. Throughout the first three-quarters of the nineteenth century, American physicians and educators depended partly on cadavers "resurrected" by body snatchers and grave robbers. (A detailed account of American resurrectionists is presented in chapter 10, which deals with body snatching in both its historical and modern settings.) The point here is the gap between the strong need for cadavers within the medical education system and the reluctance of the public to fill that need.

State legislatures in the nineteenth century gradually moved to increase the supply of legally obtained cadavers. From 1832 to about 1885 the majority of American states statutorily authorized the use of unclaimed bodies for dissection and anatomical study.[29] These nineteenth-century "anatomy laws" usually provided that a body unclaimed after twenty-four hours could be used as a subject by anatomists.[30] Because unclaimed bodies most frequently came from public institutions like poorhouses, workhouses, and hospitals, the statutes were "effectively substituting the poor for the executed."[31]

Surprisingly, unclaimed bodies today supply only a small percentage of cadavers for dissection. Ninety percent of the corpses now used in U.S. medical schools are donated.[32] The remainder are supplied under state statutes that continue to authorize the utilization of unclaimed bodies for educational purposes.[33] The transition from expropriated to donated corpses occurred over the course of the twentieth century. As medical science progressed, more and more people responded to the refrain of physicians that a corpse could make a significant contribution to science and human advancement. More and more decedents willed their remains to science. By the 1940s, voluntary bequests accounted for approximately 40 percent of medical school cadavers; that percentage rose to 70 percent by the 1970s and to 90 percent today.[34]

The transition to donated cadavers for dissection was encouraged by medical schools' concerted efforts to display greater respect and less disdain for donated cadavers. It is no secret that anatomy labs and their silent teachers had traditionally been a subject of coarse humor in medical school yearbooks—posed photos, cartoons, and crude jokes. Over time, though, medical school culture became much more respectful toward the donated cadavers in anatomy labs. Gestures of respect include keeping faces and private parts covered, collecting dismantled body pieces and holding them for appropriate respectful disposition, and conducting an annual ceremony of reflection and gratitude.[35] The accompanying message to medical students is that they should be grateful for the altruistic gift bestowed on them by each anonymous cadaver donor.

Altruism may not be the only motivation for dedicating one's cadaver to science. One person making an anatomical gift to Harvard Medical School wrote: "I couldn't make it to Harvard as a youngster, but I'm coming now."[36] That message from the donor was somewhat presumptuous, as not every applicant cadaver gets into Harvard Medical School's anatomy lab. Harvard could again have rejected this aspiring donor if his corpse had been unfit—too emaciated, too obese, too old, or too ravaged by prior surgery to furnish good material for dissection. Presumably, though, that donor's cadaver did get into Harvard.

Some controversy exists about whether donated corpses are really voluntarily donated for use in dissection. The concern is that a donor is not informed enough about the ultimate uses of the cadaver—especially the mutilation involved in dissection.[37] By the 1980s institutions were well aware that a body donation required informed consent, but solicitors of such consent were typically advised not to go into detail about the dissection process.[38] The common institutional excuse was that such detail would create unnecessary stress and anxiety. A 2001 survey of the twenty-two largest American medical schools discovered that in their cadaver donation forms only two described dissection and only seven mentioned the word "dissect."[39]

## Autopsy and Medical Knowledge

The role of a cadaver as an educator or transmitter of knowledge reaches its pinnacle in the postmortem process of autopsy. An autopsy is performed by a pathologist or another physician and is aimed primarily at determining a cause of death and adding to medical knowledge about illness. The process correlates the postmortem anatomical condition with symptoms and other attributes of disease. In the history of medicine, autopsy has contributed enormously to medical science and knowledge.

Autopsy has historical roots going back to the ancient Egyptians. Around 1500 an innovative Italian physician, Antonius Benivieni, sought to use the autopsy process to explain preceding deaths.[40] In 1605 the French explorer Samuel de Champlain ordered barber-surgeons to open and examine the corpses of sailors in an effort to trace the cause of the scurvy that had claimed many victims.[41] (The examinations did not uncover vitamin C deficiency as a cause.) While physicians during the seventeenth and eighteenth centuries had progressed in matching the pathological changes seen at autopsy with clinical symptoms, diagnostic and curative medical science remained at a primitive level. Belief in the four humors as causes of disease and death had paralyzed medical theory for centuries.[42] Giovanni Batista Morgagni, the father of clinical pathology, made a great stride by associating pathological factors rather than humors with death and disease. His 1761 book *The Seats and Causes of Diseases Investigated by Anatomy* based its theory of physiological causations on seven hundred autopsies that Morgagni had performed.[43] In Vienna in the mid-nineteenth century, Karl Rokitansky advanced the discipline of medical pathology by prescribing regularized procedures for autopsies.[44] (Rokitansky claimed that in his lifetime he performed thirty thousand autopsies—two a day, seven days a week, for forty-five years. He left behind tens of thousands of anatomical specimens.) However, it was in the twentieth century that autopsies and pathology made their greatest contributions to the advancement of medical science and public health. However, before we consider the contributions of autopsy to medical science, it may be helpful to know what an autopsy entails.

An autopsy is most frequently performed in a hospital that has its own morgue and autopsy room. A pathologist is in charge. The pathologist may be assisted by aides or lab technicians and medical records staff while performing the two- to three-hour procedure.[45] The first step is to examine the body surface for lumps, bruises, or other signs of trauma or disease.[46] A long Y-shaped incision is then made from both armpits to the bottom of the breast bone and downward to just above the genitals. After some ribs and bone are cut, the sternum and adjacent ribs are withdrawn, exposing most of the thoracic and stomach cavities.[47] Internal organs are then removed en masse, cut free, and individually weighed and examined. A technician takes specimens from each organ, as well as from major viscera and tissue, for later lab analysis. The stomach is removed and the contents are spilled onto a stainless steel tray.[48] The heart is opened to examine the valves and inner walls. Small incisions are made in the coronary arteries. A section of intestine is pulled out and sliced open to check for tumors, blockages, or other abnormalities.[49] The kidneys, urethra, bladder, and testes are removed and examined. Fluid samples are extracted from the cadaver—including urine, blood, and liquid from the gallbladder—to be analyzed for alcohol, drugs, or other chemical or biological agents.

In a full autopsy, the brain is removed and examined. This begins with an incision across the scalp, starting behind one ear and going up across the back of the head and down to the other ear.[50] The pathologist then pulls the front section of the scalp over the face and the back section over the nape of the neck. A saw is then used to open the skull. After a portion of the skull has been sawed and lifted, the exposed brain is examined. Following observation of the brain in place, the pathologist removes and further examines the brain, ultimately slicing it into sections. The pathologist fans out the sections to examine its composition, looking for signs of infection, swelling, or deterioration.[51]

Toward the end of a full autopsy, the corpse looks like Humpty Dumpty after the fall. Yet at the conclusion, organs, tissue, and bone are returned to the cavities and the incisions are loosely sutured. Small tissue samples are held for toxicological testing. Within a few hours, a funeral home can tighten and glue the sutures and perform its cosmetic tasks so that a tranquil viewing will be possible despite the pathologist's intrusive interventions.[52]

The invasiveness and disruption of autopsies seem repulsive. Important reasons must exist for such gross medical interference with the quiet repose of a corpse. A perennially important rationale is to allow government authorities to investigate the cause of death in unusual circumstances—those involving suspected crime, apparent suicide, or simply unexpected and unexplained demise. Every state authorizes a medical examiner's office to perform a forensic autopsy in such circumstances. (I focus on the subject of forensic autopsies in the section of this chapter titled "The Cadaver as Witness.")

In the absence of statutory authorization for an autopsy, the decedent (while still alive and competent), and later the next of kin, control whether an autopsy can be conducted. Why would anyone choose to subject his or her cadaver to the violence of an autopsy? Why, other than a wish to vent accumulated anger against the departed, would a next of kin consent to have a corpse subjected to the intrusive bodily explorations involved in an autopsy?

There are many good reasons for consent to an autopsy. One is the self-interest that survivors might have in clearing up uncertainty surrounding a particular death. Family members might be concerned about the possible impact of a suspected genetic or contagious element. Or certain family members might be seeking verification that a surrogate's decision making concerning the departed's end-of-life care had been well grounded. Recall the *Schiavo* case in Florida in 2006. Family members bitterly disputed the mental condition of the unconscious patient whose husband had authorized withdrawal of life support. Her husband contended that the patient was permanently unconscious, while her parents insisted that she could recover her mental function. Florida courts upheld the husband's position, allowing removal of artificial nutrition and hydration, which resulted in Ms. Schiavo's death. An autopsy verified that the patient's brain had indeed deteriorated to a point where no further consciousness was possible, so her husband's decision had been morally and legally well grounded.

Another explanation for consent to an autopsy is the suspicion of medical malpractice. Many a towel, sponge, or other detritus has been found by an autopsy following a surgical procedure in which the patient unexpectedly died. Or an autopsy can dispel the cloud of suspicion by showing that the unexpected fatality could not have been avoided.[53] Keep in mind that consenting kin can limit the scope of an autopsy. Instructions such as "heart and lungs only" or "omit the head" can limit the intrusiveness of an autopsy when only certain body parts are under investigation.

Traditionally, the most important reason for consenting to an autopsy has been altruism—a desire to advance medical science. The cumulative impact of millions of autopsies has been an enormous boost to medical science and public health. Autopsies have been critical in identifying the presence, nature, and progression of numerous maladies, often leading to successful treatment.[54] For example, peritonitis was a mysterious, often fatal condition in the late nineteenth century. Around 1885, after having conducted 257 autopsies, pathologist Reginald Fitz identified the appendix as the source of infection and advised that early surgery was essential.[55] A staggering number of lives have been saved by that discovery alone. Of course, autopsies have not always produced beneficial results. Over the course of the nineteenth century, pathologists sometimes became a source of contagion rather than a curb to its spread. Physicians at that time performed autopsies without gloves. Afterward they moved freely about the hospital, transmitting infections from the dead to the living.[56] Pathologists also contracted tuberculosis from cadavers well into the twentieth century.

Over the course of the twentieth century, autopsies were key to identifying many potentially fatal afflictions (such as heart attacks and various pulmonary diseases). Between 1950 and 1988 alone, autopsies accounted for the discovery and investigation of eighty-nine diseases.[57] More recently, autopsies were integral to the identification of causative elements of asbestosis, toxic shock syndrome, Legionnaire's disease, West Nile virus, Ebola virus, and AIDS.[58]

The link between autopsy and public health is expressed in many additional ways. Autopsies assist epidemiologists by identifying disease patterns and providing vital mortality statistics.[59] Epidemiological data then help to identify and track health hazards of environmental, occupational (e.g., asbestos), or medicinal (e.g., Vioxx) origins. Autopsies provide crucial information in the assessment of treatment modalities.[60] In the case of cancer, autopsy examination of the impact of radiation therapy and chemotherapy in varying doses has greatly facilitated treatment advances. In the study of infectious diseases, the efficacy of various forms of antibiotics has been determined in part by the results of autopsy. The effectiveness of various new surgical techniques is determined in part by autopsy. This was certainly true with regard to advances in laparoscopic surgery, implantation of medical devices, and repair of aneurysms. Toxicological results from autopsy show whether medications have been overdosed or underdosed or have caused unexpected reactions.[61]

At one time autopsy also served as an important quality control over hospital practice. As a percentage of hospital deaths occurred without initial identification of the cause, autopsies helped to identify disease and comorbidity patterns within health care institutions. By associating causes of death with institutional conditions, hospitals received warning clues about problematic conditions such as sanitary lapses, faulty procedures, or weak personnel.[62] Autopsies were useful in quality control by detecting iatrogenic injuries such as those stemming from improper in-tubations—including those involving catheter, nasogastric, and endotra-cheal tubes.[63] (Until 1971 the Joint Commission on Accreditation of Hospitals [JCAH] demanded that hospitals perform an autopsy on at least 20 percent of their fatalities.) During the first three-quarters of the twentieth century, autopsies therefore became a focal point for weekly morbidity and mortality review conferences.[64]

An autopsy was, and still can be, a highly useful test of the accuracy of medical diagnoses.[65] In 1912 Richard C. Cabot presented an analysis of three thousand autopsies at Massachusetts General Hospital, reveal-ing a shocking percentage of diagnostic inaccuracies—approximately 40 percent.[66] The Cabot study helped confirm inadequacies in medical edu-cation, as described by Abraham Flexner, and therefore helped lead to standardization of an improved medical school curriculum. However, standardization of the curriculum did not fully solve the problem of di-agnostic inaccuracy. Additional studies in the 1980s and 1990s still showed significant continuing discrepancies between clinical diagnoses and findings upon death. One review of one thousand autopsies between 1983 and 1988 found major discrepancies in 32 percent of cases.[67] A Con-necticut research study in 1985 found that the cause of death was as-sessed inaccurately in 29 percent of cases. In another 26 percent of cases, the same study found that the diagnosis correctly identified the major disease category that afflicted the patient but not the elements that caused death.[68] Also in the 1980s, postmortem analysis of brain tissue disclosed an incorrect diagnosis of Alzheimer's disease, as opposed to other metabolic or degenerative disorders, in approximately 25 percent of cases.[69] A 1993–1994 study showed that in over a third of autopsies pathologists found a major, clinically unidentified element that had con-tributed to the decedent's demise.[70]

Just as autopsy became central to the investigation and discovery of causes of disease in the early twentieth century, it also became an inte-gral part of medical education. The early-twentieth-century reforms of medical education placed both pathology and autopsy in positions of importance. The medical school curriculum included a one-year course in pathology using diseased organs removed at autopsy as teaching tools.[71] In addition, students were taught how to perform autopsies. That training was accomplished in part by participation in or exposure to actual autopsies. The pathology rotation in the fourth year of medical school included daily attendance at an autopsy.[72] Into the 1980s participation in an autopsy was still a rite of passage for all medical students. The correlation between diseased tissue and symptoms could have been learned by reading a textbook rather than by performing an actual autopsy, "but how much more meaningful and memorable the experience [is] when one can see, feel, and study the real thing."[73] This real-life exposure to a corpse, together with dissection, were also considered useful in helping students to develop empathy with and respect for human remains and to process thoughts about the meaning of death.

During the first half of the twentieth century, rates of autopsy rose as the role of autopsies in medical education increased. That upward trajectory continued until approximately 1960. The autopsy rates in Chicago hospitals increased from 10 percent in 1919, to 20 percent in the 1930s, to 49 percent in the 1950s. At New York City's Mount Sinai Hospital, the autopsy rate rose from 20 percent in 1920 to 55 percent in 1955.[74] Teaching hospitals' rates rose even higher—to 80 percent by the late 1950s. (As teaching hospitals tended to be located in urban centers, often servicing low-income populations, African Americans comprised a disproportionate share of the autopsied population—approximately 50 percent higher than the rate of white autopsies in Philadelphia and Baltimore.[75]) Apparently physicians in the 1950s were able to convince approximately one-half of mourning families to allow autopsies to be performed on their loved ones. The central theme was an appeal to altruism, and it is doubtful that solicitors spent a lot of time describing the gory aspects of the procedure.

In theory, authorization to perform an autopsy limited the pathologist's conduct to the bounds of a standard autopsy. This meant examination of body parts followed by their return to the cadaver (except for tissue samples). Organ removal and retention beyond the standard autopsy protocol, even with no malevolence or disrespect intended, constituted at common law a wrongful mutilation, making the pathologist liable to the consenting family.[76] Abuses of authority clearly did sometimes occur. In 1958 a thirty-eight-year-old lab worker at a federal installation died from a lethal dose of radiation. His widow consented to an autopsy, but thirty-five years later she discovered that government scientists had, in the course of the autopsy, removed almost nine pounds of organs, bones, and tissue. Their intention had been to study the broad effects of radiation exposure on the human body. The widow successfully sued for emotional suffering connected with her discovery of the purloined body tissue.[77]

Some pathologists did not allow lack of legal authorization to inhibit their pursuit of tissue for postautopsy retention. During the 1950s and 1960s some pathologists considered that organs or tissue withdrawn from a cadaver during an autopsy could be retained for therapeutic, research, or teaching purposes.[78] Beginning around 1963, pathologists conducting forensic autopsies commonly removed pituitary glands in order to harvest human growth hormone for therapeutic use. It was standard operating procedure in the 1970s and 1980s for pathologists who performed autopsies to remove pituitary glands for contribution to a national pool of human growth hormone.[79] It was not uncommon for tissue removed during autopsy to reappear on pathologists' laboratory shelves for educational or research purposes.[80]

The pathologists in question rationalized their unannounced removal of tissue as avoiding unnecessary distress for already traumatized relatives.[81] Perhaps they believed that no one would care about the status of tissue that was no longer useful to the deceased and not likely to be noticed as missing. In the same period, some pathologists who performed autopsies retained for further chemical analysis certain organs initially removed at autopsy. Postautopsy retention of brains was common because two weeks were needed for that body part to reach the ideal consistency for sectioning.[82] Surviving relatives were typically unaware that the postautopsy cadavers they reclaimed were missing certain internal parts.

A recent Ohio case involved parents who sued a coroner after they discovered that they had received and buried their son's cadaver without his brain.[83] The coroner/pathologist had retained the brain following a forensic autopsy. (It was kept in formalin suspension for several weeks in order to create better tissue samples.) In June 2008 the Ohio Supreme Court ruled that the son's brain had been legitimately removed for analysis and that the family had not been deprived of any protected right in the body part.[84] In Great Britain, autopsy practice up to 2004 allowed pathologists to retain tissue useful for research or educational purposes. British autopsy practice considered postautopsy tissue retention "for the greater good" to be ethical.[85] Between 1970 and 1999 British pathologists collected 21,000 cadavers' brains.[86] One institution, Alder Hey Hospital, retained 2,124 hearts removed from children who had died of heart disease. Relatives were outraged when they finally discovered the wholesale deception that had resulted in the burial of cadavers without the physical integrity that the relatives had assumed.[87]

Since peaking in 1960, the performance of autopsies has plunged both in medical schools and elsewhere. Today autopsy plays a negligible role in student or graduate education in most medical schools. Many medical students graduate without ever having witnessed an autopsy, let alone having participated in one.[88] At one time, brain autopsies were critical to teaching neuropathology. They have now been replaced by magnetic resonance imaging (MRI) scans, thus losing the dimension of full visual observation in learning about brain pathology.[89] One Harvard Medical School educator comments that MRI versus autopsy is like "the difference between looking at maps of a place and driving around it."[90] Worse, the decline of autopsy in medical education reflects the precipitous decline in the rate of autopsy generally.

Rates of autopsy dropped dramatically after the 1950s. In 1971 the JCAH eliminated its modest guideline of a 20 percent autopsy rate for accredited hospitals.[91] The American Board of Pathology lowered its requirements for board certification as a pathologist from seventy-five to fifty autopsy experiences.[92] By 1979 the average autopsy rate had dropped to 15 percent.[93] By 1988 fewer than 10 percent of cadavers were autopsied, and at least half of those were statutorily required forensic autopsies.[94] In 2008 the autopsy rate dropped below 5 percent. Autopsy is now "tangentially employed in patient care, [and] no longer central to the practice of medicine."[95] At the same time, it is doubtful that the potential utility of autopsy changed dramatically over the twentieth century. A long-time editor of the *Journal of the American Medical Association* said in 1983 that "everyone who dies in a civilized country should have an autopsy."[96]

The precipitous drop in autopsy rates is attributed to a number of factors. The biggest reason for the decline is the prevalent medical belief that sophisticated diagnostic tests and imaging make autopsy superfluous.[97] Modern premortem imaging—including x-rays, positron emission tomography (PET), computed tomography (CT), ultrasound, MRI, electrocardiography (EKG), and echocardiography—allows extensive scrutiny of the workings of the human body. In addition, modern medical technology allows chemical analysis of body fluids, secretions, and excretions of all kinds in making diagnoses. With all of these tools, clinicians feel that their diagnostic powers are fully reliable. That feeling is almost certainly misplaced, as discrepancies between diagnosis and autopsy findings are still common.[98]

Another modern disincentive exists for performing autopsies. In the minds of physicians, the specter of malpractice litigation lurks if the autopsy turns up some previously undetected causative factor. (That specter persists among clinicians despite the greater probability that an autopsy will dispel, rather than fuel, suspicion of a medical mistake.) In earlier decades, physicians sought autopsy of their deceased patients in the pursuit of self-education. Today clinicians tend to shy away from approaching a family to seek permission to mutilate their loved one's body even in the pursuit of scientifically useful information.

The prospects for a revitalization of autopsy practice seem dim. Relatively few medical students today are taught how to perform an autopsy.[99] The decline in students' interest in learning about autopsies is due in part to the erosion of the image of pathologists. The pathologist is seen as someone outside the mainstream of medical practice—working for two to four hours at a smelly morgue table and then spending hours analyzing tissue samples, as well as being constantly exposed to threats like human immunodeficiency virus (HIV), hepatitis, or other communicable diseases.[100] Meanwhile, financial incentives to become a pathologist have diminished. Autopsies are labor intensive and expensive, and the costs are not fairly reimbursed. Federal funding provides some generalized support to hospitals for autopsy, but there is no fee-for-service payment for the professional staff.[101] Most hospitals do not charge for an autopsy unless it is performed at the request of a family.[102] Hospital administrators strive to cut expenses by curbing autopsies.

The sharp drop in autopsies almost surely reduces quality control and diagnostic accuracy in hospitals. Clinicians' convictions about their diagnostic abilities, which rely on sophisticated technology, are probably misplaced. Clinicians are likely operating under a "vast cultural delusion" that their sophisticated imaging tools allow a definitive antemortem diagnosis.[103] The discrepancy rate between the diagnosis and the actual cause of death may still be surprisingly large, though the issue has not been well researched.[104] In addition, the quality as well as the number of autopsies performed may be in decline. The rate of discovery of new diseases and new cures may be lower than it would have been had autopsy procedures not steeply declined.

Additional negative consequences accompany the large decline in autopsy rates. Accuracy of vital statistics and epidemiology data are affected. Postmortem assessment of treatment modalities—the impacts of medicines and medical procedures—is diminished. This is especially true with respect to elderly persons who tend to die in places where an autopsy seldom follows. The autopsy rate for persons dying in nursing homes is less than 1 percent.[105] Advances in geriatric medicine are therefore slowed by the inability to trace medication effects more accurately. (Yet advocacy groups for the elderly are not likely to complain that not enough cadavers of older persons are being opened and investigated.) Important research on dementia and brain trauma is inhibited by lack of brain examination at autopsy.

## The Neomort as Practice Tool

Cadavers that serve as subjects of dissection and nonforensic autopsy— the two teaching roles discussed so far—come to those roles primarily by means of consent. Cadaver donations now account for 90 percent of dissection subjects in medical schools. Family consent accounts for the majority of nonforensic autopsies performed in hospitals. In one context, though, cadavers have been exploited as teaching tools without having been volunteered for the role.

This context is teaching hospitals, where medical students and novice physicians have for decades been able to learn and practice certain medical procedures on the newly dead—even without consent. Those procedures include endotracheal intubation, placement of central venous and other catheters, liver biopsy via needle, and bone needle placement.[106] The relevant institutional policy is often "don't ask, don't tell."[107] A 1999 study of emergency departments in teaching hospitals indicated that 76 percent "almost never" obtained consent to such practice exercises.[108] A 1994 report on critical care training programs indicated that 40 percent of them used newly dead bodies for training and that only 10 percent of that 40 percent required the family's consent.[109]

Tolerance of these postmortem corporeal interventions is rationalized primarily by a utilitarian balancing of the social gain in training fledgling doctors versus what is perceived as a relatively minor disturbance to a cadaver.[110] The physical intrusion is justified, it is argued, by the considerable benefit to medical patients who will subsequently undergo similar procedures performed by the former trainees. Physicians and emergency personnel must be proficient in lifesaving procedures, it is said, and live patients should not have to bear the inevitable mistakes of novices. Supporters argue that the physical intrusion from practice procedures is brief and nonmutilating—no more obtrusive than the embalming to which families typically consent. (While consent is required for an embalming, the next of kin give cursory approval without much awareness of the physical intervention involved.) No permanent harm is done to the corpse during the minor physical impositions of practice on neomorts. The corpse remains fit for any subsequent exposure entailed in a wake or viewing. The need for medical proficiency in performing lifesaving procedures, coupled with the quick, unobtrusive bodily invasion, it is asserted, warrants omission of prior consent. Just as some states have permitted routine harvesting of corneas (during forensic autopsies) in order to bring sight to blind beneficiaries, or authorize autopsies in cases of strong public interest, the public interest warrants the modest cadaveric invasion involved.[111]

Efforts to articulate legal justifications for practicing medical procedures on the newly dead are unconvincing. Unconsented touchings are generally a legal wrong—a battery. Mere utilitarian gain (as in improved medical training) does not normally provide a legal rationale for disturbing cadavers; otherwise, routine recovery of vital cadaveric organs would have long ago become accepted practice. Another argument supporting the legality of practice procedures is that cadavers, as nonpersons, have lost all legal rights.[112] I believe that this claim is transparently wrong. I have argued strenuously (in chapter 3) that cadavers do have rights to deferential, respectful treatment even if those rights get enforced by a next of kin or a public agency. Another possible legal rationale is that patients who use the facilities of a teaching hospital have implicitly agreed to allow their cadavers to be used for minor postmortem training procedures.[113] That argument seems inappropriate when applied to people who have been forced by emergency or necessity to use the hospital facilities in question without any consideration of options or consequences. Nor is the so-called implied consent consistent with the actual wishes of dying persons. According to one study, only 10 percent of patients themselves would consent to postmortem invasions, even for educational purposes.[114]

Legislative bodies could decide that practicing medical procedures on neomorts is legally permissible—that the gains to medical education warrant the relatively minor impositions on the dead. Such a statutory regime authorizing practice on cadavers has analogous precedents. For example, public needs—such as discovering the causes of mysterious deaths—have been found by legislatures to justify forensic autopsies both morally and legally. Also, legislatures have sometimes established that the public benefit suffices to uphold interference with cadavers' quiet repose, as in jurisdictions that permit, absent any known objection, the harvesting of corneas and/or pituitary glands in the course of forensic autopsies. For those people who unsentimentally believe, like the 1830 Massachusetts committee quoted by Laderman at the start of this chapter, that corpses are inanimate objects appropriate for service to humanity, the solution is clear. For them, the importance of training emergency personnel warrants the temporary, relatively unobtrusive, and usually unnoticeable intrusion on a newly dead body—even without consent.

Concerning the practice of procedures on the dead, the strength of the utilitarian argument depends on the answers to two questions relating to "necessity." That is, the public benefit rationale for authorizing practice procedures should fail if there is no necessity to use cadavers for educational practice exercises. The first necessity question, then, is whether alternatives to practice on the newly dead exist for training medical students in the procedures involved. The two most promising candidates are lifelike mannequins perfused with red fluid that simulate bleeding and virtual-reality computer programs that simulate the medical procedures involved.[115] These alternatives to cadavers for training purposes are not fully satisfactory; many physicians claim that practice on the newly dead is the best way to teach the procedures because the artificial models cannot adequately mimic flesh.[116] The texture of the material and the consequences of mistakes are supposedly too different. In short, the available alternatives have not convinced medical educators to replace their preference for fresh cadavers as teachers.

The other necessity issue is whether sufficient practice cadavers could be obtained by compelling medical personnel to secure consent from the next of kin. That issue has provoked a lot of debate. Some authorities contend that the next of kin will give consent if sensitively approached.[117] Empirical studies appear to yield conflicting results about the willingness of survivors to consent to practice exercises on their loved ones.[118] Some physicians argue that the consent process entails unwarranted stress and trauma for surviving families. The notion is apparently that unannounced teaching exercises harm no one and avoid the aggravating confrontations that would otherwise regularly ensue.

The medical establishment has waffled for approximately twenty-five years on whether to make consent a prerequisite to practice on cadavers. Uncertainty has prevailed about the potential for a consent regime to provide enough cadavers for students to practice on. In 1983 the President's Commission for the Study of Ethical Problems in Medicine and Biomedical and Behavioral Research concluded that physicians "should" make a reasonable effort to get consent for postmortem practice procedures "whenever practical."[119] The commission thus implied that impracticality would be a sufficient excuse for failure to obtain survivors' consent. As previously noted, many teaching institutions have continued to dispense with family consent up to the present. In 2002 the AMA *encouraged* institutions to get preauthorization for practice procedures.[120] In 2003 the AMA Council on Ethical and Judicial Affairs *urged* that prior consent be sought from surviving family members before performance of training procedures on the newly dead.[121] The council cited family sensibilities, public trust in the medical profession, and discomfort of medical trainees as the conclusive factors. It suggested that hospital authorities could explain to family members the importance of providing training to novice practitioners and could ask the family to envision what the decedent would have wanted. (As to the projected wishes of a typical decedent, the solicitors of family consent would have to cope with one survey reporting that only 10 percent of seriously ill patients wanted such procedures performed on their own cadavers.)

The issue of postmortem practice procedures still seems up in the air. The medical profession seems more and more aware that performance of unconsented procedures on a corpse is not strictly legal. No medical instructor or student is legally entitled to poke or probe a corpse in an effort to improve his or her medical skills. At the same time, emergency physicians are not convinced that sufficient practice material is obtainable via family consent. And some medical professionals are still convinced of the necessity of using unannounced practice procedures in the training of physicians. In 2003 the American College of Emergency Physicians suggested the need for further research on the feasibility and consequences of asking for consent before performing postmortem practice procedures.[122] That position reflects continued reluctance to make survivors' consent a prerequisite to student practice on cadavers.

I believe that the matter of student practice exercises can be resolved appropriately by a presumed consent (PC) framework. Decedents in teaching hospitals should be deemed to have consented to have these relatively minor intrusions performed on their cadavers unless they have made a prior objection or the family makes a postmortem objection. Just as PC could provide a framework for harvesting organs for transplant, it can provide a default position for postmortem practice procedures. To be meaningful, though, a PC framework must provide information about the system in place. In other words, there should be an easy way for hospital patients and/or their families to opt out of becoming postmortem teaching subjects. The best mechanism for informing the patient about the relevant hospital policy, and for providing an opt-out opportunity, is in the documents provided at hospital registration. That is, a checked box in the hospital entrance materials would suffice to allow the patient to opt out. Admittedly, it is somewhat unseemly to ask entering hospital patients to indicate whether they want their corpse to be subject to student learning exercises. Yet federal law already demands that hospitals inform every entering patient about the nature of an advance medical directive (AD) that becomes applicable if and when the patient becomes mentally incapacitated and subject to serious medical decisions like removal of life support. An entering patient who expects to leave the hospital alive should be no more traumatized by the mention of postmortem bodily intervention than by the mention of end-of-life medical options.

## The Cadaver as Witness

> A dead body tells no tales, except those which it whispers to the quick ear of the scientific expert.
>
> Douglas Maclaghan, Scottish professor of medical jurisprudence (1878), as quoted by Ian Burney, *Bodies of Evidence*

> Patient and silent while we live, our skeletons shout to heaven and posterity after we die.
>
> William Maples and Michael Browning, *Dead Men Do Tell Tales*

> God put certain internal organs in the human body for purely aesthetic reasons. They just look nice when the forensic pathologist opens you up.
>
> Mark Leyner and Billy Goldberg, *Why Do Men Have Nipples?*

The true end-of-life story—and sometimes even the identity of the deceased—are often shrouded in mystery. Sometimes even the deceased doesn't know what hit him. Often those persons surrounding the deceased know roughly what events precipitated death but not what the particular causative factors were. Examination of the remains, by autopsy or otherwise, provides the best means to unravel the mystery. Over time a whole science, forensic pathology and anthropology, has been dedicated to deciphering the story provided by the physical conditions of a cadaver and its surroundings.

Public investigations into the cause of death have a long history. In 44 BC the Roman physician Antistius examined Julius Caesar's corpse in an effort to pinpoint which of twenty-three stab wounds had been fatal.[123] (Antistius concluded that only one knife thrust—the one that had penetrated the chest below the first rib—had caused death.[124]) The Anglo-American system of cause-of-death investigation dates to the Middle Ages, when the Crown appointed a nonclerical official, a coroner, to make inquiries about the way in which a citizen of the realm had died.[125] The main object, apparently, was to pursue the Crown's financial interest in certain kinds of fatalities. In the event of suicide, the decedent's estate was forfeited to the Crown. In the event of homicide, the Crown had interests both in penalizing the criminals and in securing the well-being of the taxpaying public.[126]

Colonial America adopted the coroner's inquest as a part of the administration of criminal law. In the early Republic, the office of coroner typically carried no professional or educational qualifications.[127] A coroner collected fees based on the number of inquests carried out; any death suspected to be criminal, suicidal, or simply unaccounted for could prompt an inquest.[128] During an inquest, an autopsy occasionally contributed to the investigation of the death. In 1639 an autopsy of a Massachusetts apprentice revealed a fractured skull and led to the prosecutor's arraignment of the master.[129] In 1662 in Hartford, Connecticut, an autopsy was performed on an eight-year-old girl to determine if she had died of witchcraft. The autopsy revealed that the upper airway of her gullet was severely constricted, a finding compatible enough with witchcraft to prompt the suspected witch to flee the colony.[130] In 1691 in New York, suspicion that the Governor's sudden demise was due to poisoning prompted an autopsy. It was concluded that his death was probably attributable to a pulmonary embolism.[131]

Until the mid-nineteenth century, an American inquest was still conducted by a nonprofessional person who had authority to convene an inquest jury or to seek an autopsy. Over the course of the nineteenth century, medically trained persons participated more and more in forensic investigations and trials. And forensic specialists began to emerge. Forensic anthropology drew wide attention in an 1849 trial in Boston. There a murderer was apprehended and convicted despite having dismembered the victim and hidden the pieces in scattered locales.[132] "Expert" testimony about reconstruction of a dismantled body and about dental records was used to identify the corpse and establish the time of death.[133] That use of a medical expert helped spur more widespread integration of medically trained people into the coroner system. The argument became that medically skilled postmortem investigators would be more objective and more detached from popular pressures in making inquiries into the cause of death.[134] In 1890 Baltimore appointed two physicians as medical examiners—medically trained officials charged with conducting autopsies and inquests.[135] However, it was only in 1937 that the first formal training program in forensic pathology was established at the Harvard Medical School.

The primary tool for investigation of a cadaver concerning the cause of death is a forensic autopsy. As mentioned earlier in the context of autopsies conducted to promote medical knowledge and education, the physical process is gruesome. After close external examination of the body's surface and drawing of fluid samples from various body sites for toxicological analysis, the corpse is sliced open from collarbone to groin, temporarily eviscerated, temporarily debrained, and its viscera and their contents examined in minute detail.[136] Major organs are removed, studied for abnormalities, and partially sectioned for later microscopic study. Major blood vessels are opened for examination, as are major structures such as the trachea and the esophagus. The opened cadaver reeks as blood, stomach contents, and colon contents are spilled out.[137] This spectacle of the splayed cadaver is, to say the least, undignified. And though the audience is small and professional, the cadaver may still be subjected to "hideously improper remarks."[138] The crime victim's battered head may prompt an observer to remark, "This man will never again find a properly fitting hat." A large penis may prompt the comment "His wife will certainly miss *him*."

The whole autopsy process is obviously in tension with the tranquility and dignity of a cadaver. Most people are not eager to commit their future cadaver to an autopsy, nor are their next of kin eager to have them subjected to one. Nonetheless state legislatures have uniformly established that there are good public reasons for performing some autopsies, even without any consent.

Legislation in every state lists circumstances in which an official—a coroner or a medical examiner—can dictate the performance of an autopsy despite family opposition. Though the details of forensic autopsy laws vary from state to state, there are common elements. Suspicious deaths—in circumstances that indicate homicide or suicide—are universally deemed to warrant an autopsy. These include deaths involving trauma, alcohol, drugs, or other toxic substances. Other circumstances triggering a possible forensic autopsy include a sudden, unaccounted-for death; a suspected contagious disease; an unidentified body; an inmate in a public institution; and anyone in police custody. In some states an autopsy can be required for deaths in accidents—including those occurring in the workplace or in traffic—where issues of liability and the proximate cause of death are likely to be disputed.[139]

Though medical examiners or coroners may be authorized to perform autopsies in all of the above circumstances, they often—for a variety of reasons—choose not to do so. Sometimes a sudden death may not be accounted for with precision—for example, the death of a very old nursing home resident—but it is clear that natural causes are involved, not crime. Or the cause of death may be clear, as in alcoholism-related cirrhosis, AIDS, or suicide, but the medical examiner wishes to spare the family embarrassment and therefore fabricates a cause of death such as a heart attack.

In the case of crime victims, the possibility of incriminating and punishing the perpetrator supports an assumption that the decedent would not object to having his or her cadaver examined, including the gross invasion of an autopsy. For centuries in England, efforts were made by a coroner's jury to enlist the limited communication abilities of a crime victim's corpse. In the seventeenth century a suspect was required to approach or touch the corpse to see if the corpse reacted in the presence of a murderer by foaming at the mouth or bleeding at the touch.[140] In the nineteenth century inquests employed another form of inquiry involving nonverbal communication. A coroner's jury looked at the corneas of murder victims in the hope of finding an imprint of the murderer's image.[141]

The subject of a forensic inquest may be so "bloated, burned, buggy, rotted, gnawed, liquefied, dismembered, mummified or skeletonized" as to prevent prompt identification.[142] Forensic teams use a variety of tools—DNA, dental records, tattoos, fingerprints, skin markings, and metal implants (such as pacemakers)—to identify badly disfigured or decomposed human remains. Dental records confirmed the identify of Adolph Hitler and Eva Braun, whose charred remains had been found in a bunker in Berlin. DNA analysis has enabled quantum leaps in ability to identify human remains. After the 1988 disintegration of Pan Am flight 301 over Lockerbie, Scotland, the remains of 253 of the 259 passengers were identified even though they were scattered over an area of 845 square miles. Identification of military deaths rose from 58 percent of Civil War fatalities to 97 percent of Korean War dead to virtually all fatal casualties in the Vietnam War.[143] Military personnel now provide DNA samples as genetic dog tags. This system has come a long way from the use of agents hired by distraught families of Civil War soldiers to comb through battlefield casualties with photos of the missing son, husband, or other relative in hand.

Even when human remains have been reduced to skeletal remnants, some important information about their identity can be gleaned. A femur can indicate gender, height, age, and weight.[144] A skull's distinctive features (usually a jaw or teeth) can lead to a positive identification; sometimes computer modeling from a skull can lead to reconstruction of a victim's visual image. All this is not to say that most skeletonized remains can be identified, only that bones sometimes do lead to a positive identification. Work with bones and skeletons also contributes enormously to knowledge about human anthropology and cultural history. Human remains consisting mainly of bones or skeletons are constantly being unearthed. Scientists have become more and more skilled at interpreting the history of such findings, as in the case of the seventy warrior prisoners ritually sacrificed 1,400 years ago at Huaca de la Luna on the northern coast of Peru.[145] There carbon isotopes supplied the age of the bones, carbon and nitrogen values in the bones disclosed the diet, fractures and wounds revealed the cause of death, and nearby wall frescoes show the procession of prisoners with ropes around their necks.

The common techniques of forensic investigation are well known, especially now that crime scene investigation (CSI) has attracted a mass television audience. A careful forensic examination can disclose a lot about the victim's end-of-life story. It can establish whether a decedent's injuries were caused by a fall or by an assailant's blows. Wound patterns can reveal the type of lethal instrument and help identify the murder weapon. The size and shape of entrance and exit wounds can show the distance and location of a shooter (the controversy surrounding the Warren Commission's conclusion about a lone shooter of President John F. Kennedy notwithstanding). Toxicological testing of fluid and tissue can show the presence of poisons, drugs, or other foreign substances. Patterns of injuries in multiple victims can help reconstruct puzzling accidents, such as a plane crash. Victims sitting close to an explosion are more shredded and retain bomb shards if a bomb has in fact exploded. Wounds of accident victims can sometimes show whether a driver braked before the accident.

Establishing the time of death is a forensic challenge and is crucial to innumerable homicide investigations.[146] Did the victim die on the day he was last seen together with the suspect? Was the victim killed on the day the suspect was viewed hefting red-stained bundles into a rented U-haul van? Did the murder take place while the suspect was at work or during a period of time the suspect cannot account for? Were Nicole Simpson and Ronald Goldman murdered within the one-hour period for which O. J. Simpson had no confirmed alibi?[147] If a corpse can establish the time of death, homicide investigators have a valuable forensic tool.

The classic indices for assessing a cadaver's time of death were rigor mortis (stiffness), algor mortis (temperature), and livor mortis (color). Until the mid-twentieth century, these factors underlay any pronouncement of the time between death and discovery of a body. Yet the factors were relevant only within about forty-eight hours after death, and even then they were imprecise tools. Imprecision was due to the multitude and fuzziness of variables underlying the expert judgments, despite the confident testimony of the so-called experts.[148]

Rigor mortis generally sets in within twenty-four hours of death and lasts for twenty-four to thirty-six hours.[149] The stiffness results from a chemical compound that forms in a corpse's muscles—adenosine triphosphate (ATP). The presence, amount, and time of the appearance of ATP are affected by variables such as stresses to the body and the extent of exertion before death. The stiffness of the body therefore can provide only a rough basis for pronouncing the time of death.[150]

Algor mortis—the temperature of a corpse—long served as a basis for pronouncing the time of death. Use of a thermometer to measure a corpse's temperature began in the early nineteenth century. In 1868 a professor of forensic medicine in Glasgow conducted studies of the rate of corpses' cooling in an effort to develop a general formula for measuring the time interval after death.[151] In 1887 a London pathologist also devised a body temperature formula purporting to measure the time of death within minutes. For almost one hundred years, forensic testimony relied on these simplistic formulas in criminal trials.[152] The problem is that heat loss is affected by multiple variables, including the normal body temperature of the decedent, the ambient temperature, wind, humidity, and the decedent's type of clothing.[153] So, algor mortis—which in any case could only be useful within about twenty-four hours of death—had too many variables to be a truly reliable indicator of the of time of death.[154]

Livor mortis—the color of a corpse—also has too many vagaries to be an accurate index of the time of death. The settling of blood in a corpse does produce purple stains in portions of the body nearest the ground. (Also, postmortem chemical changes affecting a corpse's blood can produce visible shades of green, blue, and black in various parts of the body.[155]) Despite sophisticated light meters for measuring lividity, the variability of color change as well as differing perceptions of color prevent livor mortis from being an accurate measure of the time of death. In short, even during the first forty-eight hours after death, multiple variables encumber all three traditional bases for assessing the time of death.

Since the 1970s anthropologists have tried to use the degree of cadaveric decomposition to measure the time of death. The problem again has been the multiplicity of variables that affect the rate of bodily decay—temperature, humidity, state of dress, and even soil acidity. Anthropologists, especially William Bass at the University of Tennessee, recognized that in order for their time projections to be accurate, systematic studies of rates of cadaver decomposition would have to relate to a variety of conditions. Professor Bass had himself demonstrated the imprecision of time-of-death assessments during an incident in 1977 when he misjudged a time-of-death estimate by 112 years.[156] Bass had been called in by law enforcement officials to help in an investigation surrounding a Civil War grave that had been opened and tampered with. The grave initially belonged to the Confederate Colonel William Shy, who had been buried in 1864. In the incident in question, a partial corpse had been found on top of Colonel Shy's lead coffin, and the police wanted Bass to determine when that corpse had died. Bass, looking at the pinkish intact flesh, estimated its age to be a few months, not more than a year.[157] But it turned out that the partial corpse was that of William Shy himself—113 years old.

William Bass's egregious error could be explained. An attempted grave robbery had created a hole in the casket through which part of Colonel Shy's corpse had been withdrawn—the part that Bass had opined was less than a year old. Colonel Shy's corpse had been extraordinarily well embalmed and placed in a sealed lead casket. Because the casket had been impervious to air and water, the corpse had resisted bacterial putrefaction and remained somewhat pliable and pinkish. While Bass's erroneous estimate was explainable, he still became fair game for defense counsel whenever he was called as a prosecution witness about the time of death. Defense counsel would inevitably ask in cross-examination: "Mr. Bass, isn't it true that you once made a misjudgment of the time of death by 113 years?"

William Bass got over his embarrassment. In fact, the Colonel Shy incident helped spur Bass to launch a systematic study of rates of bodily decomposition at the University of Tennessee.[158] In 1981 Bass set up a research facility—called the anthropological research facility (ARF), sometimes known as BARF (Bass anthropological research facility) or The Body Farm—to measure bodily decomposition under a variety of conditions.[159] Bass charted the decomposition rates of hundreds of corpses—at varying temperatures, locales (in woods, in fields, and within vehicles), depths of dirt, and even depths of submergence in water. Other researchers did parallel decomposition studies. However, their research used pig carcasses rather than human remains; the Department of Justice therefore funded studies to correlate the decomposition of pig carcasses with that of human cadavers. All of these research efforts have presumably improved time-of-death assessments well beyond Bass's 1977 effort.

Another tool for time-of-death analysis is called "forensic entomology."[160] In this method the corpse speaks indirectly through the bugs that occupy its remains. By the end of the nineteenth century, entomologists were well aware of the waves of cadaver-feeding insects descending on any accessible corpse. The presence of various flies, maggots, mites, and beetles—coupled with information about the duration and timing of their various life cycles—could help date a corpse's time of death.[161] In 1894 a book by Jean Pierre Megnin described eight distinct waves of insects and their time intervals. In the 1930s and 1940s, an American, David Hall, developed timetables for the life cycles of a variety of North American flies, eggs, larvae, and maggots.[162]

Despite Hall's efforts, the forensic utility of cadaver-eating insects has been limited. Although more American research followed Hall's lead on insect development as a gauge of the time elapsed since death, law enforcement officials into the 1980s still regarded maggots largely as a disgusting nuisance rather than as a forensic tool. By then, forensic entomological experts were occasionally testifying on insects as a gauge of timing, but their testimony was vulnerable because multiple variables— weather, heat, geographical area, and soil composition—challenged their laboratory-based research. In the 1990s, field research sharpened analysis of these variables, as well as the effects of burial or submersion or closed spaces. Even today, however, forensic entomology still gives rough assessments—fudging estimates by hours or days.[163]

In short, forensic science since the mid-twentieth century has regularly sought more exact ways to assess the time of death. Researchers have tried to examine various elements of bodily decay and to measure their breakdown rates. One effort used the level of potassium in the eyes' vitreous humor—an effort that has failed because of multiple variables such as heat, humidity, state of infection, and sampling techniques.[164] Rates of breakdown of amino acids within cells have been another focus of research.[165] In all of these areas of research, imprecision persists. Nonetheless, forensic science continues to give cadavers an opportunity to communicate nonverbally about their time of death and about their entire end-of-life story.

### Safety Research and the Sturdiness of a Cadaver

Despite the gruesome physical damage to the integrity of a cadaver, dissection in a medical school and autopsy in a morgue are regarded not only as tolerable but also as praiseworthy contributions to the advancement of medical education and science. Dissections and autopsies are not the only ostensibly revolting uses of a cadaver that have benevolent justifications. Other praiseworthy manglings of a cadaver take place in the course of so-called scientific research. Mary Roach ably recounts the historic role of human cadavers in research using crash simulators to measure the success or failure of automobile safety devices.[166] Corpses as crash test dummies contributed to the development of more effective seat belts, air bags, collapsible steering wheels, and dashboard padding. Not only were the corpses subjected to powerful disfiguring trauma, but they were then autopsied to assess the internal damage. In other words, those particular research cadavers were twice mangled.

Cadavers as research subjects have also been mauled while contributing to military assessment of munitions capabilities and the effectiveness of protective countermeasures. In the 1950s, federal government scientists analyzed cadavers to measure the effects of atomic radiation. In 1999 the army placed various kinds of protective footwear on uniformed cadavers and strapped the cadavers into harnesses above a blast center to measure the protective capacities of the footwear.[167] Similar experiments occurred in military evaluation of body armor.[168] In other words, some corpses were blown to smithereens in the course of weapons research.

Law enforcement objectives can also provide reasons for conducting otherwise gruesome research on cadavers. An example is the previously mentioned research on rates of cadaveric disintegration carried out for decades at The Body Farm at the University of Tennessee. Forensic expert William Bass, seeking to sharpen his frequent testimony about crime victims' time of death based on the extent of bodily disintegration, laid out cadavers in various outdoor settings to study the rates of body decomposition from natural decay and from insect devastation under diverse conditions. He measured the degree and speed of bodily disintegration into what was ultimately a moldy, stinking mess.[169] Bass's Body Farm research drew some criticism as a "ghastly affront to human dignity," but it was highly praised and assisted by forensic students and by state and federal law enforcement agencies. The cadaveric research material in all of these studies consisted of unclaimed bodies rather than volunteer contributors. The social utility (advancement of forensic science) of the research projects was sufficient to overcome concern about the disgusting physical treatment of the cadaver. The decedents' survivors were unaware of the exploitation of their loved ones' cadavers.

How much physical abuse is tolerable in the course of research on cadaveric subjects? The yuck factor, the instinctive revulsion toward physical disturbance of a cadaver, cannot alone be determinative. In 1993 thirty-nine-year-old condemned prisoner Joseph Paul Jernigan donated his future corpse to science. Upon Jernigan's execution, his body was frozen and sliced into 1,871 sections; the sections were digitally photographed and the photos were posted on the Internet for use by scientists.[170] Some people called the action ghoulish or questioned the voluntariness of Jernigan's consent, but most people saw it as a modest, commendable gesture toward human progress. The acceptability of the previously described military weapons and law enforcement research, despite the revolting physical consequences for cadavers, reinforces the notion that the yuck factor cannot be determinative.

The Jernigan episode underlines a few relevant factors in assessing the moral bounds of dismantling a cadaver for purposes of research. One factor is the importance of autonomy—consent—in determining the acceptability of exploiting a corpse in a messy, if not disgusting, fashion. Individuals can to some degree define personal dignity and weigh for themselves the value of medical science versus the ostensible mistreatment of their cadaver. Mr. Jernigan did not think that being sliced like a cucumber was intolerably demeaning, because he apparently valued medical science and was not revolted by his salami-like role. People who will their bodies to medical schools (for dissection in anatomy lab) or to the general advancement of science apparently believe that the physical mangling of a cadaver is not intrinsically disrespectful or degrading. Also, people who contribute their corpses to a Body World exhibition do not think that the flaying and displaying of their inhuman-looking remains is a desecration, given the educational value of the display. In the early nineteenth century, Americans' outrage toward anatomists was fueled in part not by revulsion toward dissection, but rather by the knowledge that the cadaver subjects had likely been snatched from quiet repose or otherwise obtained without anyone's consent.

Mr. Jernigan's donation also shows the relevance, in assessing indignity, of a researcher's purpose and attitude in exploiting a human cadaver. Normally, picking a corpse's brain apart would be a sacrilege. But when the picking is being done by a scientist studying the causes of Alzheimer's disease, Parkinson's disease, or Huntington's disease, one can readily understand a family's willingness to have their afflicted loved one's cadaver dismantled. Maliciously disemboweling an enemy's corpse is very different from extracting an organ as a holy relic (as done after the death of numerous Roman Catholic martyrs) or as a transplant organ to save a needy human. As Mary Roach thoughtfully points out, virtually any use of a cadaver (as opposed to simple repose) can potentially be upsetting to observers.[171] The yuck factor of mutilation of a corpse is overcome when an authorized donor makes a reasonable judgment that the disfigurement is not intrinsically demeaning and that an important justification (such as expanding scientific knowledge) exists.

The respectful or disrespectful attitude of researchers toward cadavers can sometimes be reflected in the way the cadaver is treated. Anatomists conducting public dissections in the Middle Ages showed little respect for their human dissection material. The detached innards of purloined cadavers were slung into buckets to be dumped unceremoniously after the event as trash. By contrast, medical students doing dissections today are supposed to be highly respectful toward their cadavers (though in the real world, some banter about the corpse's features is an almost inevitable part of the nervous enterprise).[172] Contemporary rules of the anatomy lab promote postmortem dignity. Such rules prevent the moving of body parts away from a dissection table in an effort to ensure that the remains of each cadaver are kept separate and identifiable for ultimate disposal.[173] A family donating a corpse for medical use has the option of reclaiming the dissected remains in order to arrange their ultimate disposal.[174] Unclaimed dissected remains are supposed to be separately incinerated or buried, not mixed with hospital waste. Body parts removed for examination during autopsy are supposed to be reinserted into the corpse or, after lab analysis, disposed of in a respectful fashion.[175] A medical school typically holds an annual service to honor the memory of the men and women who contributed their remains to science. Even when a cadaver is about to be used in a crash test, it is clothed in a way that avoids unseemly exposure or leakage. All of these are gestures of respect for the human connections of a cadaver—acknowledging it as a very special, albeit inanimate, object.

In sum, the degree of physical destructiveness accompanying postmortem handling is only one relatively minor element in assessing the moral acceptability of research on cadavers. Dignity and respect are key elements, and those elements are measured, in most postmortem research contexts, by a variety of factors other than the degree of bodily invasion involved. Ordinarily a corpse and its survivors are entitled to maintain absolute cadaveric integrity. Minor bodily intrusions, as well as major ones, are impermissible without appropriate consent (or justification). As law and custom entitle the next of kin to receive a cadaver in the same condition in which it existed at death, the removal of corneas from the surface of the body is a breach of the corpse's expected bodily integrity just as removal of the heart would be. Sometimes any bodily intrusion, regardless of its depth, will violate important religious or cultural beliefs that are entitled to respect. Both the Uniform Anatomical Gift Act

(UAGA) and the common law uphold interests in the integrity of a cadaver even in the face of strong justifications for invasion, such as saving an organ donee's life. Yet reasonable legislative judgments can and sometimes are made that—at least in the absence of an objection by a decedent or by his or her representative—some cadaveric tissue (such as corneas) can be harvested at the time of a forensic autopsy.

The ability to cause children to come into existence long after the
death of a parent is a recently acquired ability for human society.
There are probably wise and wonderful ways in which that ability
can be used. . . . There are, I think, ethical problems, social policy
problems and legal problems which are presented.

> Judge Reginald Stanton, in *Kolacy*, N.J. Superior Court
> (2000)

Worrying about who owns a dead man's sperm is almost obscene
in a nation that lacks universal health care, in which 20% of our
children . . . are hungry a significant part of the year and in which
a large percentage of people . . . no longer remember what hope
might look like.

> Erich H. Loewy, bioethecist, Medical College of
> Wisconsin Ethics Listserv (December 2004)

*Chapter 9*

# The Cadaver as Parent

It is not easy for cadavers either to become or to function as parents.
Though necrophiliacs may try all sorts of sexual stimulation, the inert
cadaver will not respond. Normal means of sexual reproduction are out.
Nor can cadavers serve as the nurturing, directive parents that child
rearing demands. There are other ineffective parents in the world, but
none so dormant as a cadaver.

These obstacles to parenting, though, do not prevent a cadaver from
becoming a genetic parent. The most prosaic scenario is one in which a
male impregnates a female and then dies during the ensuing pregnancy
that leads to a birth. Some males have thus become posthumous fathers
without knowledge or intention.

Artificial means of reproduction—originally used to assist infertile
couples—can also be used to make a cadaver a genetic parent. A common technique for assisting infertile couples is to extract ova from
the female and fertilize them with sperm (usually from the male partner) to create preembryos to be implanted in the woman's uterus.[1] The

extraction of ova can be arduous, involving intramuscular injections to stimulate the ovaries and a needle or laparoscope to remove the ova. To avoid repetition of the burdensome extraction process when an initial implantation fails, backup preembryos are usually created and frozen for later use if needed. Tens of thousands of such preembryos are frozen and stored each year in the United States; they are usable for up to fifty years. Disputes about the fate of frozen embryos usually arise in the context of divorcing or separating couples—with both progenitors still alive.[2] But a gamete provider's death before implantation of a preembryo creates the potential for posthumous genetic parenthood and for disputes over the use of stored preembryos.

Postmortem parenthood can occur when a live person's sperm or unfertilized ova are frozen and later used in posthumous fertilization.[3] (Cryopreservation of sperm dates to 1949.) The usual motivation for storing sperm is to facilitate a pregnancy while the male progenitor is still alive—either because a couple is struggling to reproduce or because the male faces a disease or condition threatening future sterility or another form of inability to reproduce. Though the typical impetus for cryopreservation is parenthood while the male is still alive, the technique is also available for postmortem fatherhood. Widows or bereaved lovers have successfully used a deceased partner's frozen sperm to generate a subsequent pregnancy. Cryopreservation of unfertilized ova has been successful in isolated cases, but it is not yet standard practice.[4] Ultimately, though, females will be able to leave frozen ova as a means of posthumous genetic motherhood.

Another technique can also produce postmortem fatherhood. Since 1980 it has been possible to extract semen from a fresh corpse, freeze it, and use it within ten years to make a woman pregnant.[5] The sperm is generally retrieved within twenty-four to thirty-six hours of death.[6] Most reports about posthumous extraction are anecdotal. The first instance, in 1981, related to the retrieval of sperm from a thirty-year-old male who had just been killed in a motorcycle accident. In 1987 two incidents involved sperm removed from accident victims at the initiative of their families—one by the parents to preserve the biogenetic heritage of their only child and one by a father who somehow wanted to be consoled by knowing that his dead son's sperm had been stored.[7] In the mid-1990s widows sometimes succeeded in convincing doctors to extract semen from their late husbands.[8] One instance in 1994 involved a twenty-two-year-old husband killed in an auto accident sixteen days after marriage. In all of these instances, no report of childbirth exists; the ultimate fate of the extracted sperm is unknown. However, one incident is recounted in which a widow successfully used retrieved frozen semen for insemination six years after its removal from her late husband.[9] There are indications that posthumous sperm retrieval has occurred a few hundred times, so it seems likely that dozens, if not hundreds, of children have resulted from postmortem sperm retrieval.[10]

Female cadavers can also become postmortem parents. This usually occurs when a woman carrying a viable fetus is killed and doctors, acting within minutes of the crime or accident, salvage a premature infant. But dead women have also given birth long after the moment of death. To the utter surprise of doctors and scientists, cadavers of pregnant women who have died according to total brain death criteria have been connected to cardiorespiratory machinery and have successfully gestated fetuses for as long as 107 days. The birth is performed by a surgical procedure. The typical scenario involves a pregnant trauma victim who experiences total brain death but whose corpse is kept tethered to machines in order to preserve the fetus. The machines, coupled with the cadaver's autonomic body reactions, provide enough sustenance to produce a healthy infant. The people seeking to use the brain-dead female corpse as an incubator are usually either the genetic father or the dead woman's parents.

Eventually another technique will allow both women and men to become postmortem parents—cloning. We all know about Dolly the sheep and a variety of other cloned animals. To date, no human has been created by cloning. The very idea of a human clone is currently anathema—in part because of the potential harm to innumerable experimental humans in the course of perfecting a human cloning process and in part out of fear of the eugenic consequences. Yet in the somewhat distant future, cloning might "become an accepted reproductive technology."[11] The technique would then be another tool for postmortem parenthood, assuming that the cloned descendant is deemed to be a child.

Legal and moral issues surround all forms of postmortem parenthood. Who controls the gametes or fetus that a decedent has left behind? An executor of the decedent's estate? A survivor previously designated by the decedent as an intended recipient of the stored gametes? Or the same next of kin normally entitled to control the disposition of the cadaver? When, if ever, is it permissible to use gametes for postmortem reproductive purposes? As to postmortem bodily invasions, is the consent of the decedent a prerequisite to harvesting life-generating bodily materials? Is inferred consent a sufficient foundation? What is the decedent's responsibility toward any after-born child? How strong are the conflicting interests of survivors other than a bonded former mate—such as the parents of the semen producer or his preexisting children? Legal intervention to resolve such issues has been sparse. Perhaps that scarcity of binding authority from either courts or legislatures relates to the relative rarity of engineering postmortem parenthood or perhaps the paucity of cases stems from agreement among survivors, physicians, and sperm banks concerning the proper utilization of the stored gametes or embryos. The lack of binding authority leaves plenty of room for speculation about the resolution of the hard moral and legal issues surrounding survivors who seek to make a cadaver a parent.

## Using Prefrozen Sperm for Posthumous Procreation

A variety of reasons might prompt a male to deposit sperm with the intention that it be used for posthumous procreation. The most common scenario involves a male facing a terminal illness or threatening condition who wants to reproduce with a bonded mate—married or unmarried. The motive for pursuing posthumous parenthood might be to express love for the mate, or simply a desire to make the mate happy, or a wish to leave a biological legacy.[12] A person's presence on earth can be marked and remembered by an after-born child, even if the sperm depositor will not be able to nurture and enjoy that child.[13] Perhaps the depositor, while still alive, is consoled by the prospect of his continuing vicarious presence in the world. Sometimes the pride of family lineage is at stake—the presumptuous notion that the world will be a much better place if the sperm depositor's biological heritage is preserved.

Could the sperm depositor be entitled—as a matter of constitutional liberty—to posthumous reproduction? That is, would the cadaver (or someone acting on its behalf) have a federal constitutional right to have a willing female partner use his sperm to become pregnant and give birth to his child? Could there be a constitutional right to prevent government interference with the reproductive wishes of a now-dead gamete producer? This is highly doubtful. The U.S. Supreme Court has acknowledged a male's fundamental liberty interest in procreation.[14] But that interest in reproduction was first recognized when a male had already created a fetus and when the potential father was willing and able to enjoy the benefits of child rearing; even then, the male's interest was trumped by a pregnant female's right to decide whether to carry a fetus to term. Access to contraception as a means to control reproduction has also been deemed to be a protected liberty, but that is still a long way from any putative constitutional right to become a parent by posthumous use of stored gametes.

The interest of a sperm donor in posthumous reproduction is somewhat attenuated when compared to the acknowledged constitutional right to procreate. A decedent cannot enjoy the benefits that customarily accompany parenthood—child rearing and companionship.[15] More importantly, any recognized right to procreate (or not) has not yet embraced all artificial means of reproduction. Becoming a father by posthumous use of sperm does not meet the judicial formula for identifying fundamental constitutional liberties—acceptance in "the traditions and collective conscience of the people."[16]

A potential recipient of stored sperm might assert her own constitutional interest in procreation.[17] She, unlike the dead sperm provider, can still enjoy all the benefits of parenthood. Nonetheless any constitutional claim to posthumous use of sperm to create motherhood is still far from the currently recognized liberty interest in procreation. The potential recipient's constitutional claim is especially undermined when the aspiring mother already has other children or has the ability to have children with another male.

While the Constitution might not compel legal acceptance of posthumous utilization of preserved sperm, this does not mean that states cannot or should not choose to recognize and enforce posthumous parenthood interests. States have leeway to adopt a public policy that allows a willing and able woman to advance her procreation interests by using preserved sperm. So long as the deceased sperm provider has not objected to becoming a genetic father, who is hurt by this policy? The woman will benefit. Any potential offspring will benefit. (No matter how dismal their circumstances while growing up, the offspring are better off existing than never having existed.) A male decedent benefits from the posthumous use of his sperm for conception if that decedent indeed wanted to promote his biological legacy or to advance the well-being of a bonded female. (A decedent's interest in *not* becoming a genetic father will be touched on momentarily.) Government interests are satisfied so long as the prospective child will be supported and cared for. A state might be concerned about the inheritance interests of the decedent's existing heirs, but that interest can be handled by statutes relating to estate settlement.

Not surprisingly, the express intention of the sperm producer has governed in the few legal cases dealing with the efforts of females to obtain and use stored sperm after the death of the producer. This policy is consistent with the tendency of law to give broad autonomy to mentally competent people in shaping the postmortem fate of their cadavers (as well as their belongings). People generally have the opportunity to determine their means and place of cadaver disposal, to determine what uses can be made of their body parts (e.g., tissue donation), and to direct by a will the distribution and fate of their property. Deposited sperm is not strictly a body part, like a kidney. Nor is it necessarily property, like a car or a wristwatch.[18] Because of sperm's procreative potential, it is a special kind of material—even more special when its usage is being considered after the death of the producer. Nonetheless the courts have given broad scope to the wishes of the decedent sperm producer in determining the postmortem fate of this special material, deposited sperm.[19]

The plea to use a decedent's preserved sperm in postmortem conception usually comes from a female with whom the deceased had a strong bonded relationship.[20] That scenario appeared in *Hecht v. Superior Court of Los Angeles*, the most well-known case in this area.[21] There the decedent, William Kane, a middle-aged divorced father of two adult children, had prior to his death been in a five-year live-in relationship with Deborah Hecht. During that period he deposited fifteen vials of sperm in a sperm bank. Mr. Kane also expressed the intention that the sperm be available to Ms. Hecht to produce a child after his death. That intention was expressed in several ways—the sperm bank's form, a bequest in his will, a statement within the will, and a letter to his children.

Two weeks after sending the letter to his children, he lost $20,000 in Las Vegas and committed suicide. When Ms. Hecht sought access to the sperm vials, Mr. Kane's existing children objected, arguing that his wishes had been uttered under undue influence from Ms. Hecht. A California court found that Ms. Hecht was entitled to use the sperm for reproduction if that is what the deceased had intended. According to the court, while the sperm was not considered to be inheritable property, its disposition and use should be controlled by the deceased's wishes. A judicial hearing concluded that Mr. Kane's declarations had not been coerced; Ms. Hecht obtained her late lover's sperm.

Other courts have also ruled that where the deceased clearly indicated that his female partner should be allowed to use the deceased's stored sperm for posthumous conception, that wish should be respected.[22] Barry Hall deposited fifteen vials of sperm after being diagnosed with cancer. He later sought to convey his interest in the frozen sperm to his female friend, Christine St. John. Almost a year later Mr. Hall died; Ms. St. John had not pursued artificial insemination during that period. When Ms. St. John sought the vials after Mr. Hall's death, Mr. Hall's mother (the executor of his estate) objected. The mother/executor contended that her late son had never intended his deposited sperm to be used for postmortem conception. She relied, in part, on the absence of any mention of a posthumous child in her son's will. The court ruled that if Mr. Hall did express an intention to give the sperm to Ms. St. John, she was entitled to use the sperm for procreation. A judicial hearing would determine and enforce Barry Hall's actual wishes. In short, courts seem willing to uphold the prior instructions of a now-dead sperm depositor to have his sperm used for conception by a bonded female.[23] Opposition from family members does not prevail against the decedent's demonstrated wishes.

In all of the litigated cases involving postmortem use of stored sperm, the decedent/donor had given express consent to postmortem conception. The harder question is how to proceed when no such express direction has been left by the decedent concerning the disposition of his frozen gametes. Sometimes the wishes of the deceased can be inferred from his lifetime actions and circumstances. Consider, for example, a father who donates sperm in the hope of creating a child who will provide matching tissue to aid an already existing stricken sibling.

One could reasonably assume that the father would want to have the critical conception take place even after his death.[24] Or a male might be deemed to have wanted deposited sperm to be used posthumously when it would preserve inherited trust benefits that otherwise would lapse without an heir.[25] One could also infer a wish to have deposited sperm used posthumously if it was deposited by a married astronaut or soldier going off on a dangerous mission. The depositor must have been well aware of the mortal dangers, not just of the risk of becoming sterile.

What if there are no illuminating circumstances like those in the examples just given? What presumption should prevail when a surviving spouse or partner seeks to use the sperm left in a sperm bank by her now-deceased husband or lover? When a male makes a sperm deposit, his willingness to become a father can be inferred, at least absent other explanations (such as the intention to provide research material). And if the donor is married or bonded to a female at the time, a reasonable inference is that the donor wants to procreate with that mate. A common scenario is that the male partner is trying to take precautions in the face of an illness or a condition that threatens to produce sterility, preventing normal conception. But does the willingness to procreate and raise a child with a mate entail a similar willingness to become a posthumous father—given that the sperm depositor will never participate in child rearing or even know that he has become a progenitor?

In the absence of express instructions, a default, rebuttable presumption could go either way—in favor of or against conception using frozen sperm. In favor of conception, one can argue that a man who wanted to procreate with a bonded partner—and went so far as to deposit sperm for preservation—would want to bring a child into the world even after death.[26] Most people want to be remembered, and leaving a child is one way to promote that goal. A surviving partner who wants to use the preserved sperm is both advancing the couple's mutual interest in procreation and creating a legacy that honors the memory of the departed male.[27] From the after-born child's perspective, he or she is no worse off than a natural child born into a one-parent household; a difficult childhood is better than the alternative (nonexistence). Of course, any presumption in favor of fatherhood could always be rebutted by circumstances—including friction between the partners or unwillingness of the surviving partner to act as the parent of any after-born child.

A presumption against the posthumous use of predeposited sperm could also be justified. The claim would be that most people who deposit sperm do not actually expect it to be used postmortem.[28] A further justification would be that people have an interest in *not* becoming genetic parents absent child-rearing opportunities. Several cases in the context of disposition of frozen embryos take that stance (though there, a gamete producer was still alive and expressing opposition to becoming a genetic parent). Arguably there is no strong social interest in facilitating postmortem conception via frozen sperm.[29] (Sperm is not like a lifesaving organ harvested from a cadaver.) The surviving woman's interest in procreation can ordinarily be met by finding another male gamete producer after her mate's death.

The only thing that is clear is that courts do promote the efforts of a surviving partner to use the decedent mate's deposited sperm when the decedent expressed consent to postmortem conception. Also, judges are prone to accept as true a surviving female's representation that her partner had expressed a wish to have her use his stored sperm to bear a postmortem child.[30] In other words, a female who desires to use her partner's sperm postmortem has a strong incentive to "remember" his expressions favoring posthumous fatherhood.

While either default presumption (absent any express wish from the decedent regarding postmortem parenthood) is defensible, I am, for once, pro-life. I would favor a pro-procreation default presumption in favor of a bonded partner, knowing that circumstances could rebut the putative wish for postmortem parenthood. No invasion of cadaveric integrity is involved. I do not think that a cadaver's abstract interest in not being a genetic parent (absent undesirable economic consequences) is strong. And if a wish to avoid postmortem parenthood can be discerned, that express or implied wish prevails.

## Extracting Sperm from a Cadaver

Various techniques exist for harvesting usable sperm from a corpse within thirty-six hours of death.[31] These include artificial electro-ejaculation via a rectal probe, "micro surgical epididymal sperm aspiration," and testicular sperm extraction after cutting into the vas deferens.[32] The extracted sperm can promptly be frozen and used to fertilize ova even years later.

In 2005 the mother of an Israeli soldier killed in a war in Lebanon against Hezbollah asked the Israeli army to permit removal of sperm from the corpse of her only son. Her intention was to find a surrogate female who would undergo implantation, gestation, and birthing; the soldier's mother would then raise her genetic grandchild. While extraction of usable sperm from a cadaver was possible, Israeli policy clearly opposed allowing a soldier's mother to engineer the process of making her son a postmortem parent. Ministry of Health regulations prohibited the taking of sperm from a male corpse (or ova from a female corpse) except at the initiative of a bonded partner who was able to show that the couple's mutual intention had been to procreate together. Absent that circumstance, Israeli authorities considered the disturbance of a corpse to extract sperm to be an intolerable offense to the dignity and repose of that corpse. A prospective grandmother's interest in her son's procreation was deemed not to warrant that disturbance.

In the United States, virtually no formal legal precedent exists regarding extraction of sperm from a cadaver. While the Uniform Anatomical Gift Act (UAGA) entitles the next of kin to dispose of a cadaver and its parts, the disposal of a cadaver's sperm for reproductive purposes has not generally been considered part of those established prerogatives. (An argument that the UAGA authorizes the harvesting of sperm will be considered momentarily, but it is not likely to prevail.) Medical institutions and medical organizations dealing with assisted reproduction have had to make their own way in establishing a policy to handle the sporadic requests for postmortem extraction of sperm.

American social policy clearly supports the fulfillment of a person's express prior request to become a postmortem parent via a bonded partner—even if sperm or ova are to be extracted from the person's corpse. The decedent's wish is probably not within a constitutional right to procreation (see p. 215). Even without that legal foundation, emerging public policy supports respect for the wishes of a gamete provider concerning postmortem parenthood. The notion is that fulfilling express procreation wishes postmortem is a means of respecting and honoring the humanity (including the autonomous choice) of a deceased.[33] Any speculative harm to the resulting offspring is insufficient to frustrate the autonomous procreation wishes of a male and a bonded mate. (Being raised in a single-parent household is not necessarily a detriment to a prospective child, and it is by no means a harm compared to the alternative fate of nonexistence.) Any associated physical disturbance to a cadaver appears to be tolerable. The bodily invasion of sperm extraction is no more disruptive of a corpse's quiet repose than organ retrieval, autopsy, or embalming (options generally available to the next of kin or to another party in control of the disposition of a cadaver).

The question is what policy prevails in the absence of express consent to postmortem sperm retrieval. Some American urologists take the position that such sperm retrieval should take place only pursuant to a decedent's express wishes.[34] Yet the issue of postmortem sperm retrieval usually arises in the context of victims of sudden trauma; the decedent's express wishes are seldom available for guidance.[35] For these urologists, a spouse's bare request to have her late husband's sperm retrieved should be rejected. One urologist reportedly turned down eighteen of twenty-two requests over the years for lack of sufficient evidence of the decedent's wishes regarding postmortem parenthood.[36] These urologists reject the premise that any male who had wanted to be a parent "would have wanted to father children from the grave."[37] They would strongly reject any premise that an unattached male normally wishes to become a postmortem father with an unknown woman later to be selected by his parents—and to have the child raised either by his parents or by the unknown woman.

American medical practice does not mirror the strict consent approach adopted by the cited urologists. A number of major medical centers have adopted internal protocols concerning sperm retrieval from cadavers.[38] While a few protocols insist on explicit consent from a decedent, others accept "reasonably inferred consent." This means that the postmortem decision makers project the decedent's unstated wishes by relying on various indices, including the decedent's general wish to have children with the partner, the closeness of the partners' relationship, the presence of other children, and the input of the decedent's parents.[39] The American Society of Reproductive Medicine advises medical personnel that they do not have to honor a spouse's request absent the decedent's prior consent.[40] This position implicitly allows physicians to agree to requests from spouses even in the absence of a deceased's known wishes.

Anecdotal information supports the thesis that some physicians, sympathetic to a mourning spouse (or even a parent), are willing to retrieve sperm from a cadaver.[41] In one previously mentioned incident, a physician extracted sperm at the request of a widow whose spouse had died in an auto accident sixteen days after the wedding.[42] This tendency of physicians to yield to the wishes of a distraught mate (or even a parent) is understandable. It is hard *not* to cooperate with survivors, given their heartrending pleas and given the modest physical invasion of a cadaver entailed. Especially if the survivor who is seeking sperm retrieval is the bonded partner of the deceased, the survivor is desperately trying to honor a loved one and preserve a biogenetic reminder of that person's prior existence.[43]

Yet it is harmful to molest a cadaver in this way unless one can reasonably infer that the decedent would have wanted his sperm to be retrieved. Any disturbance of a corpse contrary to the decedent's projected wishes is a harm to that decedent's interests in prospective autonomy (control over postmortem fate) and in quiet repose. The fact that the decedent wished to someday be a parent does not, by itself, support an inference that he wanted to have sperm extracted from his fresh corpse in order to become a postmortem parent. An inferred wish for postmortem sperm extraction may be more plausible when a bonded partner testifies to a mutual determination of herself and the decedent to procreate together. Even then, some people relish parenthood for the benefits of child rearing and would eschew genetic parenthood without participation in bringing up the child. And when the petitioner for sperm extraction is a prospective grandparent who is searching for an egg provider and a surrogate mother, the claim to be implementing the decedent's wishes is particularly unconvincing. Do young men really want their own parent or parents to choose the mother and nurturer for a never-to-be-known future genetic child?

In September 2007 a twenty-three-year-old Iowa resident was hospitalized moribund following a motorcycle accident. His parents requested that the hospital harvest their son's sperm for subsequent implantation in his twenty-three-year-old fiancée. The wedding had been planned for the summer of 2008, and the engaged couple had intended to have two children. The woman was anxious to become the mother of her fiancé's genetic child; she had spurred his parents to seek retrieval of their son's gametes. The hospital was unwilling to harvest sperm absent an indication of the moribund patient's consent. The hospital also was dubious about whether Iowa law permitted sperm retrieval for reproduction. The parents and fiancée went to court, and an Iowa judge ruled that Iowa's version of the UAGA permitted the parents as next of kin to harvest and donate their son's sperm. The hospital complied with the court's ruling.[44]

The Iowa court's interpretation of the UAGA is surprising and is unlikely to be extended beyond Iowa. The UAGA authorizes the next of kin to make gifts of body tissue for purposes of "transplantation" or "therapy" (the most relevant of the statutory reasons). Commentators had always assumed that a gift of sperm for egg fertilization and implantation did not meet the UAGA's terms—that is, that transplantation was meant to save existing lives, not create new lives.[45] The law professor who was a principal drafter of the UAGA contended in an affidavit in the Iowa case that the UAGA was intended to encompass sperm harvesting within permitted tissue "transplantation." (Even that representation doesn't really show that the Iowa legislators themselves had a similar understanding in mind.) The Iowa case is likely to stand alone—that is, to be *sui generis*, as lawyers are fond of saying. For the UAGA would probably give next of kin too much discretion in giving consent to postmortem sperm retrieval and should not be interpreted to cover cadaveric sperm retrieval.

Going beyond the UAGA as a possible source of a next of kin's authority to request harvesting of sperm from a cadaver, why can't the traditional common law right to control the disposition of a corpse and its parts provide a legal basis for the next of kin? One counterargument is that the next of kin's common law control extends only to final disposal of a corpse (usually burial) or some other explicitly approved use, such as medical research (autopsy) or medical education (dissection), as provided in the UAGA. And a fair reading of the UAGA (especially outside of Iowa) would be that it does not endorse sperm harvesting for reproductive purposes.

As a matter of historical development, though, it appears that the next of kin *did* have a broader common law prerogative in the control of a cadaver than just prompt disposal. Consents by the next of kin to autopsy, dissection, participation in research, taking of bodily mementoes (e.g., a lock of hair), or taking of other relics were apparently honored even before any explicit statutory authorizations of such practices. In other words, the next of kin probably did have the prerogative to dispose of the decedent's body parts in a variety of ways, some of them useful to others, so long as the next of kin were neither violating the decedent's wishes nor unconscionably desecrating the deceased's remains in some fashion. From such a common law legal perspective, it can be argued that the next of kin should be able to control sperm harvesting so long as it does not contradict the decedent's express or likely wishes.

This is probably the actual legal framework applicable to postmortem sperm extraction in the United States today. The UAGA is not dispositive on the issue. As long as the next of kin are not contravening the decedent's explicit or reasonably inferred wishes, they can seek sperm retrieval from their loved one's cadaver. At the same time, such retrieval is a medical procedure, and the next of kin have to convince medical personnel that the extraction is ethically appropriate in the circumstances at hand. Medical professionals will do well to adhere to the policy that postmortem sperm extraction is *unethical* absent a fair inference that the now-decedent would have consented to the postmortem procedure if asked.[46] Normally this means, at the least, a showing of the decedent's bonded relationship with a partner and their mutual intention to procreate together.

The consequences of this narrow policy can be harsh when the decedent is an only child, offering the only hope of grandparenthood and of continuation of a particular biogenetic heritage. To make this hypothetical scenario even more heartrending, add the fact that the decedent's parents have found a willing and able potential surrogate mother (previously childless) who wants very much to use the decedent's sperm and be a mother to his children. Despite the disappointed prospective mother and grandparents, the harsh result seems consistent with preserving a cadaver's postmortem human dignity. Mere speculation about the decedent's likely wishes in such circumstances is too little to warrant interference with the cadaver's quiet repose. Keep in mind that the next of kin in control of the cadaver whose sperm would be harvested often have their own strong personal interests at stake.[47]

**The Female Cadaver as Gestator of a Fetus**

Talk about a cadaver that looks a lot like its live source! Still connected to cardiopulmonary machines, a totally brain-dead cadaver remains warm and pink as a result of continued blood circulation. The chest heaves as the lungs are artificially pumped. And if the female cadaver is carrying a live fetus, the cadaver's artificially maintained organs are capable of gestating that fetus for some period—sometimes to the point where a viable fetus can be removed surgically from the cadaver's womb and saved.

Marie Odette Henderson died three days after surgery for a brain tumor.[48] She was then six months pregnant by her fiancé, Derrick Poole. While Ms. Henderson's parents wanted her cadaver to be disconnected from the life support machinery and buried, Mr. Poole wanted to maintain life support in the hope of salvaging his child. A court supported Mr. Poole. Fifty-three days after her death, Ms. Henderson gave birth to a healthy girl to be raised by her father.

There are approximately a dozen known instances in which a brain-dead pregnant cadaver gestated a fetus for weeks or months until the fetus could be delivered.[49] The earliest one occurred in 1983. The two longest periods of postmortem gestation were 100 days and 107 days.[50] So far as is known, the newborns were generally healthy, though at least one died within days of birth.

Resolving the legal fate of the pregnant cadaver pursuant to constitutional jurisprudence is rather complicated. While alive and mentally competent, a pregnant woman has a fundamental constitutional right to decide whether to carry her fetus to term. That precept of *Roe v. Wade* has prevailed for thirty-seven years. Yet the circumstance of a pregnant cadaver may alter the constitutional picture. A live woman's wish for an abortion prevailed in *Roe v. Wade*—against the father's right to procreate (interest in preserving the fetus) and the state's interest in protecting a prospective life—because of the woman's strong liberty interests in avoiding the burdens of pregnancy and child rearing.[51] A pregnant woman's postmortem interests in parenthood (or its avoidance) are not the same as her premortem interests. The pregnant cadaver will never sense the burdens of gestation and will never have to rear the child in progress. These factors *might* alter the constitutional calculus—giving the biological father a stronger claim to his prospective progeny or giving the state a stronger interest in protecting a prospective life. (In fact, even under *Roe v. Wade*, the state's interest in a prospective life prevailed against a live woman's abortion preference once the fetus had reached viability. Arguably the state's interest in a prospective life might prevail even earlier in a pregnancy when the fetus is within an insentient cadaver—especially when the state's interest is reinforced by that of a biological father who wishes the fetus to be born.)

States have in fact sought to assert their interest in preserving fetal life when a pregnant woman is no longer competent to make her own abortion choice. In at least thirty-six states, statutes purport to invalidate any provision in an advance medical directive (a living will) that dictates a now-pregnant woman's rejection of life-sustaining medical intervention.[52] The object is to keep the fetus alive in the mother's womb even when the pregnant woman had expressed a preference to be allowed to die. The constitutionality of those statutes—at least prior to viability—is dubious and has never been tested. Nonetheless the statutes reflect legislative interest in preserving fetal life in the face of waning maternal life.

One state court precedent acknowledges and upholds paternal and governmental interests in fetal life in the context of a pregnant cadaver.[53] In 1986 a pregnant woman, Donna Piazzi, was found unconscious and not breathing in the restroom of a Georgia mall. She was removed to a hospital, where resuscitation efforts failed. After Ms. Piazzi was pronounced dead in the hospital, her husband requested that her body be disconnected from all medical machinery. But a man claiming to be the biological father of Ms. Piazzi's fetus objected to the disconnection. In the ensuing judicial proceeding, the judge could not discern any prior preference of Ms. Piazzi about continuation of the pregnancy in the current postmortem circumstances. The judge then relied on the state's policy in favor of fetal life, coupled with the biological father's interest in procreation, to order continuance of the medical machinery. After the cadaver spent another six weeks on machinery, a premature baby was delivered, but it died of multiple organ failure within forty-eight hours.

The judge in the case asserted that Ms. Piazzi's constitutional privacy right (meaning the right to end her pregnancy) died with her.[54] That seems to be a highly dubious assertion. If Ms. Piazzi had decided, before her death, that her pregnancy should be terminated in the event of her death, that choice would still be a cognizable aspect of liberty. A decedent has a strong autonomy interest at stake in having personal choices concerning the postmortem disposition of her fetus honored. (Of course, as was the case in *Piazzi*, a now-dead pregnant woman—often the victim of sudden, unexpected trauma—is not likely to have made an actual choice regarding postmortem procreation.) Moreover, a pregnant cadaver has other continuing interests—besides avoidance of the sensed burdens of pregnancy—that were not acknowledged by the judge in *Piazzi*. A pregnant cadaver, like any other cadaver, has traditional interests in bodily integrity, in quiet repose, and in dignified disposition according to her actual or inferred preference. The machine maintenance of a pregnant cadaver entails significant and ongoing bodily intrusions. Weeks or months of insensate functioning as an incubator might also be contrary to some women's concept of a dignified disposition of their corpse. As a matter of constitutional law, there is as yet no authoritative resolution of an insensate pregnant cadaver's interests arrayed against the procreative interests of a biological father and/or an asserted state interest in preserving fetal life.

Resolution of the fate of pregnant cadavers will come not from constitutional dictate but from judicial and/or legislative weighings of the competing interests. One abiding interest is the potential life of the fetus. That interest exists even though the fetus is unborn and perhaps not even viable. (Detection of severe fatal defects destined to result in a brief and tortured existence if the fetus is brought to term might diminish the interest in prospective life, but that would be a very rare scenario.)

A pregnant woman ought to be entitled to determine whether her cadaver will be used to make her a postmortem parent.[55] A policy deferring to a pregnant decedent's actual or reasonably inferred wishes would be consistent with the long American tradition acknowledging a person's prerogative to shape his or her cadaver's handling. A decedent is traditionally entitled to control a cadaver's place of disposition, mode of disposition, availability as a teaching or research subject, and transfer of body parts for transplantation. Similar deference should be accorded to the pregnant decedent's preferences about postmortem gestation and parenthood. Just as the next of kin who are entitled to dispose of a cadaver are expected to implement a decedent's wish to be or not to be an organ donor, or to be or not to be a sperm provider, a similar expectation favoring a decedent's wishes should govern regarding a cadaver's extended gestation of a fetus.

The problem is how to determine the pregnant woman's wishes for disposition of her pregnant cadaver when, as is common, those wishes are not explicit. Because the fatal event is usually unanticipated trauma, the pregnant woman will seldom have thought about, let alone communicated, her attitude toward postmortem gestation and parenthood. And just because the potential mother had become pregnant and had not aborted her fetus up to the time of the fatal trauma, it cannot be assumed that she wanted her cadaver to function as an insensate incubator for weeks or months in order to produce a child that someone else would raise.[56] A number of factors must be examined in projecting the potential mother's attitude toward postmortem gestation. It is necessary to consider the closeness of her relationship with the biological father, her confidence in the economic and emotional parenting ability of the biological father, the prospective family's economic circumstances, the biological father's willingness to undertake single parenthood, the prospective health of the fetus, the potential mother's concept of dignity, and that concept's application to circumstances delaying the quiet repose of a cadaver for weeks or months.[57]

Some circumstances might prompt the conclusion that the prospective mother would want to become a postmortem parent. Her closeness to her spouse or partner and their mutual desire to create a living legacy would support such an inference. A wish to promote a beloved partner's happiness would provide an index of her willingness to continue a pregnancy postmortem.[58] The biological father's eagerness and ability to raise the coming child would be relevant.[59] Also important would be the strength of the prospective mother's confidence in her partner's parenting ability. Or perhaps the pregnant decedent's religious beliefs deemed all fetal life to be sacred. Or perhaps she had strongly wanted to benefit a particular childless couple. All of these factors might tend to support the attribution of a wish for postmortem parenthood to the pregnant decedent.

Other circumstances might point to the conclusion that the pregnant decedent would *not* have wanted to become a postmortem parent, at least not at the expense of bodily exploitation of her cadaver for a period of weeks or months. Perhaps the decedent had a religious belief dictating that all corpses should be promptly buried. Perhaps the biological father was a rapist or simply an irresponsible person ostensibly incapable of raising a child properly. Perhaps the biological father had no interest in supporting and raising the potential infant. Perhaps the financial costs of a lengthy hospital gestation period coupled with additional child-rearing expenses would have a negative impact on the well-being of existing children. Or perhaps the decedent had a strongly developed sense of postmortem dignity that would forbid weeks of mechanical ministrations to an inert cadaver. And what if a sonogram disclosed that the fetus would be born with conditions that would ensure a lifetime of pain, dysfunction, and distress? Such factors could prompt a conclusion that this pregnant decedent would not have wanted her corpse to be suspended in a prolonged limbo resulting in postmortem childbearing.[60]

Attributing to the decedent a position on postmortem gestation would be easier if the prolonged, unremitting medical ministrations to an insensate human cadaver were widely considered per se demeaning and disrespectful. Some people think so. Postmortem gestation has been branded "a mechanical and pharmacological mimicry of what pregnancy should have been."[61] John Robertson speculates about a "dehumanizing effect of allowing a brain-dead woman to serve as an incubator."[62] Some women might view the extreme and lengthy postponement of quiet repose as a degrading reinforcement of a woman's image as primarily a child bearer. If this vision of indignity can be attributed to the pregnant cadaver at hand, an inference could be drawn that this decedent would not want prolonged medical intervention.

While some people might feel that prolonged mechanical invasion of a cadaver is intrinsically degrading, not everyone concurs. Rebecca Bennett argues that because the gestator is now an insentient corpse, the bodily impingements involved are no longer a serious affront to cadaveric integrity.[63] There are indeed situations in which prolonged mechanical connections of a cadaver have at least been tolerated. Families have occasionally refused to acknowledge medical pronouncements of death and have insisted on taking their dead loved ones home tethered to life support machinery for whatever period elapses until the cadaver undergoes cardiac death. I have argued (in chapter 7) that it is acceptable to keep a totally brain-dead potential organ supplier tethered to perfusion machinery for a period until consent to transplant is confirmed and transplantation is undertaken. If the pregnant deceased woman likely would have regarded the mechanical maintenance of her corpse in order to preserve her offspring as a desirable outcome, no offense to intrinsic dignity would exist.

Even if machine maintenance of a pregnant cadaver is not intrinsically undignified, any significant impingement upon the cadaver's integrity is offensive if it is contrary to the deceased's actual or reasonably inferred preference. That is the customary approach to postmortem bodily invasion, as illustrated by organ harvesting. American policy does not override actual or presumed opposition to tissue transplantation even if the invasion would be brief and would result in saving a human life. A major exception is forensic autopsy. There government has decreed that a corpse must answer certain questions even though the interrogation entails gross cadaveric invasions. Keep in mind, though, that in many instances of forensic autopsy the approval of the decedent might be implied because the intrusive autopsy is aimed at apprehending and punishing a murderer.

### Postmortem Parenthood via a Frozen Embryo

The couples involved in creating frozen preembryos are usually seeking to procreate and raise a child or children together. If the gamete producers' relationship breaks down before frozen preembryos are implanted, disputes arise about the fate of the stored preembryos. Usually such disputes occur between parties who have separated or divorced.[64] Typically one party wishes to go ahead and use the frozen embryo for reproduction and the disenchanted other party no longer wants to become a biological parent with this partner. In the cases reported to date, both parties were still alive. But there are also situations in which one of the partners died before a frozen embryo was successfully implanted. In such cases implantation of a frozen embryo—whether in the egg contributor or in a new partner of the sperm contributor—can make the deceased a postmortem biological parent. Fertility clinics then need legal guidance about the disposition of the stored preembryos.

Because of its potential to become a human being, a frozen embryo is judicially regarded as a special entity.[65] An embryo is not considered a

piece of property to be disposed of at the whim of a possessor or a putative owner. Rather, the two gamete contributors are jointly entitled to
determine the fate of the embryo.[66] Even though the female egg contributor has undergone the more arduous process in producing the preembryo, the male sperm provider (a potential biological father) has equal
status in determining the embryo's fate.

The point at which the two gamete producers are allowed to express
their joint wishes for the disposition of extra frozen preembryos generally comes when the fertility clinic agrees to perform an artificial fertilization and implantation process and to store extra frozen preembryos.
The clinic's form lists several options for disposition of the preembryos
in the event of the separation, divorce, or death of one or both parties.
These options typically include continued access to the preembryo for
procreation by one of the parties, destruction, donation to a childless
couple, use in research, or indefinite storage.[67]

This variety of options is appropriate. While the basic object of in
vitro fertilization is for a couple to produce and raise a child together—
an object frustrated by intervening death—subsidiary motives might
prompt agreement to any of the above options. For example, one gamete
producer might want to facilitate the surviving party's access for implantation and procreation, even postmortem, because of a desire to promote
the other party's happiness or to create a biological legacy for public remembrance. Or the producers of a preembryo might favor donation of
excess preembryos to a childless couple, either to altruistically enhance
the lives of others or to prevent destruction of what they consider a life
in being.

One approach to resolution of the fate of a stored preembryo is to
view the documents provided by a fertility clinic and signed by the two
gamete producers as a binding contract. Formation of a binding contract
for the disposition of frozen preembryos has considerable appeal. A
binding agreement might foster certainty and reliance by all parties
without resort to costly, distasteful litigation. It might also prompt
thoughtful deliberation at the outset by the signers. Contracts have been
supported by some commentators.[68] A few courts have expressed willingness to enforce them.[69] The American Society of Reproductive Medicine also urges couples to reach a written agreement (in conjunction with
a fertility clinic) on the subject of ultimate disposition of preembryos.

Such a written agreement would be a way of exercising a person's normal right to decide when and if to become a biological parent.

A contract approach for settling the fate of a preembryo after the death of one of the gamete producers cannot produce absolute certainty in results. Any contract can be subject to legal challenges concerning flaws in formation. A signatory who later resists the contract can contend that the relevant terms were buried in small print, or expressed in unclear language without an explanation, or secured by means of a threat.[70] One fertility clinic's form for cryopreservation took up seven single-spaced pages.[71] Another objection to a contract approach is based on the intensely emotional nature of decisions concerning reproduction.[72] The argument is that certain personal matters—including marriage, surrender of a child for adoption, and surrogate motherhood—are so emotionally sensitive that courts are reluctant to enforce agreements to these matters absent some postevent waiting period for reflection.[73] That argument is then extended to the matter of biological parenthood in order to oppose binding contracts governing the disposition of frozen preembryos.

These arguments against upholding a contract for the disposition of frozen preembryos are not convincing. Contracts have always been salutary devices even though they are subject to challenges concerning flaws in formation. Fertility clinics can learn to present and explain the relevant postmortem provisions in understandable terms. The emotional state of parties who sign a contract for the preservation of preembryos is not so overwrought or delicate as to prevent sensible consideration of the available options. A contract for the disposition of stored embryos is, to my mind, roughly akin to a prenuptial agreement—an emotional subject that nonetheless can and should be the subject of deliberation and agreement. While certain bodily invasions (such as abortion) might not be appropriate subjects for contract and compulsion, no such compelled bodily invasion is involved in a contract governing the disposal of stored preembryos after the death of one of the parties. This is so even if the agreed-upon disposition allows ultimate implantation of an embryo. In the event of a sperm provider's death, a woman can choose to have a preembryo implanted. Her decision to become pregnant at that point is a matter of choice, not compulsion. Nor is compulsion involved following the death of a woman who has contracted to allow her husband to use stored preembryos. The widower might seek to fulfill the contract by recruiting a willing surrogate mother, but no woman (certainly not the dead female) will be forced to gestate or give birth to a child. The widower has an option, not an obligation, to use the stored embryos to become a parent.

The main obstacle to reliance on a contract by gamete producers and the fertility clinic is the judicially created notion that no one should have to become a genetic parent against his or her will. Several courts have expressed this notion in the context of a live party to a contract for disposition of an embryo who is now seeking to change his or her mind and prevent the implantation of the embryo and the birth of a genetic child. These courts have announced a "public policy" against what they call "forced procreation."[74] This public policy supposedly dictates that "individuals shall not be compelled to enter into intimate family relationships."[75] Under this approach, even if a gamete producer had previously agreed to permit implantation of the preembryo, any change of mind should be upheld. Note that these courts do not rely on the financial implications for the now unwilling genetic parent. The judicial objection applies as much to a different infertile couple using the preembryo as to a former partner (cogamete producer). The harm that the judges seem to find is the supposed psychological trauma of being a now-objecting genetic parent (despite having given previous consent).

This notion of psychological damage resulting from being a genetic parent seems silly. I agree with Glenn Cohen that this projected harm is a product of judicial imagination.[76] By analogy, no research shows that women who sell eggs for $8,000 later suffer from being anonymous genetic parents. But even if psychological trauma were in fact associated with genetic parenthood by courts dealing with divorcing or divorced couples, that objection does not apply when the potential objector is dead and postmortem use of a stored embryo is at issue. The decedent who had previously agreed to a life-preserving option for the stored embryo is not afflicted with any guilt or responsibility for being a genetic parent. (Nor can that decedent be harmed by an agreement to allow the preembryo to be used for scientific research.)

In short, the postmortem fate of a stored embryo ought to be determined by mutual agreement of the progenitors at the time when they enlist the services of a fertility clinic. The only real question is what to do when no agreement exists or when an existing agreement is invalid because of flaws in the contract. The answer, I suggest, is already provided in the previous discussion in this volume about the postmortem fate of a decedent's voluntarily stored sperm.

The actual or constructive wishes of the now-dead gamete producer should, if discernible, prevail. In the absence of a decedent's explicit agreement to postmortem genetic parenthood, a frozen preembryo could still be used for procreation so long as the embryo is sought by the bonded person with whom the decedent had, for procreative purposes, produced the preembryo. In the absence of contrary indications, a now-dead embryo producer would be presumed to accept postmortem genetic parenthood. This result seems acceptable because the decedent had at least intended to procreate with the person who is now seeking the embryo for implantation and because no postmortem bodily invasion is entailed.

Other positions have been suggested. One is that if a female is the survivor, she should always have the option of using the stored preembryo for procreation.[77] The justification for this stance is apparently that a female gamete provider has invested more effort in the procreation process—having undergone burdensome uterus stimulation and egg extraction procedures. Moreover, the egg provider may have relied on the prospect of procreating with the now-deceased partner when they entered into their partnership.

Another possible position is pro-life, automatically favoring postmortem utilization of preembryos for procreation. This position can go beyond giving the surviving partner the option to use the preembryo, even to the point of requiring the surrender of the preembryo to a potential adoptive couple. Louisiana has a statute forbidding the destruction of frozen embryos and requiring that disputes about them be resolved in the "best interest" of the embryos—that is, adoptive implantation if available.[78] Of course, a state that elects this strong pro-life policy will likely impel infertile couples to limit the number of extra preembryos created in any in vitro fertilization procedure.

In at least one circumstance, the case favoring access to preembryos for postmortem procreation is strengthened. That is the circumstance in which a surviving gamete producer has no other possibility of becoming a genetic parent.[79] In Israel, Mr. and Mrs. Nachmani had created frozen preembryos in the course of fertilization treatments. An initial implantation failed, and the couple became estranged after the wife underwent a hysterectomy in the course of treatment for an illness. Despite the marital breakdown, Mrs. Nachmani sought access to the couple's preembryos in order to have them implanted in a surrogate birth mother who would turn over the resulting child to Mrs. Nachmani for rearing. The estranged husband objected, but the Israeli Supreme Court ruled in favor of Mrs. Nachmani. Because Mrs. Nachmani had no other way of becoming a genetic parent, the court deemed her interest in procreation to outweigh Mr. Nachmani's objections. The court conditioned Mrs. Nachmani's access to the preembryos on her waiver of any claim to economic support from her resistant spouse. The Tennessee Supreme Court also hinted that it might allow a gamete producer access to preembryos when the prospective parent has no other way to become a genetic parent.[80] The proparent position adopted in the *Nachmani* case is partially attributable to the strong Israeli cultural sympathy for procreation. In England a different approach prevailed. In the wake of a broken relationship, Mr. Johnson withdrew his consent to any procreative use of the preembryos he had created with Ms. Evans. Ms. Evans nonetheless sought access to the stored preembryos because intervening illness had made it impossible for her to become a genetic parent by any other means. She contended that denial of access would violate her fundamental human right to procreation. Ms. Evans's claims were rejected both by the British courts and by the European Court of Human Rights.[81] Those judicial bodies upheld Mr. Johnson's objection to becoming a genetic parent.

In the context of a postmortem dispute about the use of an embryo, I would favor the Israeli approach. When a surviving gamete producer now has no other means of procreation, the survivor's claim for postmortem use of a frozen embryo should prevail—absent proof that the decedent had objected to any prospect of postmortem parenthood—even without the decedent's prior explicit or implied consent to becoming a postmortem genetic parent. Postmortem use of a previously frozen embryo involves no invasion of a cadaver. So long as no economic or social consequences affect the decedent's estate, the minimal "harm" of being a genetic parent is warranted by allowing the survivor access to the only remaining way to become a natural parent.

So much for the diverse ways in which a cadaver can become a genetic parent even without the joys of parenthood. We now turn from the elevated status of postmortem parent to the dismal status of a desecrated cadaver and consider the many ways that people have found to abuse human remains.

# Part IV

# Abuses of the Cadaver:
# What Does Decency Demand?

*Chapter 10*

# Body Snatching, Then and Now

## The Offensiveness of Disturbing Human Remains

The archetype of cadaver abuse is grave robbing. Purloining a human
body or its parts is a serious offense to all interests associated with human remains. While the corpse may not physically sense disturbance to
its sepulcher, "rest in peace" has always been considered an appropriate
approach to disposal of human remains. And because the cadaver is a
powerful symbol of the decedent, its mistreatment strongly affects the
feelings of survivors.

Most Americans have chosen sepulcher—below or above ground—
as a dignified means of final disposal. That a corpse, once decently buried, is entitled to quiet repose is a sacrosanct principle of the American
"legal and cultural fabric."[1] Quiet repose for the cadaver protects the
symbolic presence of the deceased, an undisturbed haven for the soul or
other spiritual presence, and peace of mind for the survivors. In many
subcultures the fate of a soul is affected by the treatment of bodily remains. That is, a soul is deemed to be attached to the body for an un-
specified period after death, so abuse or disinterment interferes with the
deceased's spiritual journey. In America, "Christian sentiment endorsed
the need for permitting the natural decay of the integral body and for its
protection during the process."[2] "Whether or not physical resurrection
would actually take place, [integrity of a buried corpse] served as a met-
aphor for the possibility of providing a secure future for the soul."[3]

Unconsented removal from a chosen resting place clearly breaches
quiet repose, disrupting the integrity of a cadaver and shattering the
peace of mind of close survivors. The offense is exacerbated when, as

was often the case following grave robbing, the purloined body was then mutilated by dissection. Being publicly dismembered and disembow-eled after being maliciously exhumed was an outrage. The desecration continued when dissected remains were cast away as garbage, as often occurred after a dissection. (Note that few physician/anatomists ever do-nated their own bodies for dissection—though philosopher Jeremy Ben-tham did instruct that his body be publicly dissected.) Stealing a cadaver from a grave or snatching cadaver parts was undoubtedly a gross form of cadaver abuse.

## The Legal Response to Body Disturbance

Acts that disrupt traditional norms of respect and dignity for cadavers are not only in bad taste but also are subject to serious legal conse-quences. The first line of legal protection is for the path to the grave—assurance that the surviving family's effort to provide respectful disposal of a corpse is not disrupted. Improper handling that disrupts the funeral routine is traditionally subject to legal liability for the mental anguish caused to survivors. Tort law covers a variety of derelictions that involve negligence in the handling of a cadaver. Any funeral director who loses a corpse—whether by carelessness in transportation or by turning the corpse over to the wrong person for disposition—wrongfully denies the surviving family their opportunity to honor and mourn.[4] A funeral di-rector who forced postponement of a scheduled funeral by preventing a cadaver's transfer to another funeral home for final disposition (while insisting on payment for services rendered) was liable in tort for the mental anguish caused to the next of kin.[5] A pathologist who misidenti-fied remains found after a fire as those of a family's pet rabbit rather than their child (resulting in mutilation of the human remains by animals) was also subject to damages.[6] A funeral home's mistaken release of a ca-daver to his ex-wife (who then cremated the body) rather than to his children for burial was also deemed to be the kind of outrageous wrong-doing that could lead to damages for emotional distress. Indeed, any disposal of human remains contrary to the wishes of the next of kin, even a respectful cremation, constitutes an impermissible interference with the right of sepulcher.

Preventing the next of kin from disposing of remains is a serious harm. Yet in earlier times, such conduct was permissible as a tool for debt collection. Under the British common law, the creditors of a deceased debtor could seize the debtor's cadaver as collateral, hoping that the deceased's family and friends would pay in order to bury the body.[7] Pursuant to the common law's tolerance of this debt collection technique, poet John Dryden's body was seized by debtors in 1780.[8] By the early nineteenth century, though, this device for extracting payment from mourners was no longer legal in England. The distaste for exploiting a cadaver had prevailed.[9]

In America there was little tolerance for the seizure of corpses as debt collateral. Early efforts were apparently made to seize and hold corpses for debt collection in Massachusetts and Rhode Island.[10] Those states and many others then banned that debt collection technique.[11] Judges also deemed funeral parlors to be acting improperly when they sought to delay burial until the funeral expenses were paid. In 1925 in Washington State, such conduct subjected a funeral director to tort liability for infliction of emotional harm and to criminal misdemeanor charges as well.[12] In 1976 a Louisiana court ruled that a funeral home could not hold a corpse until the relatives had paid the $125 fee for preparation of the corpse for burial.[13] Undertakers' charges do become a liability payable by an executor or administrator of a decedent's estate, but the undertaker cannot legally hold the deceased's body to secure payment.

Body snatching was both outrageous—because of disrespect toward the deceased and injury to survivors' feelings—and unlawful. The common law had always deemed disturbance of a grave or a corpse to be an offense against public morals. The precise legal offense might have been abuse of a corpse, desecration of a grave, vandalism, or a disorderly person's violation, but such conduct was always a public offense. Grave robbing was criminally punishable in most jurisdictions from the early nineteenth century on. During the nineteenth century some states made grave robbery a felony, subjecting it to even stiffer penalties than those previously imposed.[14]

American law permits exhumation of corpses, but only for "good and substantial reasons."[15] Adequate justifications for disinterment include investigation of a crime and resolution of civil disputes over insurance or inheritance. Family reasons for exhumation and transfer may also be adequate—for example, if all of the mourners are now located far from the initial resting place. Or a burial place may be shifted to provide a more honorific location, as with memorials for public figures. Land uses may change over time, and burial plots or whole cemeteries may be displaced by roads or public buildings. Respectful transfer of remains is then demanded from public authorities, and descendants can collect for emotional harm if remains are lost or damaged in the process. A man whose sister's and two aunts' remains were lost in a cemetery relocation accommodating a new highway was entitled to damages.[16]

Criminals and poorhouse occupants were deemed to be less entitled to quiet repose than other persons, either because their criminal acts had harmed the public welfare or because indigents had sucked excessively from the public teat. A 1789 New York State statute allowed anatomists access to the cadavers of people who had died in prison or to those of indigents whose representatives could not afford to pay burial expenses.[17] A 1790 federal statute allowed federal judges who imposed the death penalty to add dissection of the remains as a further punishment.[18]

### The Cadaver Shortage That Triggered Grave Robbing

The close relation between medical education and dissection has been recounted in chapter 8. In the early nineteenth century, clinicians who had gone to Europe to further their medical education became the founders of America's first medical colleges. As in Europe, anatomy and dissection became central to medical education. During the considerable expansion of American medical education later in the nineteenth century, an anatomical understanding of the body (achieved in part by dissection) remained important to the medical school curriculum.[19] In addition, practicing physicians and surgeons needed cadavers to improve their own skills.

The continuing emphasis on anatomy and dissection in medical education resulted in a chronic shortage of cadavers in the United States from approximately 1780 to the late nineteenth century. At the outset, the corpses of hanged criminals were the main legitimate source of cadavers for dissection. This source supplied some cadavers each year, but the demand for cadavers was in the hundreds. In 1807 New York's College of Physicians and Surgeons alone needed two hundred cadavers per year and Philadelphia's University of Pennsylvania medical school needed four hundred. (Keep in mind that embalming was at a very primitive stage in that period, and medical students therefore needed more than one cadaver per semester.[20]) In each of the twenty years between 1820 and 1840, Vermont medical schools alone needed approximately four hundred cadavers—of which only about forty could be obtained from executions, leaving a shortage of several hundred to be met by other sources.[21] By the time of the Civil War, eighty-five medical schools (to say nothing of practicing surgeons) needed cadavers for medical training. Between 1865 and 1890 the number of medical schools doubled and the demand for cadavers rose accordingly. It is estimated that by 1878 American medical students needed five thousand cadavers per year.[22]

The unmet need for cadavers in teaching and continuing education meant that some unsavory supply practices had to be undertaken. The most notorious practice was body snatching. People who participated in this practice were variously known as "grave robbers," "resurrectionists," "snatchers," "ghouls," "fishermen," and "sack-em-up men."[23] None of these nicknames was complimentary. The general public regarded body snatching as an abomination.

## The Methodology of Body Snatching (and the Defenses)

Resurrectionists used a variety of methods to procure dissection material. The classic grave robbery took place in the first hours or days after a burial. (After that time, putrefaction hampered or precluded dissection.) Sometimes a fake mourner accompanied the funeral cortege in order to mark the grave (in the face of survivors' efforts to camouflage any recent burial).[24] That night, at the grave, the robbers dug down to the coffin with short wooden spades (to muffle the noise). They then knocked off enough of the lid to drag out the corpse, quietly refilled the hole, and smoothed out the surface dirt to hide the theft.[25] Sometimes the hole did not have to be very deep; a sexton or grave digger had been bribed and had buried the body in loose dirt near the surface.

In some instances resurrectionists were able to avoid the dirty job of grave digging by accessing the corpse before it reached the grave. One way of taking early delivery was by paying a sexton or undertaker to remove the cadaver from the coffin and to substitute weighted sacks. Another early access technique was for the wives of grave robbers to arrive at an almshouse and claim to be long-lost relatives intent on providing a decent burial.[26] The almshouse staff was happy to get rid of the cadaver without adding another resident to its potter's field. Anatomists were happy to receive the corpse without asking questions about its provenance.

After the surreptitious removal of a corpse from its burial place, grave robbers would truss up the corpse, stuff it into a satchel, and transport it as if carrying a sack. That was not the only means of transport, though. The infamous William Cunningham (Old Cunny) of Ohio was a surly, hard-drinking body snatcher whose daytime job was that of a wagon driver. Old Cunny sometimes dressed a stolen corpse in old clothes, sat it upright on his wagon seat, and "conversed" with it on the trip from the cemetery. He successfully marketed bodies to Cincinnati medical schools until he maliciously delivered the corpse of a smallpox victim to student customers. That misstep ended his career. After Old Cunny died, his wife sold his corpse to the Medical College of Ohio for dissection.[27]

The economics of cadaver selling were so appealing that some body snatchers streamlined the process by murdering people in order to market their remains. The model for such an operation was created by the laborers William Burke and William Hare in Edinburgh, Scotland. Over a period of months in 1827 and 1828, the two periodically lured a waif or homeless person to their boarding house. In approximately fifteen instances, Burke and Hare then got the visitor drunk and suffocated him before transporting the remains to anatomists.[28] This process became known as "Burking" people (not to be confused with "Borking," a modern American process of verbal assault and browbeating used by U.S. senators to smother nominees to the Supreme Court). Burke and Hare were caught in 1828 when they murdered Mrs. Doherty, a recent arrival to their boarding house. Scottish authorities tried, convicted, and hung Burke and then handed his body over to physicians for dissection.[29]

Americans also sometimes Burked people. In the early nineteenth century one enterprising funeral director generated business by kidnapping and killing a person before collecting a burial fee from the family.[30] This kind of practice impelled government authorities to require a medically issued death certificate before any disposition of a body. Prospective Burkers were supposed to be deterred by this required medical scrutiny of any corpse. The deterrent did not always succeed. In Cincinnati in 1884 a murderer delivered three victims' bodies to the Medical College of Ohio, receiving $100 in return. In 1886 two men murdered a woman and, posing as funeral directors, delivered the corpse to the University of Maryland's medical school for dissection.[31]

The primary victims of nineteenth-century body snatching were poor people. Anyone who died in a poorhouse or other public institution became fair game for dissection.[32] The supervisors of some poorhouses could be bribed to hand over cadavers for ultimate dissection. These bribed public officials did not necessarily feel guilty about their exploitation of indigents' corpses. Some of them sympathized with the idea of retribution for paupers' drawing from public treasuries,[33] while others emphasized the public gain from receiving cadavers for medical education.[34] By handing over the corpses of indigents, these officials also thought that they were doing a good deed by saving church and private cemeteries from plunder.

Even if the corpse of an indigent made it to the potter's field, its stay was often limited. Paupers tended to be buried in shallow graves with no coffins—easy prey for body snatchers.[35] Unhindered access was assured if the caretaker of the potter's field had had his palm greased in advance.[36] An 1831 Rutgers medical student reported that "whoever bid the highest to induce the keeper of Potter's field to tie up his dogs, get drunk, and go quietly to bed was allowed to monopolize the pauper bodies."[37] Not all of the purloined bodies came from potter's fields. Rural churchyards, scattered family plots in the country, and African American cemeteries were also frequent targets. The low-quality coffins in African American cemeteries, along with civic indifference to African American outrage over body thefts, made these cemeteries more vulnerable than the typical white cemetery.

Americans used various means to defend against body snatchers. All of these measures required some expenditure of resources and so were used primarily by the affluent. When Dr. Philip Syng Physick died in 1837 in Philadelphia, he left instructions on how to thwart grave robbers. His will requested that his corpse be left in a warm room until putrefaction became noticeable and that a guard be assigned to his grave for six weeks.[38] The protective measure of posting a cemetery guard yielded the term "graveyard shift."[39] Another protective device was to install heavy impediments to digging in the vicinity of a grave—a wooden plank or iron slab over the coffin or an iron cage (called a "mortsafe") around the coffin.[40] Inventors came up with all sorts of reinforced coffins using materials such as wrought iron; most of the reinforced coffins, though, were still vulnerable to grave robbers' sledgehammers.

Some cemeteries set up small buildings called "watch houses" where corpses could be stored for weeks until putrefaction made them unusable for dissection. Then the corpses could safely be buried. The houses themselves had to be guarded, but that was easier than guarding a whole cemetery.[41] Poor families adopted a variation on the watch house theme. A family would keep the corpse at home long enough for putrefaction to make it less appealing to dissectors.[42] When the stench became intolerable, the family would bury the body. A good strategy for avoiding grave robbers was to die in summer, when medical classes were not in session and heat accelerated the decomposition of the body.[43]

Attempted theft and ransom prompted extreme measures to protect the remains of Abraham Lincoln. In 1876 a plot to abscond with Lincoln's coffin was foiled only when the coffin had already been partially extricated from its stone sarcophagus. For the next twenty-five years the remains were hidden in cellars and secret burial spots while the public paid homage to an empty sarcophagus.[44] Finally, in 1901, the casket was immunized against virtually any attack by embedding it in steel and concrete six feet below the floor of Lincoln's memorial.[45]

## The Participants in Body Snatching

Medical educators and practitioners were not as offended as the public by the purloining of bodies for educational and scientific purposes.[46] Medical educators saw the corpses as inert, unfeeling objects whose exploitation would make a vital contribution to the advancement of medical education and science. In the minds of some physicians, the only way for an otherwise worthless corpse to recapture some value would be "as an instrument for the advancement of medical knowledge."[47] Said one physician in 1885: "The science of medicine demands the right to dissect human remains to guide it in the relief of human suffering."[48] Medical students shared that belief. Consider this quote from an 1855 medical student: "In the absence of spirit, the body is but the material tenement of man, from which the spirit has fled. . . . It is a piece of inanimate clay that cannot be preserved from instant decay . . . [and should be used to benefit mankind]."[49]

The result of this preoccupation with obtaining cadaveric material was that for approximately 110 years, between 1780 and 1890, medical students as well as medical practitioners sometimes became either direct participants in body snatching or employers of grave robbers.[50] In 1818 Thomas Sewell, a personal physician to three American presidents, was convicted for digging up the body of a young woman for purposes of dissection.[51] In the same period Boston physicians John Warren and Joseph Warren founded and operated a gang of resurrectionists.[52] In New York the founder of Bellevue Hospital and several presidents of the New York Academy of Medicine were implicated in body snatching.[53] In Philadelphia in 1882 authorities exposed a gang of resurrectionists that included physicians and cemetery administrators.[54] By the 1880s body snatching had become a part of the culture in some medical schools—a medical rite of passage.[55] More than one student was caught in the act and bloodied by outraged citizens. In 1824 a Yale medical student was almost tarred and feathered after a stolen body was located in a basement at the medical school.

Many anatomists who needed cadavers would not take the physical and legal risks involved in grave robbing. For them there was always a cadre of professional grave robbers like Old Cunny who could be paid for the goods.[56] During most of the nineteenth century the economic incentives were sufficient to attract some people to grave robbing. A reasonably fresh corpse could bring between $10 and $30—at least a week's wages for an average laborer, even a skilled laborer.[57] The typical grave robber could easily rationalize his misdeed: "People have feelings about it [grave robbing] but if they don't know that the grave is empty they are just as well off and we are a great deal better off."[58] As noted, the economic incentives to provide corpses for dissection were so strong that some cadaver suppliers murdered beggars or other homeless persons to keep the supply flowing.[59]

The economic incentives also prompted entrepreneurship. Some grave robbers developed business networks that shipped cadavers to medical sources in undersupplied states. In 1873 George Christian, a government clerk in the Surgeon General's office in Washington, D.C., operated a grave-robbing and cadaver-shipping business along with four other persons.[60] The stolen bodies were packed in brine in whiskey barrels, rolled to the Army Medical Museum, and shipped to Virginia and Michigan. Christian was caught and sentenced to a year in jail.

**Public Distaste**

During the heyday of body snatching—between 1780 and 1890—the American public considered the practice to be a gross and despicable abuse even if its object was the enhancement of medical knowledge and performance. By instinct, religion, and law, Americans thought that corpses were entitled to quiet repose, so dissection was a sacrilege, a practice contrary to burial customs and morals. They also saw dissection— the cutting up and exposure of a cadaver in front of an audience—as a highly demeaning act.[61] Sometimes the conduct of anatomists reinforced the public's perception of dissection as degradation. In 1835, at the dissection of a hanged pirate, the anatomist gratuitously demonstrated to the audience how an electrical charge could produce twitching in the corpse's lips, fingers, and toes.[62] Some anatomists sold tickets. In 1836 P. T. Barnum arranged a public dissection of an aged African American woman whom Barnum had previously presented live to the public as the 161-year-old former nurse of George Washington.[63] Barnum collected fifty cents per spectator.

American law always reflected the strong public distaste for unauthorized disturbance of a grave. (Authorized disturbance existed because there were a few legitimate reasons, such as public construction projects, for respectfully moving a grave from one place to another.) Criminalization was one mark of public distaste for grave robbing and its accompanying mutilation of cadavers by dissection. Public outrage against anatomists took other forms as well. In 1765 in Philadelphia, when physician/anatomist William Shippen was suspected of grave robbing, a mob stoned his house.[64] Shippen promptly published a disclaimer saying that his corpses for dissection had been obtained from executions, suicides, and "now and then" a potter's field—as opposed to a church cemetery or another private burial ground. In 1788 mobs seeking to reclaim bodies from potential dissectors ransacked the College of Physicians and Surgeons in New York City as well as a medical school in Baltimore.[65]

During the nineteenth century public outrage over dissection continued. There were dozens of riots or ransackings in protest against medical school dissections and/or grave robbing.[66] In 1807 in Baltimore a mob burned down the anatomy hall at the University of Maryland. In 1824 mobs rioted every night for a week against barricaded Yale medical students after a purloined body was found at the medical school.[67] Rioters destroyed medical school buildings at Worthington Medical College in Ohio (1839), McDowell Medical College in Missouri (1844), and Willoughby Medical College in Ohio (1847).[68] In short, the detested scourge of body snatching plagued every state with a medical school at some point during the period from 1807 to 1890 and often produced an outraged public reaction.

## The End of Grave Robbing

The body-snatching business ended by the late nineteenth and early twentieth centuries. Gradual state adoption of "anatomy laws" ensured a lawful supply of cadavers, reducing body snatching "to the level where the interred remained in the ground."[69] The anatomy laws allowed medical schools to take possession of unclaimed cadavers from poorhouses, workhouses, and other public institutions. In other words, paupers continued to be the main source of dissection material, but their corpses no longer had to be stolen from the grave.[70]

Massachusetts enacted the first anatomy law in 1831. Over the next 120 years other states gradually adopted similar laws. The medical establishment pushed for such laws, emphasizing the need to end grave robbing and touting anatomy laws as the solution. In 1878 a scandal erupted when the body of John Scott Harrison, the seventy-four-year-old son of President William Henry Harrison and himself a former congressman, was stolen from its mausoleum. It reappeared at the Medical College of Ohio.[71] The ensuing uproar helped spur Ohio to adopt an anatomy law in 1881; Vermont and Virginia followed in 1884. As of

1958, forty-four states provided that unclaimed corpses could be delivered to a state anatomical board, a medical school, or a physician for study.[72] Many states still authorize the transfer of unclaimed cadavers to institutions for the "advancement of health science."

Isolated grave robbing continued into the twentieth century. By 1913 among the only states without an anatomy law were four states with large African American prison populations—Alabama, Louisiana, North Carolina, and Tennessee.[73] Even there, executions or deaths in custody did not meet anatomists' needs. As late as the 1920s, grave robbers still sold bodies to Nashville's four medical schools.[74] (Tennessee passed its anatomy law only in 1947.) But the widespread phenomenon of grave robbing had been rendered obsolete by the nineteenth-century anatomy laws. Today most cadavers for medical education and research are willed by decedents, or contributed by relatives, or legally expropriated by medical schools pursuant to still-existing anatomy laws.[75]

**Modern Body Parts Snatching**

The demise of grave robbing to supply dissection material did not end all efforts to steal bodies and body parts for personal gain. In scattered instances, people have continued to try to remove buried human remains. Sometimes the motive has been to extract a ransom for return of the remains. In 1977 four men attempted unsuccessfully to steal the remains of Elvis Presley from its marble mausoleum and ransom them.[76] Occasionally body snatchers have had spiritual rather than financial objectives. In 2004 members of an occult religious sect were arrested for breaking into graves in two Newark, New Jersey, cemeteries and stealing skulls and other bones.[77] Cult members wanted to use the purloined remains in their religious rituals.

A modern version of body snatching has surfaced in the context of supplying cadaveric tissue for transplant. Over the last twenty-five years crooks have found ways other than grave robbing to divert corpses from their intended dispositions and to steal body parts for the purpose of sale. Recall (from chapter 7) that advances in immunosuppressive drugs and transplant techniques have created a thriving market for transplant tissue removed from cadavers—a market supplemented by the demand for body parts from researchers, educators, and sellers of medical technology. Though the sale of tissue for profit is supposedly prohibited, middlemen/tissue processors extract considerable sums by charging the ultimate users for testing, processing, storage, and transport. While transplant tissue from cadavers is usually obtained legitimately by donation from testators or relatives of the deceased, some people with access to cadavers steal whole cadavers or body parts in order to increase the flow of marketable tissue. This practice has gone on since the 1980s, and the perpetrators tend to be people who work in medical schools, morgues, funeral homes, or crematories.[78] A diener (helper at an autopsy), a person in charge of donated bodies at a medical school, an owner or worker at a funeral home, and any worker at a crematory has many opportunities to purloin body parts and cover up the theft.

A notorious funeral home owner, David Sconce, was convicted of stealing body parts in 1986 in Pasadena, California. He used two techniques. He either carved up and plundered bodies destined for cremation—after the wake or funeral ceremony had been held—or he tricked family members into signing consent forms and then harvested tissue from the deceased. Affected customers did not sense any deficiency in the ashes they ultimately received or did not notice the alterations to corpses in closed caskets.[79] Another notorious figure in the funerary industry was Michael Brown, owner of a crematory in Lake Elsinore, California. Between 1999 and 2001 Brown and his staff systematically disassembled cadavers that were handed over for cremation. In one of his back rooms, Brown had freezers filled with various body parts (including heads, torsos, and knees). In 2003 Brown plead guilty to sixty-six counts of mutilation of human remains.[80]

Managers and workers in willed body programs at several medical schools have, over the years, diverted corpses for sale to research facilities or other customers. In the mid-1980s two employees at the University of Pennsylvania medical center were disciplined for selling human heads for $150 each to a local ear, nose, and throat doctor.[81] Between 2000 and 2003 Allan Tyler at the University of Texas Medical School in Galveston sold dozens of donated corpses to middlemen tissue processors, who cut them up and sold the parts. Tyler reported to the university's administrators that the corpses were damaged and unusable.[82] A similar operation was uncovered at the UCLA Medical School in 2004. Between 1998 and 2004 Tulane Medical School sold donated bodies to the U.S.

Army for research even though they had been donated for medical school purposes.[83] Outraged relatives of affected decedents sued for fraud, breach of contract, and intentional infliction of emotional harm.

The uncontested champion of twenty-first-century body snatching is Michael Mastromarino. He is a former New Jersey dentist who in 2001 set up a company, Biomedical Tissue Services (BTS), in Fort Lee, New Jersey, to exploit the contemporary demand for body parts of cadavers. BTS, through Mastromarino, made deals with numerous funeral directors in New York City, Rochester, New York, Philadelphia, and northern New Jersey. BTS paid the funeral director a "facility fee," and in return the director notified BTS when an appropriate cadaver was available.[84] BTS then dispatched a crew to the funeral home that carved up the cadaver in the embalming room. The crew substituted PVC pipe or other materials in order to deceive any subsequent viewers of the corpse. Funeral home owners or employees were paid to forge both death certificates and donation consent forms. BTS sold all sorts of raw tissue to tissue processors in a national network supplying body parts to surgeons, hospitals, and researchers. One of those processors was Regeneration Technology Inc. (RTI), a major player in the field. Between 2001 and 2006, BTS cut up hundreds of cadavers and sold thousands of body parts.[85]

The BTS body parts operation was particularly heinous because of the health risks for tissue recipients. BTS did not properly screen tissue for communicable diseases and infections, creating the risk of transmitting hepatitis, syphilis, cancer, or HIV. False blood samples further masked the presence of possible disease. BTS also gave the processors/distributors false information concerning the age of the "donor," the cause of death, and the time that had elapsed between death and tissue harvesting—variables that could affect the suitability of tissue for transplant. One well-known victim was former media personality Alistair Cooke. Cooke died at age ninety-five from lung cancer. Bone was harvested from his corpse by a BTS operative, and the documents accompanying the transfer stated that the bone came from an eighty-five-year-old man who had died of a heart attack.[86]

Once BTS was exposed in 2006, no one had trouble perceiving the horror of its operation. Criminal charges were filed against Mastromarino and more than a dozen funeral home operators. Mastromarino initially pleaded not guilty and was released on $1.5 million bail. In March 2008 he changed his plea and in May of that year he received a sentence of eighteen to fifty-four years in prison. At least seven funeral home operators have also pleaded guilty and face prison terms.[87] The criminal charges included body stealing, forgery, mutilation of a corpse, and grand larceny. One funeral director who cooperated with BTS approximately seventy-five times—Stephen Finley of Newark, New Jersey—pleaded guilty to one count of desecrating a corpse and was sentenced in June 2009 to five years in prison.[88] Beyond the criminal charges, hundreds of civil suits seeking money damages have been filed against BTS and RTI, the main processor of BTS-supplied tissue. Some claimants are family members who seek damages for the emotional upset from the knowledge that a loved one's corpse had been carved up and body parts taken without authorization. Some claimants are tissue recipients who seek compensation for the emotional anxiety associated with having received possibly defective tissue. Nine claimants allege that they contracted hepatitis from the transplanted tissue.

It is doubtful that these disgruntled transplant recipients or relatives of plundered cadavers will get much monetary relief from the body snatchers associated with BTS. BTS and Mastromarino, while unquestionably guilty of tortious conduct, are probably judgment proof—that is, without assets to pay off prospective financial recoveries. Nor did insurance cover their misdeeds. The major tissue processor, RTI, is a defendant accused of negligence in accepting the false documentation, including consent forms, from BTS. RTI contends, however, that it has always used a sterilization process that prevents transmission of harmful tissue. If this is true, it might diminish the recovery for emotional anxiety associated with the implantation of possibly contaminated tissue.

> To desecrate a corpse is, in an intangible way, to desecrate a
> person, even though the person we knew is no longer "there."
>
> D. Gareth Jones, "Use of Bequeathed
> and Unclaimed Bodies"

*Chapter 11*

# Desecration of Human Remains

Since time immemorial, the human cadaver has been regarded as a sacrosanct entity entitled to dignity and respect. Because of the human aspects of cadavers—whether due to their human origin or to the continuation of a deceased's memories in survivors—the concept of dignity has extended to the treatment of cadavers. As noted in chapters 2 and 3, society protects interests in postmortem bodily integrity as an element of postmortem human dignity. In the Anglo-American tradition, families take possession of their relative's cadaver for the purpose of providing a respectful final disposition—usually after funerary rites (such as a wake, visitation, or memorial service) mourning and honoring the departed. The family is normally entitled to receive the body in the same condition in which it existed at the time of death, that is, without disturbance by incisions, punctures, or probes. Mistreatment that communicates debasement of the main symbol of the deceased is the antithesis of the respectful treatment supposedly due to every cadaver.[1]

### Disrespectful Neglect

Even without active physical disturbance of human remains, various types of conduct can degrade the dignity of a corpse enough to qualify as abuse. Simply failing to dispose of a cadaver in a decent way is an offense to social sensibilities that subjects the (non)actor to damages and/or criminal prosecution. The well-meaning intentions of the actor do not excuse the conduct. There are many stories of families keeping the cadavers of loved ones at home for excessive periods in the vain hope that a miracle would restore life. An Illinois family kept the father's corpse in their house for eight years (presumably with the aid of air fresheners), and an Oklahoma man kept his mother's body at home for four years.[2] A religious cult leader in New Mexico believed that corpses must be kept in their natural state in order to facilitate reincarnation.[3] When a nineteen-year-old congregant died of natural causes, the leader kept the unembalmed body in a house for eight days wrapped in plastic sheeting, followed by twenty-two days in a shed in the yard. The court conceded that no mutilation or physical mistreatment had occurred, but it found that the cult leader's well-meaning conduct violated standards of public decency and was criminal. The judge would not accept "sincere but erroneous religious belief" as an adequate justification for the improper handling of the corpse.

Neglect rather than purposeful physical mistreatment can also be a criminal offense for a professional who is supposedly engaged in disposing decently of cadavers. Lewis Howell, owner of a mortuary in Jackson, Florida, left forty-four decomposing bodies stacked in closets. His explanation for the mishandling—that paperwork had backed up, delaying correct disposition—was unconvincing to authorities.[4] The record for professional neglect belongs to Ray Brent Marsh, the manager of Tri-State Crematory in Georgia. Marsh left hundreds of moldering, uncremated bodies scattered and stacked in woods and structures on his property. He was indicted on 787 felony counts, pleaded guilty to fraud, theft, and abuse of a dead body, and was sentenced to twelve years in jail.[5] His attorney, pointing out that Marsh had not physically abused the corpses and that they were not live humans, called the sentence "a bit of overkill." The families of the 226 identified corpses meanwhile sued for $80 million. The insurers of funeral homes that had used Tri-State Crematory paid $36 million. There was no word on recovery from Marsh's own insurer.

Professionals responsible for the decent disposition of human remains sometimes make unintended mistakes so injurious to the dignity of a cadaver that the offended loved ones can collect for the mental anguish suffered. In one case, a New York City embalmer so botched his job that the corpse appeared at the viewing decomposed, swollen, and distorted. Shocked relatives collected damages for the trauma. In another case, staff at Brooklyn State Hospital in New York City mislabeled the cadavers of two elderly patients, Ms. Lott and Ms. Tumminelli, who had just passed away. The Jewish Ms. Lott was embalmed, laid out for a viewing, and decorated with a crucifix at a Roman Catholic funeral home. The Catholic Ms. Tumminelli ended up wrapped in a plain shroud in an Orthodox Jewish funeral home. Each family collected damages from the state for the mental anguish flowing from the offense to their respective creeds and emotional sensibilities.[6] In such instances the careless actors had no malicious intent to demean the human remains being handled, yet the attendant indignities were offensive enough to be actionable.

The same principle prevailed in numerous other cases where mishaps affecting a corpse resulted in indignity to the corpse and anguish to the relatives. Bodies can roll out on the floor when a casket lid is insecure, or a casket falls apart, or the handles fall off, or pallbearers carelessly drop the casket. Even though the actors have no malice toward the cadaver, the mistake may be deemed to be egregious enough to allow mourners to collect damages for emotional suffering. In many jurisdictions damages for mental anguish from unintentional mistreatment of a corpse depend on whether a jury labels the mistreatment "outrageous."[7] Juries are less prone to grant such awards when the mishap only causes the corpse to tumble within its casket (as opposed to spilling out on the ground or otherwise being abruptly exposed). For example, when mishaps occur and the coffin is pitched headlong into the grave, juries tend to forgive the disarrangement of the corpse within its container.[8]

## Mutilation of a Corpse

Physical destruction of a cadaver often carries some distasteful connotation. With the possible exception of cremation, virtually every mutilation of a corpse evokes an initial sense of disgust that sometimes helps to identify abuse. Even an anatomy student dutifully dissecting a donated cadaver may be troubled by a gnawing sense of wrong in destroying a human body.[9]

Perhaps the ultimate offense to postmortem human dignity is mutilation of a cadaver in a contemptuous way. Over time physical abuse of a cadaver as an expression of contempt has appeared in numerous contexts. Military history is replete with soldiers mistreating fallen enemy soldiers—not just by leaving their bodies to rot or piling them into unmarked pits, but also by desecrating their corporeal remains. Victors in battle have cut up a dead enemy's corpse in order to disgrace the fallen foe, or to distribute morale-boosting memorabilia to the victorious soldiers, or to publicly brandish symbols of a military accomplishment.

Carving up an enemy's cadaver in order to take home a corporeal souvenir has been an accoutrement of much American warfare. Soldiers have kept ears, noses, fingers, penises, and other body parts for such memorabilia.[10] In the nineteenth century Native American warriors were notorious for sometimes scalping their victims. Sioux and Cheyenne warriors beheaded some of General George Armstrong Custer's dead troops and flaunted the severed heads on stakes during victory celebrations.[11] During the Civil War some soldiers shaped the skulls of fallen enemy soldiers into bowls or cups.[12] During World War II, marines in the Pacific made letter openers and rings out of Japanese soldiers' bones. That unfortunate conduct prompted a 1942 Pacific command communiqué warning against such desecration of enemy remains.[13]

While not strictly classifiable as military conduct, sectarian violence motivated by religious or racial hatred often results in gross mistreatment of victims' corpses. In 2006 in southeast Nigeria, Christian youths butchered Muslim residents with machetes and then burned the corpses in piles. Sectarian killing has also often prompted unceremonious dumping of bodies into unmarked pits, as occurred in Rwanda, Kosovo, and Croatia not many years ago. Nazis' atrocities toward their victims' corpses are well documented, with mass burning in crematoriums being a favored methodology. The Nazis sometimes disposed of the remaining ashes by combining them with other substances to form road paving material. In the United States, racist southern lynch mobs sometimes burned African American victims after cutting them down or dismembered a victim's corpse after beating the victim to death.[14] In late-twentieth-century "lynchings," racially motivated killers dragged African American victims' corpses behind vehicles until they were totally mangled.

One might think that murdering a person would sufficiently vent the rage, jealousy, or whatever obsession motivates a killer or killers. Clearly this is not so. Innumerable American episodes show murderers exacerbating their crimes by physically dismantling or otherwise defiling their victim's corpse. Sometimes a murderer dismembers a corpse in an effort to hide the *corpus delicti*. Rory Thompson dismembered his wife's corpse and flushed the remains down the toilet. (Recall also the ex-wife mentioned in chapter 5 who, after arranging a brief church service over her ex-husband's ashes, promptly flushed the ashes down the church's toilet.) The murderer Ivan Poderjay smuggled his wife's corpse into his cruise ship cabin, which was strategically located just above the waterline. He then spent his honeymoon slicing pieces from her body and feeding the flesh to the fish; later he dumped the skeleton overboard.[15] A Tennessee murderer, seeking to make the victim's cadaver disappear from the victim's home, tried a variety of ways to dismantle it. First, he sought to feed the corpse to a resistant Doberman, then he tried to dynamite the remains (but only split them in two), and finally he doused the house with gasoline and set it on fire.[16] Despite this herculean effort to disguise the murder, bones remained among the cinders and the killer was apprehended.

Serial killers have frequently aggravated their misdeeds not only by sexual exploitation of victims' cadavers (necrophilia will be addressed shortly), but also by various other forms of physical defilement.[17] Serial killers, like deranged victorious soldiers, have cut off body parts as useful or decorative souvenirs—including ears as bookmarks, female breasts as paperweights, and human lips on a string. Serial killer Ed Gein fashioned clothes from the skin of female victims and constructed furniture from the bones of victims.[18]

## The Variables of Postmortem Human Indignity

While an overriding principle in the disposal of human remains is to uphold what I call postmortem human dignity—a modicum of respect for human remains—maintaining a modicum of dignity does not always require preservation of the physical integrity of a cadaver. From an aesthetic perspective, there is no pleasant way of disposing of a human corpse. Various forms of disposition—including the most common, burying or burning—are all "a little disagreeable," to quote Mary Roach.[19] The prospect of physical disintegration, whether by putrefaction or other means, is not the main determinant of a cadaver's dignity. While malicious dismemberment of a cadaver (as by a murderer intent on hiding or defiling a victim's remains) is an abomination, not all mutilation of a cadaver is performed in a degrading manner and not all dismantling of a corpse constitutes desecration. The mangled physical state of a cadaver—even if a seemingly repulsive sight—cannot be the sole factor in assessing the dignity or indignity of a form of body disposal.

Postmortem human dignity, like many aspects of human dignity, is in large part a construct of social mores. In most instances, the *acts* of disposition (including destruction of a cadaver) are neutral and are labeled as dignified or undignified in the context of the acts, the motives and messages of the actors, the preferences of the deceased, and the traditions and practices of the relevant culture.

Burning a corpse is a good example of how diverse factors determine the dignity and acceptability of destruction of a corpse in the course of its disposition. Cremation can be a perfectly suitable mode of disposal when it is desired by the deceased or the next of kin and conducted in a respectful manner. Without such authorization and respectful treatment, the burning of a corpse can be an outrage. If burning is done in a disrespectful manner, the conduct may be unlawful. After Frank Bradbury's sister died of natural causes at his home, Bradbury shoved her body into his basement furnace, where it was consumed. A Maine court found the conduct to be a criminal offense not because of the burning, but because the manner of disposal outraged the "feelings and natural sentiments of the public."[20] Rioters who torch the bodies of their victims are adding a gratuitous desecration to their crimes. Incineration of body parts (even after an authorized autopsy) may violate the creed of the deceased and his or her family (i.e., a religious belief requiring the integrity of cadaver parts) and may constitute a significant legal wrong causing compensable emotional harm.[21]

The history of dissection of corpses for educational purposes illustrates how ambiguity can attach to destructive disposal of a corpse even in its most ostensibly repulsive forms. The cultural perception of the practice has changed remarkably over the centuries. Dissection (anatomization) was, from the fifteenth century on, widely regarded as a repulsive form of body disposal. The public process involved mutilation, dismemberment, disembowelment, and tossing of the effulgent remains into large buckets. The stench was horrible. The spilling of excrement and blood was disgusting. The dissection process was considered utterly degrading and was reserved for the dregs of society—executed criminals, Jews, other infidels, or foreigners. Later, in America, the process utilized prisoners who had died in jail or in some other institution, including almshouse residents whose bodies were unclaimed. In 1885 a physician commented that no self-respecting physician would donate his own body for dissection, given the degradation of lying naked and being probed before a crowd of vulgar, joking students.[22]

The mangling of a corpse by dissection has, over time and circumstance, achieved a measure of dignity and respect. Dissection is no longer intrinsically undignified if performed with appropriate authorization and in accord with the protocols now governing medical education. The modern version of dissection in medical school instruction is still a violent process of slicing, sawing, shearing, and cutting, ultimately reducing each cadaver "to a shambles of muscle and bone, cut away and divided."[23] Despite the gross dismantling of the cadaver, modern dissection is not considered a particularly degrading or undignified process. Today enough people donate their remains to science so that the cadavers reach the anatomy lab with the consent of the great majority of the deceased. Decedents' willingness to consent flows from continued recognition of the importance of the educational mission and from steps now taken to respect the postmortem human dignity of the corpse.

Today every American medical school strives to respect the cadavers donated for dissection. Anatomy students are supposed to show constant respect to their dissection subject and to its disassembled parts. The naked cadavers are covered whenever exposure is unnecessary, and the investigated body parts are held for respectful disposal rather than careless discard. Clearly a respectful student attitude cannot always prevail. Stories are legion about the jokes and pranks that medical students traditionally engaged in—often posing the subject cadaver in positions or with accoutrements that were demeaning. Humorous photos, cartoons, and jokes about anatomy labs appeared in medical school yearbooks until the mid-1970s. Laughter in an anatomy lab may be inevitable as students seek to relieve their tension, but there is a fine line between easing tension and disrespecting the humanity of a corpse.[24] Medical schools make a concerted effort to educate students in decorum, and a common practice today is for each class to conduct a formal ceremony of remembrance and thanks to the donors and their cadavers. The educational or scientific objects, along with consent and respectful treatment, render a corpse's ostensible abuse in the anatomy lab tolerable. The evolution of dissection shows how the annihilation of a corpse can still be done with consideration for cadaveric dignity.

## Justifications for Ostensible Mistreatment

Certain circumstances can justify the rough physical treatment of a corpse. For example, violent efforts at resuscitation after cardiac arrest may end up battering a corpse and breaking bones. That rough physical treatment is warranted (in the absence of a Do Not Resuscitate, or DNR, order) because the object is to salvage a person not yet known to be dead. (By analogy, consider how open-heart surgery damages a person's physical structure but is justified by the life-preserving objective.)

A variety of public interests have traditionally justified what would otherwise be intolerable mutilation of a cadaver. One example is the forensic autopsy authorized by state laws when the cause of death is uncertain. As described in chapter 8, these autopsies involve severe violations of bodily integrity; pathologists open the torso, cut loose and examine internal organs and tissue, open the skull, and remove the brain for examination. Yet these disturbing corporeal invasions and disfigurement are legally and morally sustainable as tools in solving crimes and investigating important public health conditions. A forensic autopsy is not done routinely just because the cause of death is uncertain. It is undertaken when public inquiry is particularly warranted, such as when criminal conduct needs to be investigated.

The bodily intrusions of forensic autopsy are not only limited to certain justifications, they must also be performed in a manner consistent with the stated justifications. That is, the dismantling of a cadaver is supposed to be limited to the steps necessary for the particular forensic purposes at hand. A forensic autopsy does not ordinarily include removal of tissue beyond the small samples necessary for forensic testing purposes.[25] Tissue kept for evidentiary purposes in later legal proceedings can only be retained as long as needed for the proceedings. Most body parts examined at autopsy are supposed to be returned promptly to their body cavities (albeit tied in a bundle). The cadaver can then be reclaimed by the next of kin for respectful disposition—usually interment of the cadaver with all parts still inside.[26] Unnecessary removal, retention, or destruction of cadaver parts can subject pathologists to significant liability to distressed relatives.[27] Professional standards of medical examiners define the scope of necessity.[28] If the autopsy goes beyond authorized bounds, the offense of "impermissible mutilation" has been committed even if the pathologists intended no disrespect toward the cadaver or the family.

Another possible justification for "abuse" of a cadaver might be necessity—a situation in which the offensive conduct is critical to save a life. Ordinarily a mass anonymous burial of corpses is an atrocity. The Nazis, aiming at efficiency and degradation in the disposal of human remains, desecrated despised corpses by burying them in mass graves. In numerous wartime ghettos, people daily collected piles of bodies in wagons and transported them for mass burial. At Andersonville, a Confederate military prison during the Civil War, a mule-drawn wagon dumped twenty to thirty prisoners' bodies per day into burial trenches, closing each trench when it contained one hundred corpses. The name and unit of each corpse were supposed to be noted, but this seldom happened. Thirteen thousand soldiers' corpses received this degrading mass disposal at this one location.

Mass burial can sometimes be necessary to avert lethal dangers. When the unidentified victims of mass disasters are placed in a common grave, the message and meaning are very different from those of the degradation accompanying atrocities. Avoidance of contagion rather than disrespect for the victims then accounts for the mass disposal of remains. Sometimes a memorial marking the site of a mass burial is ultimately erected as a belated gesture of respect for the anonymous victims.

Another situation in which repulsive disposition of cadavers might be considered necessary is when starving survivors devour the flesh of dead compatriots. Eating dead human flesh is not intended as degradation when stranded survivors take that step as a last means of survival. Can such necessity justify the otherwise deplorable action? (In order to avoid a further moral dilemma, assume that the eaten survivor had died of natural causes.) In a number of instances in famine-stricken countries, starving residents overcame their normal abhorrence of cannibalism in order to sustain themselves by eating the flesh of dead neighbors. This occurred in China, India, the Ukraine, and Nigeria at particular moments in the last 250 years.[29] More isolated instances of cannibalism for survival purposes have occurred among plane crash victims or others stranded without means of sustenance.

A starving person's ingestion of the flesh of other humans who have died of natural causes is understandable and probably forgivable. Killing and then eating a victim, even as a means of self-preservation, is much more problematic. The action is at least theoretically defensible under a legal doctrine of unavoidable necessity. The legal claim is that otherwise unlawful behavior can be excused if it is shown to be the result of a genuine and immediate threat to an actor's life. The question of whether this form of homicide under duress—cannibalism by a starving cosurvivor—is legally excusable has seldom been addressed. In one classic British case, the court ruled that the killing and eating of an already dying raft occupant was not excusable. The court's fear was that all sorts of necessitous circumstances could be imagined and that no legal system could reliably demarcate the boundaries of a necessity defense for killing. That conclusion has been criticized, but no authoritative decisions have upheld a supposedly necessary cannibalistic killing.

## Motives and Messages of the Mishandlers of Cadavers

Ostensibly repugnant modes of cadaver disposal can vary in acceptability according to the intentions of the people disposing of a cadaver and the cultural understandings surrounding the conduct. Exposing a corpse as prey to animals provides an illustration. When the intention of the conduct is to degrade and disrespect the decedent, the appropriate reaction is revulsion. What could be more vile than gibbeting—hanging an executed criminal's naked cadaver exposed in an iron cage until birds of prey and insects devour the remains? In ancient Egypt, the corpses of slaves, cripples, and the poor were carried into the desert and left as prey for the hyenas, wolves, and jackals. In such circumstances, delivering the corpse to animals of prey seems to be a rather demeaning disposition.

Yet a number of cultures, with no connotation of disrespect toward the deceased, have used exposure to animals and the accompanying skeletonization as an efficient way to dispose of human remains and speed the soul's journey onward. Over time, cultures have used sharks, fish, hyenas, vultures, termites, crocodiles, dogs, and alligators as facilitators of the last journey. Some Native American tribes placed their dead on high platforms to be eaten by birds and animals. Some Parsees of India place corpses on high towers in order to have the flesh devoured by vultures within hours. The point is that the dignity of the corpse and acceptability of the means of disposal can vary greatly, depending on the attitudes or intentions of the people carrying out the disposal process and the cultural beliefs underlying the conduct.

There have been societies in which survivors' ingestion of the decedent's body parts—particularly the heart and the brains—was a mark of respect. The survivors were seeking to absorb the positive attributes of the diseased by ingesting the flesh of the cadaver—"to incorporate the essence of a loved one into [a successor's] body."[30] Buddhist monks have been known to ingest flesh as a tribute to a fallen comrade and in an effort to incorporate some of the prized qualities of the deceased. Tribes in the Amazon and in New Guinea have had such funerary customs. The practice backfired for one tribe in New Guinea in the 1950s. By eating the brains of deceased relatives, the tribe passed on a lethal disease and prompted a wave of deaths. The brain-eating practice promptly ended.[31] Public health might dictate that the practice of ingesting remains be forbidden. But it is interesting that the practice is not necessarily intended as a desecration of human remains; in certain circumstances, it could be intended and even understood as a compliment to the deceased.

Motives matter in the handling of cadavers, but motives that are thought to benefit the interests of the cadaver may not, by themselves, salvage what would otherwise be unacceptable cadaver abuse. An example is the dismantling of a corpse in order to preserve it, or parts of it, for enshrinement as an object of veneration. Extraction of bodily relics from the cadavers of saintly figures has a long religious history. Many churches in Italy house ancient hearts, hands, bones, blood, or skin preserved as an act of exalting and honoring a departed personage (to say nothing of the object of attracting tourists to the local cathedral).[32] Religions other than Roman Catholicism have given similar treatment to body parts. When the cultural tradition accepts the taking of cadaveric relics as an honorific form of cadaver disposal, and if the "honored" decedent would not have objected to the dismemberment of his or her corpse, the taking of relics is not intrinsically demeaning. So long as the now-deceased figure was an adherent of the religious tradition expressed, it is probably safe to assume that he or she would not have objected to having a body part become a religious relic.

The benevolent intentions of admiring survivors who seek relics or mementos of the deceased probably make the practice tolerable, but there has to be a limit. Suppose that a deceased's relative wants tissue from the cadaver to serve as a handy memento or as part of a prospective shrine. This occurred in 2008 in an American hospital when a young man asked for a vial of his dead mother's blood to make it part of a planned home shrine. The hospital initially worried about the ethics of extracting and handing over this corporeal tissue (blood). Upon reflection, and upon confirmation of the son's motives and intentions, the hospital fulfilled the request, assuming that the mother would not have objected to the unusual form of remembrance. Suppose, though, that the request had been for a finger, toe, or heart as a relic. Or suppose that there were many admirers or worshipers, each interested in obtaining a memento of the deceased. To my mind, a bodily memento is not per se so intrinsically undignified as to be categorically forbidden. The hospital's decision to extract and provide the vial of blood seems right. Would I feel the same way about a preserved breast or penis? Perhaps not. Yet I am not sure what, other than a sense of good taste or decorum, differentiates a lock of hair or a vial of blood from a finger.

The motives of actors in their treatment of cadavers may sometimes be ambiguous. William R. Maples recounts that a former museum curator had left his skeleton to the museum's bone collection.[33] But the museum staff did more than display the skeleton. They brought it to Christmas parties and bedecked it with tinsel and ornaments. Maples classifies this conduct as a mark of respect and affection for a departed colleague. Others might see it as demeaning and disparaging. Did the testator/curator want his bones only to be a lasting part of an educational exercise and would he therefore be offended by the frivolous trimmings? The actual attitude of the staff—admiring or derogatory—would go far in characterizing the acceptability of their conduct.

People with clearly malevolent motives and derogatory messages in regard to a deceased may seek to bring their vitriol directly to the setting of disposal of a cadaver. In 2006 representatives of the Westboro Baptist Church of Topeka, Kansas, sought to picket with signs at burial services for military casualties of the Iraq war.[34] Their appearances at funerals were part of a church campaign to express outrage at certain American public policies. The demonstrators sought to tell the bereaved families that their son or daughter had been struck down by God. God's wrath, in turn, had supposedly been triggered by "America's unwillingness to condemn gay people and their lifestyles."

These distasteful messages outraged not just mourners, but also the public and state legislators, who saw the demonstrators as interfering with "a right to bury a loved one in peace."[35] The legal problem with legislation to suppress the offensive demonstrators was that the U.S. Constitution protects the expression of hated ideas—even the notion that these fallen soldiers died not just because of war but as God's punishment for America's moral laxity. One state legislative approach was to ban the Westboro Baptist Church's signs as supposedly dangerous fighting words. The U.S. Supreme Court does allow suppression of "fighting words," meaning personal epithets directed at the person of the hearer, but the signs from the Westboro church do not qualify as unprotected fighting words. The content of offensive messages is still constitutionally protected.[36]

A more successful approach to protect soldiers' mourners is to regulate the time and place at which funeral demonstrators can appear. At least ten states categorically forbid the appearance of demonstrators—without reference to their messages—within a certain distance of a funeral (usually five hundred feet) for an hour before and after a funeral. The First Amendment permits "reasonable" regulation of the time and place of expression. It is probably legitimate to safeguard the sensibilities of mourners at the moment when they are burying a loved one. Maintaining the privacy and dignity of such a sacrosanct occasion serves a strong public interest. The time and place regulations described will be deemed to be reasonable and will be upheld constitutionally so long as there are a modicum of alternative channels for speakers to address their intended audience. (The constitutional test of time and place regulations demands consideration of the availability of alternative channels of communication.) As the funeral demonstrators can still express their position by phone, mail, or advertisement, as well as by demonstrations away from the immediate vicinity of an ongoing funeral, the disputed state regulations will probably be upheld as constitutional.

## The Decedent's Desires as a Determinant of Respectful Treatment

One element in defining postmortem human dignity is the decedent's own assessment of the degree of degradation involved in various means of cadaver disposal. In American tradition and jurisprudence, a competent person is generally entitled to dictate the mode of disposition of his or her cadaver. Survivors are expected to implement the deceased's wishes, even though those wishes may be difficult to enforce—in the face of the next of kin's resistance—unless some interested party undertakes to assert the deceased's preferences. In the course of controlling his or her own disposition, a person has some leeway in defining a tolerable or intolerable level of indignity. That is, an autonomous person's definition of postmortem dignity is entitled to some deference. The respect generally due to the deceased's autonomous wishes includes some respect for the deceased's value judgments about dignity.

Changing personal perspectives on indignity have accounted for a variety of changes in cadaver disposal customs over the years. Evolving acceptance of cremation is one example. Testamentary gifting of cadavers to medical schools for dissection is another. (Both of these forms of cadaver disposition were once condemned as intolerably degrading.) Willingness to consent to research protocols in which cadavers are decimated also helps to shape the evolving meaning of indignity in cadaver disposal. Hundreds of people have agreed to leave their cadavers to The Body Farm at the University of Tennessee so that their disgustingly exposed, rotting remains can be observed and the rate of disintegration measured. This ostensibly vile form of disposal is accepted as part of a commendable effort to improve forensic science.[37] Researchers who explode cadavers (in the course of weapons research) or use cadavers as crash dummies (in vehicle safety tests) are not violating moral bounds so long as they obtain appropriate consent and act in a respectful manner toward the cadaver subjects before and after the research.

The actual or likely preferences of the deceased determine in significant part what disposition of a pregnant corpse is dignified and appropriate. I argued (in chapter 9) that keeping a pregnant corpse tethered to life-sustaining machinery for weeks or months is prima facie undignified and offensive unless the deceased can reasonably be deemed to have been willing to become a posthumous gestator and mother. The benevolent motives of physicians (such as the preservation of a potential human life) would not ordinarily overcome the indignity of the incongruous display of a corpse lingering tethered to the machinery. Yet if the deceased would likely have been willing to become a posthumous mother, the display could not be considered intrinsically demeaning or intolerably undignified.

The wishes of a decedent help to determine whether certain uses of human remains are morally acceptable. Ordinarily, using cadaver tissue for utilitarian ends—as tools or clothing—carries a demeaning connotation and is unacceptable. The degrading message is that human remains are like animal remains—subject to expropriation and exploitation to improve the comfort and convenience of living humans. Condemnation has always followed when malefactors exploited cadavers for utilitarian ends. The Nazis on occasion used victims' tissue to create soap, lampshades, shoes, handbags, and gloves.[38] Some prisoners at the Dachau concentration camp were killed by blows to the head in order to preserve their skin for tanning.[39] Crematorium ashes were used in road-paving material. Serial killers, such as Ed Gein, have been known to use victims' skin to fashion vests, lampshades, or drums.[40] All of these uses of human remains constituted such repudiations of the human dignity of victims as to be deemed to be intolerable desecrations.

The wishes of a decedent can create a different perspective on utilitarian uses of a cadaver. Some people see utilitarian use of their remains as a method of perpetuating their memory, or of making an altruistic gesture, or of communicating a message. The idea of creating from human remains a remembrance, a commemorative reminder of the deceased, has often been applied in the disposal of postcremation ashes. Requested uses of cremains include pencils, artificial diamonds, artificial reefs, and fertilizer. One artistic decedent requested that some of his ashes be mixed with paint and used to create a painting. Such unconventional uses of cremains do not seem troubling, particularly when the cremains are not separable and identifiable as human remains. These formats are not per se demeaning (as opposed to flushing cremains down the toilet). Queasy survivors need not handle or use the postmortem creations.

Suppose, though, that a person wants his cadaver's skin to be made into a pair of soft, attractive boots for a beloved relative. For some people, this testamentary gift might be a touching reminder of the deceased. For others, it might be a shocking desecration of human remains. Many people have requested similar commemoration in the form of continued use of their remains. A poet requested that his corpse's skin be used to bind a volume of his verse; his idea was to add an element of physical immortality to his printed verbal legacy. A theater worker requested that his skull be used in productions of *Hamlet* staged in his former workplace. A patriot requested that his cadaver skin be used to create two drumheads—one inscribed with the Declaration of Independence and the other to be sounded each July 17 at Bunker Hill.[41]

Such requests for unconventional uses of human remains—as mementos or commemorative reminders—should probably be honored. To my mind, self-designated uses of cadaver tissue that are intended to convey lasting messages and that do not harm others ought to be deemed tolerable. Of course, the next of kin or professional morticians may refuse to cooperate with unconventional, arguably distasteful wishes as a matter of conscience. (When the poet's widow sought to implement her husband's wish to convert his skin into a book cover, a mortuary refused to perform the relevant tasks and a court refused to compel it to do so.) The self-commemorating poet could have been told that he would have to find a more conventional binding than tanned cadaver skin to preserve his collected poems. Yet if his widow did not regard the unconventional use of his skin as a sacrilege, and if the mortuary had cooperated with the deceased's wishes, no funeral decorum arbiters should prevent fulfillment of the deceased's wishes. What if the patriot's skin was made into a drum and pounded each July 17 at Bunker Hill? If the descendants felt good about honoring their patriotic forefather, should outside arbiters of bad taste frustrate their efforts? Only if the contemplated use of the remains is so starkly offensive as to intrinsically violate postmortem human dignity. Otherwise, in such cases, cooperation with the decedent's wish to leave a useful remembrance should be upheld. After all, Americans commonly donate corpses or body parts for unseemly destruction in the course of education and research—including dissection and autopsy research—to say nothing about cadaveric mutilation in the context of tissue and organ donations for transplantation. There are limits, though, to any individual deceased's prerogative to subject his or her remains to postmortem human indignity.

## Intrinsic Indignity as a Limit on Unconventional Personal Choice

Some sources deride the whole concept of intrinsic indignity as so subjective and malleable as to be unhelpful in regulating human behavior.[42] Especially in a pluralistic and multicultural community, value judgments concerning the bounds of dignity may vary markedly. Illustrations of conflicting conceptions of dignity abound. One example is the dignity of a woman asserting reproductive autonomy versus the asserted dignity of a human fetus. Another example is the decision to end life support for a person dying in circumstances of apparently intolerable indignity (e.g., a permanently unconscious patient) versus ascription of intrinsic dignity to all living humans even in an unwinnable struggle against death. The latter right-to-life position opposes any quality-of-life judgment and thus insists on continued life support.[43] The conflict between paternalism and protection of autonomy arises as well in the contexts of mandatory bike helmet use, dwarf tossing, and religious rejection of lifesaving blood transfusions. Human autonomy (based on respect for human mental capacities) is often in tension with competing elements of human dignity.

Despite the subjective nature of some value judgments underlying human dignity, modern society accepts the notion of a hard core dignity that can be governmentally and culturally protected. The European Charter of Fundamental Rights, the German Constitution, and some American state constitutions protect human dignity by terms—defining it as "the intrinsic worth, the basic humanity" of persons.[44] The definition of "cruel and unusual punishment" prohibited by the Eighth Amendment to the U.S. Constitution is largely grounded in evolving concepts of decency and dignity. Fundamental liberties protected by the Fourteenth Amendment are defined in part by the collective conscience of the people, thus incorporating human dignity.

While alive, every human being is morally entitled to a basic level of dignity—meaning a modicum or core level of respect.[45] Certain actions so degrade a human being that they are socially intolerable. In the case of living persons, slavery, torture, and rape are obvious examples of intolerably disrespectful violations of human dignity.

By analogy, certain treatments of human remains are deemed inherently intolerable violations of postmortem human dignity. In these cases, the concept of intrinsic indecency precludes acceptance of the excuse that the now-dead victim consented to or even desired the mistreatment. Ingestion of human remains, except perhaps under the duress of starvation, is a candidate for such classification. In 2004 a story surfaced in which a German citizen had advertised for a volunteer to be killed and eaten. One person did respond to the ad and traveled from Austria to Germany to cooperate. This victim was ultimately killed, and portions of his corpse were fried and eaten. Prosecution ensued. No one suggested that the conduct was less degrading because the victim had agreed in advance to be consumed. The public reaction might have been more tolerant if only postmortem ingestion of human flesh (with no preceding murder) had been involved. Or perhaps not.

The ingestion of human remains seems to be a heinous and disgusting mistreatment of cadavers, and it usually is. Primitive cannibals ate their fallen enemies as a mark of disparagement and disdain. Religious dictates sometimes prompted eating of cadavers' flesh. The Aztecs not only sacrificed tens of thousands of people by cutting their hearts out, but also cooked and ate parts of the resulting corpses.[46] Ritual cannibalism existed in Brazil as late as the 1960s.[47] It is doubtful that the victims of religious sacrifice derived much consolation from the social fact that prevailing beliefs about religious duties accounted for the killings and ingestion of their remains.

Serial killer Jeffrey Dahmer provided a modern illustration of the horror of cannibalism. The Milwaukee resident admitted in 1992 that he had, over a thirteen-year period, murdered, dismembered, boiled, and eaten seventeen young men. The cannibalism seems to have been just another expression of the distorted psychodynamic that prompted the underlying atrocities. That analysis can also be applied to the conduct of a notorious Colorado mass killer and cannibal, Alfred Parker.[48] In 1874 Parker killed and ate five members of his traveling party during a Rocky Mountain trip. Public outrage was increased by a perception of partisanship in Parker's choice of victims. The sentencing judge commented to Parker: "There was 7 Democrats in Hinsdale County, and you've ate 5 of them, God damn you. I sentence you to be hanged by the neck until you is dead, dead, dead, as a warning against reducing the Democratic population. . . . You Republican cannibal, I would sentence you to hell if I could."[49] Parker was never executed, but his cannibalism did provoke outrage.

Perhaps ingestion of human remains is, in American culture, so intrinsically undignified as to be forbidden. It would probably make no difference if a Buddhist monk ate part of a deceased colleague as a gesture of respect. The benevolent intention might not balance the ingrained insult to human remains. Musician Keith Richards claimed (though he later retracted the statement) that he had snorted his late father's ashes mixed with cocaine. For Richards this action may have been an homage and, he thought, his father would not have objected if asked. Richards stated: "I couldn't resist grinding him up with a little bit of blow. My Dad wouldn't have cared. . . . It went down pretty well."[50] For me, snorting of human ashes constitutes at least borderline intrinsic indignity. It seems implausible that Richards's father, if asked, would have accepted the snorting of his ashes. The illegality of the conduct also helps push it over the line.

At the same time, it is at least arguable that extraction of tissue from human remains might be acceptable (especially if consent of the deceased could be inferred) in order to obtain therapeutic benefits for survivors. Since time immemorial and until the late eighteenth century, the human cadaver was frequently used as a source of therapeutic agents.[51] Blood from corpses was drunk as an elixir of life. A corpse's hand was applied to a diseased body area in order to cure the disease (e.g., goiter). In the Middle Ages mummy powder was widely used for the treatment of abcesses, contusions, rashes, and ulcers, among other things.[52] The powder was either applied topically or mixed into drinks. In seventeenth-century Europe genuine mummies were in short supply and tissue of fresh corpses was sometimes substituted as a curative agent. Ground skull became a medicinal agent in nineteenth-century England.[53]

The assumed therapeutic benefit of material from corpses was apparently once viewed as a sufficient justification for the exploitation of the corpses. No one had asked the decedents, before mummification, if their remains could be harvested for therapeutic purposes. But the benefit to the living seemed so great, and the harm to the ancient remains seemed so slight, that people did not hesitate to exploit the remains. If the cultural context accepts therapeutic applications of material extracted from human remains as respectful, then a next of kin could conceivably authorize some retrieval of tissue for that purpose. Even when fresh corpses were being tapped for medicinal purposes in the nineteenth century, the harm probably seemed slight compared to the dissection that awaited unclaimed corpses.

Contemporary American law makes it clear that retrieving cadaveric tissue for therapeutic uses is permissible upon consent of the decedent or a conscientious representative of the decedent. As stated in chapter 7, the UAGA explicitly authorizes the gifting of cadaveric tissue for therapeutic purposes. If a person wants to donate cadaver bone, skin, or other tissue to a medically needy person, that donation is encouraged. Unconsented taking for therapeutic purposes is criminal, as Dr. Mastromarino discovered in New Jersey.

The archetype of intolerable intrinsic indignity toward the human cadaver is necrophilia. Regardless of an actor's motives and regardless of a deceased's actual or putative wishes, necrophilia has always been deemed to be a heinous, condemnable abuse. Defined broadly, necrophilia is a psychosexual disorder involving performance of erotic actions upon corpses.[54] Culpable conduct includes fondling or manipulating breasts or genital areas, anal or vaginal intercourse, fellatio, cunnilingus, and sexually motivated insertion of objects into body orifices.[55] Coitus is not an essential element.

Explicit criminal prohibitions of necrophilia exist only in a minority of states. Nonetheless, sexual contact with a corpse can always be classified as punishable abuse of a corpse, even in jurisdictions lacking express prohibition of necrophilia. The abuse is patent. Whatever the sexual conduct involved and whatever the motivation, the necrophiliac inflicts "posthumous indignity in its grossest form."[56] It is bad enough to be a sexual object when alive and capable of resistance. Making a helpless corpse an object of unwanted sexual attention is utterly degrading.

Not surprisingly, given the natural human aversion to cadavers, necrophilia is "a very rare and poorly understood phenomenon."[57] The most common psychological explanation is that the perpetrator feels terribly inadequate, fears rejection, and seeks a sexual partner who is totally unresisting and unrejecting. Putting aside the problems of temporary rigor mortis and gradual bodily deterioration, considerable control can be exercised over a corpse—thus giving the necrophiliac a sense of power.[58] Certain incidents of necrophilia perhaps illustrate this psychological phenomenon. In 1931 in Florida, Carl van Cassell fell in love with a young woman who was dying of tuberculosis. She rejected him. After her death from natural causes, van Cassell dug up her body and slept with it in his bed for seven years.[59] (After the authorities found and removed the corpse, van Cassell cheekily sought its return, claiming unsuccessfully that no criminal offense had occurred.) Henry Lee Lucas had sex with the cadavers of two women he had killed. After the second episode, upon being apprehended, Lucas was asked why he only had sex with women after he had killed them. His response: "I like peace and quiet."[60]

Whatever the psychodynamic of necrophilia, the conduct is often traceable to people with common access to cadavers and a certain level of comfort in their presence. Hospital orderlies, mortuary attendants, funeral home assistants, cemetery workers, an ambulance driver, an anatomy student, and a pathologist have been among the people identified as necrophiliacs.[61] Funeral home mortuary workers who do embalming sometimes exploit their jobs for the purpose of necrophilia.[62] In 1979 an apprentice embalmer in Sacramento, California, admitted to having had sexual contact with approximately forty male corpses.[63] Another female embalmer pumped hydraulic fluid through a thin plastic tube into a male cadaver's member, then hopped on and rode to climax. The majority of necrophiles, though, are males who make sexual contact with female cadavers.

Serial killers have both access to cadavers and a certain level of comfort in handling them. Their deeply disturbed psyches sometimes prompt them to sexually exploit their victims' corpses. One estimate is that 42 percent of serial killers follow this pattern.[64] Simply sexually assaulting victims' corpses is bad enough, but some killer/necrophiliacs have gone much further. Ted Bundy more than once returned to the site of a killing and sexually assaulted severed body parts—for example, ejaculating into the mouth of a disembodied head.[65] Carl Drew kidnapped and imprisoned several women in Massachusetts. He then killed a few of the victims and raped their headless bodies in front of living kidnap victims.

In 2005 Dennis Rader was sentenced for the murder of ten people. In one instance he strung a live woman from a basement pipe (after murdering her parents), strangled her, and then masturbated on her corpse.[66]

Worse atrocities in desecrating cadavers are hard to imagine. It was not enough for serial killers to murder. It was not enough for them to then decimate the corpse with utter disdain. These killers were somehow impelled to sexually exploit the victim's corpse as a final act of defilement.

*Chapter 12*

# Public Display and the Dignity of Human Remains

Since Gunther von Hagens started the Body Worlds traveling exhibitions of plastinated corpses and body parts in 1995, over twenty-five million people worldwide have viewed these displays of the marvels of human body systems. (The plastination process for extracting liquids from cadavers and creating polymer-reinforced cadaveric tissue is described in chapter 6.) In the exhibitions, various plastinated figures highlight different aspects of body function. The circulatory system, respiratory functioning, neurological networks, the gastrointestinal tract from mouth to anus, and the interconnections of muscles and ligaments are vividly reproduced—usually in contrasting colors and with clear labels and explanations.[1] Though the figures are former human beings, their plastinated appearance makes them look more like fiberglass constructs.

Each Body Worlds exhibition contains one or more action figures—plastinated human remains shaped and displayed in action poses. These action figures include a football runner, a basketball dribbler, a runner, a soccer player, a ballerina, an archer, and a chess player. They are lifelike in shape, though not in facial features, somewhat reminiscent of the statuary of George Segal, who specializes in lifelike poses of people standing in lines or in other street scenes. These action figures appear more like statues than instructive models. Several observers have suggested that Gunther von Hagens is basically a sculptor working in the medium of desiccated human flesh.[2]

That judgment seems harsh. There appears to be more than aesthetic value in von Hagens's action plastinates. First, muscles and ligaments

*276*

look different in action than when inert, perhaps casting a somewhat different light on the relevant body parts. Also, each action figure has a section cut away in order to expose and highlight some body parts. The plastinated runner's leg musculature is partially peeled away from the bone, and the goalkeeper's leaping figure has the spinal cord pulled away and exposed. A jumping dancer also has the back of the trunk exposed behind the rest of the figure. One member of a poker-playing trio has an open abdomen exposing the intestinal loops. In short, Body World's artistic action figures have at least a patina of educational value.

A rival operation, called Bodies: The Exhibition, has been running in New York City for several years in a format like Body Worlds'. At least ten other exhibitions, with titles like "Mysteries of the Human Body," have appeared on the international scene.[3] Body Worlds and its imitators are commercial enterprises. The entrance fees (usually about $25 per person) do not simply cover the costs of plastination, transportation, and display. Its millions of customers have made Body Worlds profitable and have inspired the copycat cadaver exhibitions.

Despite the lucrative nature of their displays, von Hagens and other proprietors insist that the primary goal of the plastinated body exhibitions is educational.[4] The exhibitions, they assert, promote better understanding of the complexity of the human body and its systems. The slogan of Body Worlds is "Discover the Mystery Hidden under Your Skin."[5]

Critics of plastinated body exhibitions have been many and vocal. A major complaint is the suspect origins of at least some cadavers on display. Some of the figures have been those of executed Chinese prisoners whose cadavers were sold by the Chinese government without the consent of the decedent or the family. Another accusation is that Body Worlds is "a macabre spectacle" constituting a repugnant violation of human dignity.[6] The thrust of this claim is that the public display is intrinsically "voyeuristic" — oblivious to the underlying humanity and individuality of the subjects and hence disrespectful of postmortem human dignity. The assertion is that exhibitions of plastinated cadavers are "merely feeding our inordinate taste for the macabre while masquerading as science education."[7] For these critics, the educational function of these exhibitions could be achieved by presenting artificial models without exploiting actual human remains.

The contention that plastinated cadavers are superfluous education-al tools is not convincing. Plastinates have an apparently unique capacity to show the minute details of human tissue. Hundreds of universities have purchased plastinated remains for use as teaching tools. Some edu-cators concede the advantages of plastinated exhibits over more tradi-tional educational resources.[8] As to the education of the general public, more prosaic models of body systems would not attract nearly the vol-ume of people who are viewing Body Worlds and its imitators. The pres-ence of actual cadavers (even though they do not look very cadaver-like) has aroused enormous public curiosity and interest.

Critics are right to inquire about the provenance of the plastinated corpses used in these exhibitions. Unconsented seizure and display of human cadavers, even for educational purposes, is a prima facie viola-tion of the right of every deceased to determine his or her own mode of dignified disposal (usually via sepulture and quiet repose). Chapters 10 and 11 recount the abuses committed when the cadavers of people per-ceived as the dregs of society were unceremoniously seized and used for teaching. Dissection before a public or semipublic audience was for cen-turies a degrading abuse of human remains. Today subjecting an unwill-ing deceased person to the gross decomposition and disfiguration of plastination, followed by prolonged public display, would indeed be an abuse of postmortem human dignity that warrants condemnation of the perpetrators and boycott of the exhibitions.

The provenance of currently exhibited plastinated corpses is not al-ways clear. Some of the displayed remains probably are those of execut-ed Chinese prisoners. The producers of Bodies: The Exhibition recently conceded that they could not show any form of consent to plastination for the bodies that were obtained "legally" in China from among "aban-doned" corpses.[9] Because of the unclear origins of the plastinated figures in that exhibition, the Florida Anatomical Board initially voted 4–2 to withhold permission for Bodies: The Exhibition to appear in Florida (be-fore the Florida legislature overrode that rejection).[10] But von Hagens's Body Worlds can better account for the sources of its human display material. One source is the Heidelberg Institute for Plastination—an operation that solicits voluntary donations of cadavers by means of an informational brochure available at every Body Worlds exhibit. World-wide, as of November 2005, 6,500 people, including 150 Americans, had willingly signed up to be body donors after attending Body Worlds exhibits. Given that Body Worlds has operated since 1995, it is plausible that its plastinated figures now in use were all obtained by a legitimate consent process, as claimed by von Hagens. This may be so even though one of von Hagens's processing plants for plastination is located in China.

The most troubling claim about Body Worlds is that the exhibition of plastinated figures is intrinsically undignified and hence is a moral abuse of the human cadaver regardless of the voluntary sources of display material. An indisputable fact—obvious to anyone who visits Body Worlds—is that some of the spectators do indeed come to gawk and be titillated in some fashion. At the same time, exhibitions like Body Worlds appear to have enormous educational potential, making it worthwhile to consider whether such exhibitions are intrinsically indecent or not. But before considering the morality of Body Worlds, it might be useful to review the long history of exhibitionism surrounding human cadavers.

## The Multiple Contexts of Cadaver Exposure

Display of human remains has occurred in many different settings with a variety of connotations. As recounted in chapter 11, the derogatory display of human remains has over time been a prime form of cadaver abuse. Recall the gibbeting of executed criminals and the brandishing of the body parts of fallen enemy soldiers. Consider the treatment of Oliver Cromwell's remains. In 1661 his remains were disinterred, his head removed and impaled on a stake, and carried through London while crowds pelted it with rocks and garbage.[11] After hanging on the spike outside Westminster for years, Cromwell's head later reappeared as an exhibit at a public peep show.[12]

Even without a derogatory intent on the part of exhibitors, the display of human remains poses obvious tension with postmortem human dignity. Corpses and their survivors generally have a strong dignity interest in privacy, meaning protection against unwanted exposure to strangers' eyes. A dead person, even after receiving cosmetic attention from an embalmer, does not create the same image or leave the same visual memories as a living person. Survivors often prefer to preserve the original personal images by putting a loved one's cadaver to rest without exposure of the corpse.[13] Without the permission of family, an open-casket wake would be a significant violation of this expected privacy. In 1963 Jackie Kennedy vigorously rejected an open casket for President John F. Kennedy's lying in state; she considered the practice of viewing to be barbarous. In 1921 in Naples, Italy, Enrico Caruso's widow objected to public display of her husband's embalmed corpse in a glass casket. She demanded, and obtained, the cadaver's removal to a marble sarcophagus in a private mausoleum.[14]

Photographing a cadaver can also violate the privacy of the cadaver and the family.[15] In 2005 a photographer was convicted of criminal abuse of a corpse after taking numerous unauthorized photos (ultimately intended for an art book) at a county morgue where autopsies were performed. (This photographer exacerbated his offense by using props such as a dollhouse ladder that leaned against the deceased's skull.[16]) A pathologist who was lawfully performing an autopsy incurred liability to the decedent's family by publishing, without permission, a photo of the deceased accompanying a scholarly article and by displaying the photo in an anatomy lab.[17] (The result might have been different if the photo had included removal of the identifying features by the use of a black bar.)

A corpse's (or family's) interest in privacy and nonexposure is not absolute. Countervailing public interests may override the customary maintenance of privacy. Compelled forensic autopsies are permissible despite the body's exposure to morgue workers or even to other observers.[18] It is not necessary to watch *CSI* to know that photographs at suspected crime scenes (including photos of a dead victim) are standard operating procedure in police investigations. While White House lawyer Vince Foster's family was able to prevent public access to the postsuicide photographs of his cadaver, the U.S. Supreme Court indicated that public access would have been granted had there been any evidence that the photos could have helped document "government impropriety."[19] It may be bad taste and insensitive to publish photos of cadavers observed lying in public places, even anonymous cadavers, but publications frequently do so to communicate the horrors of war, mass disaster, or crime—all in the interest of providing public information. In 2009 the Associated Press aroused a furor by publishing a photo of a specific war hero as he lay dying.

Despite the natural tendency to maintain the cadaver's privacy, a decedent or family may choose to surrender the customary privacy of a corpse and permit some exposure. Jackie Kennedy's preferences to the contrary notwithstanding, open-casket wakes have a long history. The open casket affords a stark reminder of the departed figure and may thereby facilitate the process of paying respect to or mourning the deceased individual. Some people want to touch and communicate symbolically with human remains before their final disposition. While open-casket viewing is distasteful to some people and anathema to others, some subcultures (such as the Italians and Irish) perpetuate the practice. Also, a photograph of a corpse for purposes of mourning and memorabilia was once considered highly desirable. In the mid- to late nineteenth century affluent families secured photo portraits of family members seated together with the recently departed "to freeze the [departed] into an iconic last frame."[20] This willingness of survivors to sometimes expose the remains of loved ones tends to show that public or semipublic display of remains is not inherently undignified.

Honorific postmortem displays also are known. Public displays of preserved corpses or body parts may continue for extended periods in order to honor symbols of political movements or of religious faiths. Lenin's body has lain in public view in the Kremlin for almost ninety years. Many churches in Italy and other European countries contain relics of heroic figures from many centuries past that are viewed by adoring or supplicating visitors.

The current exhibitions of plastinated corpses continue an uneven history of cadaver display to educate both lay and professional people. Recall that public dissections go back to the early Renaissance. For centuries, people seeking to learn about human anatomy gathered and observed public dissections, overcoming their aversion to the gore and foul odors. Spectators included laypeople and artists, not just the medically oriented. American medical students have, for almost two hundred years, systematically dissected corpses in order to learn about human anatomy. While the audience in an anatomy lab may be limited, the cadaver is nonetheless exposed to numerous strangers' eyes.

During the nineteenth century in the United States, a variety of display venues exhibited cadaveric material both to educate people and to exploit the public fascination with human remains. Pathological

cadaveric specimens were especially popular exhibits. Displays of medical pathologies and oddities to attract the curious public became popular
in the middle to late nineteenth century. (The phenomenon coincided
with circus side shows displaying living persons with a variety of extraordinary body features—the thin man, the fat lady, the midget, and
the giant.) One venue of display was the medical museum featuring
human remains that highlighted anomalous body parts. The first, the
Mutter Museum at Philadelphia's College of Physicians and Surgeons,
opened in 1842. It featured extraordinary remains including the skeletons of a giant and a dwarf, a preserved liver shared by Siamese twins,
and an array of human skulls.[21] In operating museums connected with
medical schools, curators could claim an educational benefit in presenting body parts that illustrated the effects of disease and the methods for
dealing with various human maladies. Anomalous or notorious body
parts later became attractions in a variety of other anatomical museums
not connected to medical schools.[22] An anatomical museum in New York
City featured body relics of notorious criminals, such as the penis of an
executed pirate.[23] A similar anatomical museum featured the head and
right arm of another executed criminal. The U.S. Army's medical museum displayed thousands of pathological body specimens, as well as
skeletons of Civil War soldiers.[24]

The anatomical museums reflect an overlap between the educational
and financial objectives connected with the display of human remains.
Commercial exploitation of the public's fascination with human remains
started early in America. In the 1760s William Schippen in Philadelphia
sold tickets to the public to witness dissections performed in a medical
theater erected for medical students.[25] In 1835 David Rogers attracted lay
spectators to his demonstrations on corpses laid out in an anatomy theater. Using the cadaver of a hanged pirate, he demonstrated to his audience that an electric current could produce twitches in a dead body.[26]
More performance art involving human remains appeared in the same
period. In 1850 Egyptologist George Glidden attracted large audiences
to "unrollings"—yard-by-yard unwinding of an Egyptian mummy's
shrouds to expose the mummy's embalmed human remains. In Boston, Glidden—based on his declared ability to read hieroglyphics—
advertised the forthcoming public unrolling of an Egyptian princess.
The princess turned out to have a penis.[27] Undaunted, Glidden contin-

ued his tour and did a more prosaic unrolling in 1852 before a New Orleans audience.

In the second half of the nineteenth century, entrepreneurs in tawdry enterprises became intent on attracting paying customers by presenting grotesque anatomical specimens.[28] These marginal enterprises, labeled "dime museums," offered sensationalized anatomical displays, including stillborn, deformed "monsters" that shocked and titillated the public. Such enterprises existed in cities like New York, Philadelphia, Boston, and San Francisco. The dime museum entrepreneurs may have claimed educational value for their exhibits, but their focus was on exploiting people's curiosity about the pathological and the bizarre. Their exhibits were more like freak shows than museums.

Physicians and medical researchers in the late nineteenth and early twentieth centuries also commonly collected and displayed body parts used in their work.[29] For example, the Wilder Brain Collection started in 1889 at Cornell University as an effort to investigate correlations between brain structures and personality characteristics—a variation on phrenology research.[30] At one point, six hundred brains were collected. Today seventy brains remain, most of them stored in formaldehyde-filled glass jars. Eight brains from identified donors to the collection are still on display to visitors at Cornell's psychology department. Harvard University also has a brain collection, and Northwestern University has a collection of fetuses and stillborn infants on display. In the late nineteenth century, physicians were advised to display in their offices anatomical specimens harvested at prior dissections in order to advertise their experience and erudition.[31]

In a number of instances, exposed corpses (originally assembled for disposal according to prevailing cultural norms) have been used to create tourist attractions for the curious public. This phenomenon has occurred primarily outside the United States. In the eighteenth century the Paris gibbet commonly held up to forty-five executed criminals whose caged remains were gradually decomposing and being picked apart. The gibbet became a tourist attraction surrounded by taverns and gardens.[32] In a later period, the Paris morgue displayed unidentified corpses behind a glass window as another crowd-pleasing diversion.[33] Some churches and monasteries have become tourist attractions by opening up their depositories of bones and skeletons, sometimes displayed in a highly decorative fashion. In the Capuchin church in Palermo, Italy, eight thousand mummified remains of friars stand in catacombs in rows, each labeled.[34] At Santa Maria della Concezione, in Rome, the remains of four thousand Capuchin friars assembled between 1631 and 1870 are displayed standing in a series of chapels.[35]

Such tourist-oriented displays have an ambiguous moral status.[36] On the one hand, the human remains are exhibited in part to attract the paying curious public. Commercial exploitation of human remains obtained without consent would normally constitute an offense to the dignity of the dead. On the other hand, there are redeeming factors. The arranged skeletons represent an historical testament to a form of disposal of human remains that began with no commercial objectives. The mummification and arrangement of cadavers was not intended to demean the departed, and the friars knew how their remains would be treated. The deceased friars gave implicit consent to their cadavers' display (though they might not have anticipated being major tourist attractions).

## Body Worlds and Postmortem Human Dignity

Are the critics of Body Worlds and similar exhibitions of human remains right in labeling these displays intolerably degrading to the dignity of human remains? Chapter 11 acknowledges the concept of intolerably abusive treatment of a human cadaver—hard-core violations of postmortem human dignity.

Some of the previously described educational displays of human remains—including some public dissections and tawdry dime museum exhibits—probably did constitute hard-core violations of postmortem dignity. Yet some of the nineteenth-century display practices provoke revulsion not because the displays were so intrinsically demeaning, but because the corpses were exploited without any legitimate authorization. The cadaveric sources for many dissections and many museum displays were executed criminals, or cadavers purloined by criminal resurrectionists, or body parts held without permission after legitimate autopsies.[37] The problematic origins of those cadavers provide a sufficient basis to condemn those displays. In the case of Body Worlds, that objection has been put aside here by assuming that informed donations are now the source of von Hagens's plastinate displays. The question becomes whether plastinate displays are so inherently disrespectful to human remains as to be intolerably undignified despite the consent of donors.

For me, the answer to that question is clearly no. Public display of a corpse need not be a degrading spectacle. That assertion applies not just to practices associated with mourning, such as open-casket wakes, but also to educational exhibits. In 1832 philosopher Jeremy Bentham successfully directed that his corpse be dissected (before a limited audience) and that his skeleton be dressed and displayed at University College, London, seated in a chair as if thinking.[38] (To this day, Bentham's remains are occasionally displayed at the college.) Presumably Bentham found none of this to be humiliating or disrespectful; rather, he perceived the dismantling and display of his remains as both educational and entertaining. Nor is a Body Worlds exhibit necessarily disrespectful. Keep in mind that more than 6,500 people worldwide have signed up to become future plastinated remains for public display.[39] These prospective donors clearly did not find the Body Worlds exhibit to be distasteful, humiliating, or disrespectful to its subjects. Plastination and display as a means of corporeal disposition appealed to some donors as an expression of thanks to their bodies by "giving [them] a shot at immortality."[40] Even if the yen for immortality seems to be a somewhat egotistical indulgence, the contribution to public knowledge about the human body seems like a satisfactory incentive. That the exhibition is entertaining as well as educational only enhances its attraction.

Some observers question whether a Body Worlds exhibit serves a real educational function. For its harshest critics, Body Worlds is a disrespectful and voyeuristic exercise in commercial exploitation of human remains—"mere gawking at the endless ways in which [body] parts can be sliced and diced."[41] My assessment is different. Yes, some of the over twenty-five million spectators come merely to gawk or be titillated in some fashion. Some observers are repulsed by the plastinated bodies on display, but a large percentage of them see the exhibition as a remarkable educational experience. In my anecdotal experience, a majority of people, both lay and professional, view Body Worlds as a constructive educational experience. According to the questionnaires circulated (albeit by the producers of Body Worlds) to exiting viewers, the general public's reaction is similar.[42] Eighty-three percent of those surveyed felt that they knew more about the human body after seeing the exhibit, and 67 percent felt greater respect for the wonders of the body. I personally was fascinated by the graphic displays of intricate body systems and learned a great deal.

Critics of Body Worlds see disrespect in the exhibit's objectifying and dehumanizing of human subjects—a "manipulation of body parts stripped of any larger human significance."[43] The objectification highlighted by these critics is certainly present. To date, plastinated remains have been displayed anonymously, devoid of identifying features. Moreover, the appearance of a flayed, desiccated, plastinated figure is that of an artifact; it does not readily trigger an association with human beings or even with human cadavers. A few critics contend that Body Worlds would be more humanizing if the donor of the plastinate display were identified and even heard in a recording.[44] Some prospective donors have expressed a willingness to be identified as the source of a plastinate figure. There does not appear to be any intrinsic dignity barrier to nonobtrusive identification of remains so that the decedent could receive credit for an altruistic gesture. At the same time, nonidentification of body donors violates no moral code. Von Hagens opposes identification as distracting from the main focus of spectators. I tend to agree that presentation of personal background information about the plastinated figures would be an unnecessary distraction in an exhibit intended to highlight universal physical characteristics.

What about the commercial aspect of Body Worlds? There can be little doubt that Gunther von Hagens's enterprises are intended to make money. In 2008 von Hagens started to market plastinated cross sections of the human body (at $250 per slice); the intended customers are not only medical schools but also private citizens. The resourceful von Hagens is clearly interested in the profitability of his work.

The profit element in Body Worlds may be distasteful and a cause for careful scrutiny of the exhibit. But the exhibit's profitability and associated entrepreneurship do not, to my mind, disqualify Body Worlds as a legitimate educational enterprise that exploits but does not demean human remains. I see no intrinsic contradiction between education and profit. Consider profit-making colleges and hospitals. These private institutions may be far from ideal suppliers of educational and health care services, but they deserve a chance to function in the market place as long as they adhere to public regulations and work within the bounds of basic human dignity.

Body Worlds elicits conflicting human reactions. While over 6,500 people want to volunteer their corpses for display, many others are repelled by the thought and the reality of an exhibit of plastinated corpses. I support the continuation of such exhibits because they are educational, they reach a wide audience, and they do not violate basic human dignity as applicable to human cadavers. The Body Worlds experience indicates that human remains can further public education while simultaneously serving as a source of entertainment and commercial gain.

The educational function and techniques of Body Worlds save that exhibit from moral condemnation. What kind of cadaver display constitutes intolerable indecency? Assuming that cadaveric displays (plastinated or otherwise) come from willing donors, what would make such displays so disrespectful to postmortem human dignity as to warrant condemnation or even suppression? The next section addresses that issue.

## The Art and Craft of Body Display

The action figures displayed at Body Worlds and its imitators have a striking aesthetic impact. One observer has wondered whether von Hagens's work constitutes "postmodern sculpture of the body in which the body itself provides the clay."[45] Von Hagens himself seems to view the action figures as sculpture. He signs each such figure, and he has asserted copyright protection for his plastinated creations. Suppose that von Hagens stopped including a micro-segment of anatomical detail in his action figures and admitted that these plastinated figures are essentially sculptures, that is, works of art. How far may an artist go in employing human remains as a medium for expression?

One can easily imagine displays of human remains so shocking as to outrage many people. Suppose that Body Worlds' action figures had been placed in other poses—in attitudes of crucifixion, masturbation, fellatio, or bodily excretion. Or suppose that, in the previously mentioned case where a photographer had photographed morgue occupants, he had received permission from the decedent to take and display photos with props like a snail crawling toward the groin or offensive items protruding from the mouth. All of these putative artistic works would shock many people as offensive to the dignity of human remains.

Keep in mind, though, that artwork is expressive and entitled to constitutional protection under the First Amendment to the U.S. Constitution. Even nude dancing is sufficiently communicative to be protected. If a person wants to become a posthumous part of an artistic statement by donating a cadaver part to an artist for use, can the display of such a body part incorporated into art be suppressed? Recall the patriot who requested that his cadaver's skin be tanned and converted into a drumhead inscribed with the Declaration of Independence. Recall the actor who wanted his skull to be used in every production of *Hamlet* in the theater where he had worked. Recall the poet who wanted to have his cadaver's skin tanned and used to bind a book of his verse. While these displays of cadaver parts may be repulsive to many observers, and while the survivors might refuse to cooperate with these modes of cadaver disposition, can government suppress such postmortem artistic expression?

Under the First Amendment, government cannot suppress expression (including artistic expression) just because it is offensive to some observers. (Recall that the demonstrators from the Westboro Baptist Church were entitled to say that a dead soldier had been punished by God; they just couldn't say it in the immediate vicinity of the soldier's funeral.) In American constitutional jurisprudence, there is no idea so outrageous that its expression can be suppressed by government. The explanation is that the offensiveness of speech and ideas is so subjective and so malleable as to make offensiveness an inappropriate basis for government to suppress speech. If the producers of plastinate exhibitions or the artists exhibiting in galleries want to engage in what some people deem to be the disgusting use of human remains, they are probably entitled to do so without government interference. If competent individuals want to contribute their cadaver's skin in order to make what they see as a postmortem symbolic statement (e.g., the inscribed drumhead), and if surviving family members and artisans are willing to cooperate, the artists and artisans probably ought to be able to work in these dubious media.

Sporadic efforts have been made to suppress the offensive display of human remains. In 1908 an Australian owner of a traveling circus displayed a stillborn fetus with two heads. He was prosecuted for "indecent exhibition of a corpse." The prosecution failed because the judge ruled that the circus owner had acquired lawful possession of the remains and could use skill to create and display something that was "not merely a corpse."[46] The incident underlines the notion that public displays of a corpse, even in bad taste, are not necessarily a basis for legal suppression.

This does not mean that entrepreneurs are free to display human remains in whatever shocking format they choose. The remedy for shocking and offensive exhibitions is condemnation of the indecent displays (thus discouraging patronage of the offending artists). Government may be precluded from suppressing offensive expression, but people can freely voice their condemnation of and disgust about outrageous displays. In May 2009 Body Worlds opened an exhibit in Berlin that included a display of two cadavers in a pose of sexual intercourse. Sharp public criticism followed. Von Hagens, in response, noted that the cadaver donors had consented to the pose and insisted that he only wanted to illustrate the full range of human functions (as opposed to provoking sexual feelings). Yet the next Body Worlds exhibit (in Singapore) omitted sexual depictions. Perhaps the episode demonstrates the clout of public condemnation of undignified cadaver displays.

Just as autonomous choices of a deceased and/or of the next of kin are generally respected in the context of cadaver disposition, so is the postmortem display of a cadaver. The bottom line is that people can allow their remains to be displayed in a museum, or exhibition, or gallery, or church, or glass sarcophagus in a mausoleum—all being closed spaces that viewers may choose to enter or not. These permissible displays of cadavers may be in bad taste and may be offensive to some people. Yet as long as displays of bodies or body parts have a cognizable communicative element—as in educational, religious, and art contexts—they cannot be suppressed by government. Again, the persons offended by these exploitations of human remains can refrain from visiting the exhibitions, they can condemn the producers, and they can discourage attendance. But if these condemnations do not persuade the viewing public, exhibitions like Body Worlds can continue to exhibit their plastinates, the Catholic Church can continue to display its relics, and the Mutter Museum can continue to exhibit its gross human remains.

## Disturbance to and Display of Ancient Remains

Archaeologists and anthropologists have long retrieved the remains of previous generations or cultures for study and ultimate display in museums. Scientific handling of human remains was apparently deemed to be a legitimate part of the exploration and documentation of the evolution and dispersion of human beings and cultures. In the case of ancient and individually unidentifiable remains, the investigators seem to have assumed that no moral harm flowed from studying, classifying, and displaying their corporeal finds. Somehow the long temporal gap between death and display, the anonymity, and the absence of known descendants diminished any offense to the dead or their descendants. The knowledge gain was thought to warrant any attendant disturbance.[47] Also, the human remains were supposedly treated with delicacy, if not deference toward their quasi-human nature, even if they were poked, transported, examined, and put on display. (Ancient remains are invariably fragile, so delicate treatment by scientists was also dictated by the goal of preservation.)

What about the dignity of ancient remains disturbed by well-meaning anthropologists or other researchers? Is it an offense to postmortem human dignity, tantamount to body snatching, when long-buried human remains are unearthed and investigated? In principle, disturbing a resting place can constitute an offense to human remains even hundreds or thousands of years after initial disposition of the corpse. Bodily integrity (even if only bones remain) is still affected. Arguably, quiet repose is the measure of the dignity and respect due to all human remains even after corporeal decomposition, and that interest in quiet repose does not terminate after any particular number of years.[48] A further harm to ancient remains can be perceived if the decedent (the origin of the contested remains) had cultural beliefs that would be offended by exhumation, research, and ultimate display.

On the other hand, shouldn't scientific and historical inquiry warrant some disturbance of ancient human remains? To some limited degree? After some time span? Exhumation and examination of ancient remains is extremely useful in studying human and cultural history. Isn't the knowledge gained from examination of ancient remains as weighty as the knowledge gained from permitted forensic autopsies and exhumations? Aren't the justifications here as strong as those commonly accepted for other exhumations and transfers of human remains—for example, to make way for a public works project, to investigate allegations of criminal conduct, or to serve the convenience of otherwise distantly located relatives? Shouldn't scientists have temporary access to unearthed remains for study before their respectful final disposition? Should the remains still be available for display to a public interested in human anthropology?

American treatment of Native American remains reflects the waxing and waning of racism. For a considerable period, Native American remains were considered appropriate items for collection, study, and display. In the 1840s Dr. Samuel Morton, an anthropologist, collected Native American skulls to try to prove by measurement that their brain size reflected inferior savages. Other researchers as well excavated thousands of Native American graves while seeking to use craniology and phrenology to establish the lower intelligence of nonwhites. In 1868 the U.S. Army's surgeon general ordered personnel to collect Native American heads; four thousand of them were transferred from past battlefields. Museum expeditions in the 1880s set out to collect relics from Native American graves. The Smithsonian Institution in Washington, D.C., once housed tens of thousands of Native American skeletons; the U.S. Army Medical Museum also held thousands of Native American skeletons.[49] Between 1957 and 1971 two anthropologists excavated between four and five thousand Indian graves in the Great Plains.[50] Some diggers had commercial motives. In the nineteenth century entrepreneurs rapaciously unearthed untold thousands of bones, skeletons, and burial paraphernalia for sale to collectors and curiosity seekers. Twentieth-century relic hunters rifled the graves of Native Americans, Civil War soldiers, and slaves for the purpose of extracting salable items. Massive numbers of Native American remains have been unearthed and moved "in the name of profit, entertainment, science, or development."[51]

Native Americans tend to believe that disturbance of their ancestors' remains traumatizes the spirit of the deceased and can bring harm to the living.[52] A disturbed spirit may restlessly stalk the earth if the remains are not returned entirely to nature.[53] Thus there is good reason to think that, historically, a Native American deceased person would have objected to research exploiting his or her remains. Contemporary Native American tribes have deemed collections and displays of anthropological remains to be a desecration. Even without any direct familial connections to remains, tribes claim a spiritual bond and a symbolic relationship between the Native American remains and current survivors. Various tribes have demanded the removal of remains from display and their reburial in line with cultural tradition.[54]

The massive offense to the dignity of Native American dead did not go unnoticed. The desecration of Indian burial sites led to protective federal legislation in 1906, 1979, and most notably 1990, when the Native American Graves Protection and Repatriation Act (NAGPRA) was adopted. In NAGPRA Congress engineered a compromise in the conflict between advancing human knowledge and giving Native American remains the respectful treatment they were due. That statute punishes removal of Native American remains and requires repatriation (from museums and other institutions) and reburial of human remains connected or "affiliated" with contemporary Native Americans or tribes. Repatriation includes respectful burial in ancestral land. Affiliation can be established by the tribe or by an individual descendant via geography, archaeology, and oral tradition. If no cultural affiliation can be shown, an institution may choose to turn over for respectful burial human remains that are being studied (but it is not compelled by NAGPRA to do so).

NAGPRA has encouraged museums to remove numerous displays of Native American remains and to permit their reburial. In one instance, a 10,675-year-old skeleton was reburied on the Shoshone-Bannock reservation even though the Shoshone-Bannock people had no connection with the site in the relevant period more than 10,000 years ago.[55] In other instances, though, tribal efforts to repatriate remains were rebuffed on the basis that the contemporary Native American petitioners could not show the statutorily required cultural link that would require repatriation of human remains. In a 2004 case, five petitioning tribes sought to rebury a 16,000-year-old set of remains discovered in 1996 in Kennewick, Washington.[56] The federal courts rejected their demand for repatriation for failure to show Native American ties to the remains. The remnants of the Kennewick man remain above ground subject to scientific study and perhaps ultimate display. In 1996 Richland Man, the skeleton of a man killed approximately 9,000 years ago, was found in Oregon. Anthropologists eagerly set out to study the remains. The Umatilla Tribe of the region then claimed Richland Man's remains for burial.[57] A federal court ultimately ruled that the tribe had not shown the affiliation of these 9,000-year-old remains and the anthropological research proceeded.

Congress's NAGPRA formula is appealing in respecting the integrity of remains that can be connected in some fashion to a tradition that demands continuing sanctity for those remains. The focus is on the likelihood or not of injury to a decedent's creed. That is, if the decedent's culture likely demanded uninterrupted burial, his or her belief system would likely be violated by disinterment and continued public display. In the absence of such a belief or tradition, gains in human knowledge probably should outweigh the temporary physical derangement of ancient human remains. If the remains are so old that cultural values cannot be postulated, the advance of human knowledge may warrant study and display of the remains.

Consistent with this framework, prehistoric remains have been treated as culturally nonaffiliated articles subject to research and display. In 1922 a prehistoric skeleton dating to the Ice Age in France went on display in Chicago. It drew twenty-two thousand visitors the first day and several million between 1922 and 1932.[58] Otzi the Iceman, a 5,300-year-old figure from the Copper Age, is on display in a climate-controlled chamber in Bolzano, Italy.[59]

How does the attempted balance between respect for human remains and pursuit of scientific knowledge play out in the context of mummies? Egyptian mummies—of which there were millions—have customarily appeared in numerous museums in many countries, with little comment about a possible misdeed or offense to the dignity of the human remains. Physical research on Egyptian mummies has been widely undertaken, including unwrapping and dissecting them for scientific purposes. Dissection of mummies has potential utility in solving mysteries of disease and parasites. One scientist alone has dissected eight hundred mummies.[60]

Modern scientists—medical researchers, archaeologists, and anthropologists—are divided in their moral appraisal of mummy dissection.

Some believe that "the pursuit of knowledge among the living takes precedence over the faith, beliefs, and hopes of the dead."[61] These scientists want to treat ancient remains as "common property of humankind" for the purpose of advancing human knowledge. Other scientists favor preserving the integrity of human remains of any person "who believed that all eternity depended on a whole, intact, preserved body."[62]

It is not easy to decide what the appropriate moral fate of Egyptian mummies should be. The now-mummified deceased's wishes and creed are still relevant, but does its contemporary display as a still-wrapped figure in a museum violate that creed? The deceased's objective was to have his or her remains preserved and ready for a postmortem voyage to an eternal promised land. Yet thousands of years have passed since his or her death. Does the passage of time dilute any projected offense to the mummy's former creed and wishes? Isn't a mummy (at least one that has not been unwrapped) still available for celestial transport even if the remains are now in a museum? Could Egyptians have expected that their remains would still be awaiting transformation thousands of years later? Perhaps the continued presence of mummies in museums results from unconcern by contemporary Egyptians about any cultural offense to remains preserved in museum exhibits.

Where does this leave mummies? Still wrapped but still on display. In 1980 then president of Egypt Anwar Sadat showed one form of consideration for the dignity of ancient human remains. He ordered closure of the mummy hall at the Cairo Museum because he did not think it fitting that visitors should stare at unwrapped mummies. President Sadat did not argue, though, that mummies should all be left in the desert rather than displaced to museums. At least the fate of Egyptian mummies is now being determined by public antiquities officials and not by the tomb robbers who exploited the mummies for so many centuries.

*Chapter 13*

# Don't Neglect the Fate of Your Remains

Now that we have examined the nature, duration, and utility of the human cadaver, it is time to consider the implications of this study. How might the fate of your cadaveric remains be affected by this book's findings?

## Corpses Are a Lot Like You and Me, Only Different

Certain commonalities and continuities between corpses and their living predecessors account for the quasi-human status attributed to human remains (see chapter 2). One of the commonalities of living humans and cadavers is appearance. A person who dies is normally readily identifiable after death as the same person, albeit in a defunct status. The cadaver contains the same brain and heart that only moments earlier constituted the essence of the cadaver's predecessor. Without artificial intervention, the physical similarity between a cadaver and its living predecessor quickly vanishes as a cadaver decomposes. With administration of artificial preservatives, usually embalming fluid, and with cosmetic attention, the physical similarity continues longer, but not indefinitely.

Another commonality between living humans and their cadaver successors is physical deterioration over time. Fortunately for living persons, their rate of decline is slower than that of their cadavers. The average living human can expect to decline gradually over a period of approximately seventy-eight years—experiencing increasing aches, pains, and slowdowns before ultimate demise. The average cadaver will undergo much quicker and much more thorough physical degeneration.

*295*

Even after typical embalming, the buried cadaver will deteriorate to a blackened hulk within two decades and to a moldy skeleton within forty years.

Cadavers are also a lot like live persons in being subject to certain social or economic disadvantages. Marilyn Yalom asserts that "differences in wealth and status are as striking among the dead as among the living."[1] She is referring primarily to ostentation in funerals, burial locales, and grave markers, as documented in chapter 5. While wealth has permitted certain indulgences in cadaver disposal, the social importance of dignified disposal has impelled efforts to mitigate economic disadvantage in that context. American experience confirms that the aspiration to achieve a "decent" final disposition affects people at all social and economic strata. Dying persons and their families, regardless of their economic status, endeavor to assure a final disposition consistent with prevailing concepts of funerary dignity. Over time, as funerary practices became more elaborate and expensive, families with few resources sought special ways to cope with the expense. In the mid-1800s people often joined fraternal and ethnic burial societies in order to ensure a decent burial.[2] In the late nineteenth and early twentieth centuries, the struggle for dignified disposition often took the form of monthly payments to secure low-cost funeral insurance to cover a decent burial. During the Depression of the 1930s, farmers' associations formed burial societies to assure decent disposition for their members. In the mid- to late twentieth century, memorial societies were organized to secure simple, inexpensive, dignified funerals by providing information about economical methods of decent disposal and by arranging special rates with cooperating morticians.[3] In 1996 the Funeral and Memorial Society of America (FAMSA) became an umbrella organization that promoted these objectives.

Military service provides another leveling effect in final dispositions. Veterans and their families have free access to a series of national cemeteries where an honor guard provides a funeral accompaniment—including a three-gun salute—and where every gravestone is twenty-four inches high and four inches thick.

Another parallel between the pre- and postmortem human conditions is in their rights-bearing status. As described in chapter 3, a cadaver possesses independent, legally enforceable rights, including the rights to decent disposal, quiet repose, and respect for postmortem dignity.

The quasi-human status attributed to the corpse entails a modicum of dignity in cadaveric treatment and disposal even in the absence of explicit directions from the deceased. Anglo-American tradition generally resists the temptation to confiscate dead bodies and exploit them for utilitarian purposes such as education and research. But a corpse's entitlement to postmortem dignity extends well beyond protection of physical integrity. Anglo-American tradition also honors the quasi-human nature of a corpse and its close identification with its deceased predecessor by giving the deceased dominion over the fate of his or her earthly remains. A cadaver is no one's property, but a deceased person's previously expressed instructions or preferences govern a spectrum of issues affecting the cadaver, including the place and mode of body disposal, usage in research and teaching, organ transplant, semen removal, and continuation of fetal gestation. Even when no explicit premortem wishes are discernible, a cadaver's fate in these matters is often governed by projecting the deceased's wishes—that is, seeking to do what the deceased would have wanted done. In sum, while a cadaver can no longer make choices, it possesses an enforceable prerogative to have its predecessor's choices or preferences regarding disposal of its remains honored.

## The Importance of Planning

The continuing personal identity attributed to the human cadaver means that the disposal of the corpse is associated with the deceased's enduring image. D. Gareth Jones and Maja Whitaker describe the phenomenon that links, in survivors' minds, the fate of a human cadaver with its predecessor. They comment: "We [the public] consider that a person and his body are inseparable. . . . While this applies supremely during life, some very important aspects of this identity continue following death. . . . While the body retains a recognizable form, even in death, it commands the respect of identity. No longer a human presence, it still reminds us of the presence that once was utterly inseparable from it."[4] This close identity between a cadaver and its predecessor dictates that anyone interested in his or her personal legacy should care about the fate of his or her successor persona (the cadaver). "A life is the sum of what has been performed and spoken by the body"[5] — meaning the body in both its pre- and postmortem configurations.

Most people are apparently content to let their survivors figure out what to do with their postmortem remains. They expect that a respectful disposal will be arranged consistent with the prevailing family or cultural traditions. Usually this means prompt burial or cremation following some memorial rites. Yet it behooves a person to articulate in advance his or her preferences for postmortem disposal. One's conception of postmortem dignity may diverge from that of one's survivors. Or the survivors may differ among themselves in projecting what the deceased's wishes would have been if they had only been expressed. And if beneficence toward fellow humans is one of your inclinations, you might well consider, in formulating instructions, the continuing roles available to the human cadaver as teacher, research subject, and supplier of used body parts. Your good deeds can continue after you die.

**Options for Enhancing Your Legacy**

Human remains can serve some useful functions. For example, an obvious beneficial impact flows from donating critical organs or tissue to medically needy living persons. Cadaveric tissue then benefits the recipient, extends the physical presence of the deceased, and adds a humanitarian element to the memories associated with the deceased. While I still favor (as described in chapter 7) a presumed consent framework that would allow the salvaging of body parts absent the deceased's previous decision to opt out of a donative presumption, such a framework is not on the immediate horizon. In the meantime, the prevailing route to organ retrieval demands that a would-be donor indicate, in advance, willingness to be a tissue donor; otherwise, the decision depends on the good will of the surviving kin.

Many other beneficial roles are open to a cadaver. In 1981 Lee Hayes of the legendary Weavers folk music group wrote a song called "Dead Earnest" documenting his instructions for postmortem disposal of his cadaver:

If I should die before I wake
All my bone and sinew take
Put them in the compost pile
To decompose a little while
Sun, rain and worms will have their way
Reducing me to common clay
All that I am will feed the trees
And little fishes in the seas
When corn and radishes you munch
You may be having me for lunch
Then excrete me with a grin
Chortling, there goes Lee again
'Twill be my happiest destiny
To die and live eternally

The fertilizer route is still available, though it generally means prompt dissolution of a cadaver rather than gradual composting (see chapter 5). For me, fertilizing radishes is not a constructive enough role for a well-meaning cadaver.

Participation in medical education seems more constructive (though not more productive) than conversion to fertilizer. Dissection of cadavers continues to be an important element of medical education. A Boston University medical student recently expressed her gratitude to the donor whose corpse provided a critical introduction to the wonders of human anatomy. She labeled the donation "an exponential gift from one man to eight future doctors to hundreds of patients."[6] Yet the modest rate of cadaver donation sometimes means that six to eight students must share access to each cadaver in an anatomy lab. There are over one hundred academically based whole-body donation programs that could benefit from increased donations, which would lower the student/cadaver ratio.[7] A decedent's recorded wishes to be a donor can smooth the anatomy lab route, which demands that a cadaver be specially embalmed within twenty-four hours of death.

A cadaver can contribute to medical education and scientific progress in other ways. Continuing medical education often requires bodies or body parts as practice material for learning or honing new skills and techniques. Researchers in both academia and industry also need cadavers or parts to help expand medical knowledge about bodily afflictions and cures as well as to measure effectiveness of safety products. Postmortem examination of the body's interior sometimes provides insights that are unavailable from living research subjects—as in brain research concerning dementia or the effects of concussive trauma. Keep in mind, though, that cadaveric donations for research or continuing education may pass through entrepreneurial operations that profit from the processing and handling of cadaveric material.[8] This does not make the ultimate contribution to medical science any less worthwhile, but people who choose to benefit research should be aware that not all of the participants are operating on a purely altruistic plane.

## On the Limits Posed by Good Taste

The good news is that living persons are entitled to shape their corpse's fate in many constructive ways. Postmortem human dignity imposes only a few constraints. Do not try to extend your sexuality beyond your lifetime; necrophilia is an intrinsic violation of postmortem human dignity even when it is based on consent. Nor is there any point in encouraging mourners, in their zeal to honor your life, to cook and ingest part of your remains. Cannibalism is a form of hard-core undignified treatment—an intrinsic desecration of human remains.

The bad news is that a corpse has an extremely limited capacity to enforce its predecessor's instructions. Implementation of controversial wishes for cadaver disposal may depend on survivors' willingness to overcome any qualms about the indignity or distaste of a chosen course. As noted in chapter 12, some people who shape their posthumous fate pursue an educational goal by agreeing to preservation and display of their remains, as in exhibits of plastinated bodies. Though some observers are repulsed by this public display—deeming it to be a crass, voyeuristic violation of human dignity—there is no consensus that such displays are intolerably disrespectful. Cooperative survivors can send a designated corpse on for plastination. Other people seek to perpetuate their memories by providing keepsakes such as locks of hair or other bodily relics. Again, there is no intrinsic bar to providing bodily mementos, but postmortem human dignity and respect pose self-enforcing limitations on this practice. That is, the people involved in the disposal of a cadaver may rebel against some bizarre efforts to perpetuate the remains, as in the case of the deceased poet who wanted his verse bound in tanned skin from his corpse.

The implementation of disposal wishes might be helped if the probable survivors are alerted to any unconventional or controversial plans and their advance cooperation is enlisted. In November 2009 an eighty-year-old Israeli man in failing health sought a judicial declaration upholding his request to have his corpse thrown to wild animal scavengers on the Golan Heights.[9] The Israeli court rejected the petition, ruling that such disposal would constitute an intolerable offense to human dignity. The result is not surprising given the religiously influenced cultural norms that prevail in Israel. Putting aside practical objections such as the unsightly debris of skeletonized remains, the question remains whether a decedent's wish to become fodder for wild animals represents a debasement that inherently violates postmortem human dignity. Is this posthumous route any more degrading than burial at sea to become food for the fish?

Instead of turning to a court, wouldn't the Israeli man have been better off soliciting advance cooperation from his likely survivors? A cooperative survivor offers the best hope for implementation of unconventional disposal wishes. If one's wishes about postmortem disposal are so morally troublesome that survivors' cooperation cannot be enlisted, chances are that the contemplated method does indeed exceed the bounds of postmortem human dignity.

# Notes

## Introduction

1. Foster, "Individualized Justice in Disputes over Dead Bodies," 1354.
2. Ibid., 1353.
3. Associated Press, "Richards," *Trenton Times,* April 4, 2007.
4. *Arthur v. Milstein,* 949 So.2d 1163 (Fla. App. 2007).
5. Webster, *Does This Mean You'll See Me Naked?,* 101.
6. Lynch, *The Undertaking: Life Studies from the Dismal Trade,* 182.
7. Harris, *Grave Matters,* 43.

## Chapter 1

1. *People v. Dlugash* 363 N.E.2d 1155.
2. Bondeson, *Buried Alive,* 136.
3. Chapter 4 traces the precise nature and timing of postmortem corporeal disintegration.
4. Bondeson, *Buried Alive,* 139–40.
5. Ibid., 146–53.
6. Webster, *Does This Mean You'll See Me Naked?,* 157.
7. Bondeson, *Buried Alive,* 138.
8. Munson, *Raising the Dead,* 180.
9. Bondeson, *Buried Alive,* 294.
10. Ibid., 121–27.
11. Ibid., 128.
12. Ibid., 134.
13. Ibid., 265.
14. Ramsland, *Cemetery Stories,* 27.
15. Webster, *Does This Mean You'll See Me Naked?,* 156.
16. Munson, *Raising the Dead,* 181.
17. Truog, "Brain Death"; Miller and Truog, "Rethinking the Ethics of Vital Organ Donations," 40.

18. Hatch, *What Happens When You Die*, 62.

19. Miller and Truog, "Rethinking the Ethics of Vital Organ Donations," 39.

20. Harrington, "The Thin Flat Line," 39–42.

21. Shemie, "Clarifying the Paradigm for the Ethics of Donation and Transplantation."

22. Truog, "Brain Death," 276.

23. Chapter 7 covers both the severe shortage of transplant organs and various proposals to increase the supply of cadaveric organs for transplant.

24. Harrington, "The Thin Flat Line," 15.

25. Fidler, "Implementing Donation after Cardiac Death Protocols," 133–34.

26. Bernat, "The Boundaries of Organ Donation after Circulatory Death," 671.

27. M. D. D. Bell, "Non-Heart Beating Organ Donation," 178.

28. Ibid.

29. Ibid.

30. Miller and Truog, "Rethinking the Ethics of Vital Organ Donations," 42.

## Chapter 2

1. Quigley, *The Corpse*, 20.

2. Lynch, *The Undertaking*, 7.

3. Quigley, *The Corpse*, 116.

4. Montross, *Bodies of Work*, 40.

5. Ibid., 24.

6. Carter, *First Cut*, 251; Montross, *Bodies of Work*, 257.

7. Carter, *First Cut*, 271.

8. Jones and Whitaker, *Speaking for the Dead*, 36.

9. Laderman, *The Sacred Remains*, 75.

10. Webster, *Does This Mean You'll See Me Naked?*, 68.

11. Laderman, *Rest in Peace*, 211.

12. Matson, *Round-Trip to Deadsville*, 65.

13. Webster, *Does This Mean You'll See Me Naked?*, 70–71.

14. Montimurro and Higbie, *Provolone in the Casket*, 98–99.

15. Iserson, *Death to Dust*, 202.

16. Ibid., 170.

17. Klaver, *Sites of Autopsy in Contemporary Culture*, 32.

18. Montross, *Bodies of Work*, 26.

19. Ibid., 29.

20. Lawrence, "Beyond the Grave—The Use and Meaning of Human Body Parts," 112–13.

21. Prothero, *Purified by Fire*, 124.

22. Richardson, *Death, Dissection, and the Destitute*, 78.

23. Webster, *Does This Mean You'll See Me Naked?*, 11.

24. Daybell, *One Foot in the Grave*, 89; Gilbert, *Death's Door*, 53.

25. Wilkins, *The Bedside Book of Death*, 13–14.

26. Richardson, *Death, Dissection, and the Destitute*, 7.

27. Dorff, *Matters of Life and Death*, 232–33.

28. Richardson, *Death, Dissection, and the Destitute*, 15.

29. Laderman, *Rest in Peace*, 207.

30. Emson, "It Is Immoral to Require Consent for Cadaver Organ Donation," 125.

31. Kerrigan, *The History of Death*, 167, 175.

32. Gilbert, *Death's Door*, 44.

33. Bahn, *Written in Bones*, 141.

34. Quigley, *The Corpse*, 86.

35. Bahn, *Written in Bones*, 141, 168.

36. Iserson, *Death to Dust*, 183.

37. Lawrence, "Beyond the Grave," 112; Colman, *Corpses, Coffins, and Crypts*, 123.

38. Quigley, *The Corpse*, 181.

39. Iserson, *Death to Dust*, 407.

40. Quigley, *The Corpse*, 90.

41. Montimurro and Higbie, *Provolone in the Casket*, 78.

42. Ramsland, *Cemetery Stories*, 50.

43. Cullen, *Remember Me*, 101–102.

44. Prothero, *Purified by Fire*, 7.

45. Laderman, *The Sacred Remains*, 4–5, 59.

46. Stannard, *The Puritan Way of Death*, 100.

47. Laderman, *Rest in Peace*, 53.

48. Yalom, *The American Resting Place*, 277.

49. Dorff, *Matters of Life and Death*, 239.

50. Laderman, *The Sacred Remains*, 29.

51. Sappol, *A Traffic of Dead Bodies*, 15.

52. Quigley, *The Corpse*, 15.

53. Saulny, "A Day of Searching, Anger and Renewed Grief in a Desecrated Illinois Cemetery."

54. *Lott v. State of New York*, 225 N.Y.S.2d 434 (N.Y. Ct. Cl. 1962).

55. Lawrence, "Beyond the Grave," 117.

56. Pedro I of Portugal sent a very different message about his late mistress via the disposition of her corpse. He had her body exhumed, placed on a lavish throne, and garbed in regal robes. How long the corpse remained in that position is unknown.

57. Laderman, *Rest in Peace*, 167.

## Chapter 3

1. Clark, "Keep Your Hands Off My (Dead) Body," 48–49.

2. *Carney v. Knollwood Cemetery Ass'n*, 514 N.E.2d 430, 432 (Ohio App. 1986).

3. Matson, *Round-Trip to Deadsville*, 44.

4. Callahan, "On Harming the Dead," 351.

5. N.Y. Pub. Health L. Section 4201.

6. Pa. Consol. Stat. Ann. Section 305.

7. *In re* Matter of *Moyer*, 577 P.2d. 108 (Utah 1978); Carey, "The Disposition of the Body after Death," 264–65.

8. *Thompson v. Deeds*, 61 N.W. 842 (Iowa 1895).

9. *O'Donnell v. Slack*, 55 P. 906 (Cal. 1899).

10. Jackson, *The Law of Cadavers and of Burial and Burial Places*, 44.

11. *Fidelity Union Trust v. Heller*, 84 A.2d 485 (N.J. Ch. 1951); Foster, "Individualized Justice in Disputes over Dead Bodies," 1376, 1390.

12. Gilbert, *Death's Door*, 272–75.

13. Ramsland, *Cemetery Stories*, 52.

14. *Sacred Heart of Jesus Polish Catholic Church v. Soklowski*, 199 N.W. 81 (Minn. 1924).

15. Taylor, "Right of Sepulture," 368.

16. *Cohen v. Cohen*, 896 So.2d 950 (Fla. App. 2005).

17. Lynch, *The Undertaking*, 8.

18. Laderman, *Rest in Peace*, 184.

19. *Enos v. Snyder*, 63 P. 170 (Cal. 1900).

20. Taylor, "Right of Sepulture," 359; Jackson, *The Law of Cadavers*, 31–33.

21. *Burney v. Children's Hospital*, 47 N.E. 401 (Mass. 1897); *Pierce v. Proprietors of Swan Point Cemetery*, 10 R.I. 227 (1872).

22. Jackson, *The Law of Cadavers*, 35–37.

23. *Larson v. Chase*, 50 N.W. 238 (Minn. 1891), 312.

24. Bray, "Personalizing Personality," 228.

25. *Nichols v. Central Vermont Ry.*, 109 A. 905 (Vt. 1919).

26. Nelkin and Andrews, "Do the Dead Have Interests?," 281.

27. Foster, "Individualized Justice in Disputes over Dead Bodies," 1396–99.

28. Jackson, *The Law of Cadavers*, 25.

29. *Pierce v. Proprietors of Swan Point Cemetery*, 10 R.I. 227 (1872); *Maine v. Bradbury*, 9 A.2d 657 (Me. 1939).

30. *State v. Glass*, 272 N.E.2d 273 (Ohio App. 1971).

31. *Pettigrew v. Pettigrew*, 56 A. 878 (Pa 1904).

32. *Silvia v. Helger*, 67 A.2d 27 (R.I. 1949).

33. Dorman, "Anger over Exhumation in Gipper's Hometown."

34. Maples and Browning, *Dead Men Do Tell Tales*, 227–28.

35. *Thomasits v. Cochise Memory Gardens*, 721 P.2d 1166 (Ariz. App. 1986).

36. *Lavigne v. Wilkinson*, 116 A. 32 (N.H. 1921).

37. *Goldman v. Mollen*, 191 S.E. 627 (Va. 1937); *Yome v. Gorman*, 152 N.E. 126 (N.Y. 1926).

38. Matter of *Elman*, 578 N.Y.S.2d 95 (N.Y. Sup. Ct. 1991).

39. Kilgannon, "Public Lives."

40. Maples and Browning, *Dead Men Do Tell Tales*, 223.

41. Ruggles, "The Law of Burial," 527–28.

42. Smolensky, "Rights of the Dead," 788.

43. *National Archives Administration v. Favish*, 541 U.S. 157 (2004).

44. Smolensky, "Rights of the Dead," 764.

45. Quay, "Utilizing the Bodies of the Dead," 905.
46. Partridge, "Posthumous Interest and Posthumous Respect," 247.
47. Ruggles, "The Law of Burial," 531.
48. *Fitzimmons v. Olinger Mortuary*, 17 P.2d 535 (Colo. 1932).
49. Jordan, "Incubating for the State," 1108–12 (discussing *University Health Services v. Piazzi*, No. CV86-RCCV-464 [Richmond County, Ga., Aug. 4, 1986]).

**Chapter 4**

1. Quigley, *The Corpse*, 4, quoting Nuland, *How We Die*, 122.
2. Sachs, *Corpse*, 17.
3. See Roach, *Stiff*.
4. Sachs, *Corpse*, 18.
5. Hatch, *What Happens When You Die*, 47.
6. Sachs, *Corpse*, 20–21.
7. Maples and Browning, *Dead Men Do Tell Tales*, 38.
8. Hatch, *What Happens When You Die*, 45; Pringle, *The Mummy Congress*, 38–39.
9. Sachs, *Corpse*, 21.
10. Laderman, *Rest in Peace*, xvi.
11. Iserson, *Death to Dust*, 41–43.
12. Laderman, *Rest in Peace*, xix.
13. Quigley, *The Corpse*, 56.
14. Mitford, *The American Way of Death Revisited*, 55–57.
15. Iserson, *Death to Dust*, 314; Ramsland, *Cemetery Stories*, 12.
16. Laderman, *The Sacred Remains*, 112.
17. Ramsland, *Cemetery Stories*, 93.
18. Pringle, *The Mummy Congress*, 40.
19. Harris, *Grave Matters*, 34.
20. Mitford, *The American Way of Death Revisited*, 135.
21. Webster, *Does This Mean You'll See Me Naked?*, 81; Montimurro and Higbie, *Provolone in the Casket*, 58.
22. Webster, *Does This Mean You'll See Me Naked?*, 91.
23. Harris, *Grave Matters*, 36.
24. Daybell, *One Foot in the Grave*, 77–78.
25. Harris, *Grave Matters*, 13.
26. Webster, *Does This Mean You'll See Me Naked?*, 100.
27. Mitford, *The American Way of Death Revisited*, 58.
28. Colman, *Corpses, Coffins, and Crypts*, 46.
29. Lawrence, "Beyond the Grave," 126.
30. Roach, *Stiff*, 77–80.
31. Wilkins, *The Bedside Book of Death*, 123–24.
32. Mitford, *The American Way of Death Revisited*, 145.
33. Laderman, *The Sacred Remains*, 114.

34. Ibid.
35. Harris, *Grave Matters*, 45.
36. Long and Reim, *Fatal Facts*, 27.
37. Laderman, *The Sacred Remains*, 8.
38. Hatch, *What Happens When You Die*, 52–57.
39. Harris, *Grave Matters*, 17–20.
40. Montimurro and Higbie, *Provolone in the Casket*, 54.
41. Colman, *Corpses, Coffins, and Crypts*, 56.
42. Harris, *Grave Matters*, 21.
43. Ibid., 20–24.
44. Montimurro and Higbie, *Provolone in the Casket*, 55.
45. Iserson, *Death to Dust*, 190–209.
46. Webster, *Does This Mean You'll See Me Naked?*, 79.
47. Mitford, *The American Way of Death Revisited*, 43.
48. Wilkins, *The Bedside Book of Death*, 138–39; Webster, *Does This Mean You'll See Me Naked?*, 73.
49. Hatch, *What Happens When You Die*, 53.
50. Montross, *Bodies of Work*, 7.
51. Montimurro and Higbie, *Provolone in the Casket*, 71.
52. Mitford, *The American Way of Death Revisited*, 55.
53. Webster, *Does This Mean You'll See Me Naked?*, 90.
54. Hatch, *What Happens When You Die*, 84.
55. Montimurro and Higbie, *Provolone in the Casket*, 40.
56. Ramsland, *Cemetery Stories*, 167.
57. Pringle, *The Mummy Congress*, 324.

## Chapter 5

1. Carter, *First Cut*, 298.
2. Lynch, *The Undertaking*, 156–57.
3. Pringle, *The Mummy Congress*, 318.
4. Richardson, *Death, Dissection, and the Destitute*, 14.
5. Ibid.
6. Laderman, *Rest in Peace*, 201.
7. Huntington and Metcalf, *Celebrations of Death*, 187.
8. Quigley, *The Corpse*, 84; Bahn, *Written in Bones*, 135.
9. Iserson, *Death to Dust*, 498–99.
10. Genesis 3:19.
11. Jackson, *The Law of Cadavers*, 8.
12. Ramsland, *Cemetery Stories*, 85.
13. Prothero, *Purified by Fire*, 4.
14. Stannard, *The Puritan Way of Death*, 100.
15. Ramsland, *Cemetery Stories*, 83.

16. Yalom, *The American Resting Place*, 95.

17. Harris, *Grave Matters*, 144.

18. Ibid., 153.

19. Bernard, *The Law of Death and Disposal of the Dead*, 79.

20. Rivenburg, "A Degree of Finality."

21. Laderman, *The Sacred Remains*, 9, 69.

22. Prothero, *Purified by Fire*, 48–51.

23. Ramsland, *Cemetery Stories*, 86–87.

24. Laderman, *The Sacred Remains*, 44, 70–72.

25. Ibid., 44.

26. Ibid., 152.

27. Kugel, "You Can Come and Go, They're Staying Awhile."

28. Brooks, "The Rich and Famous at Rest in Eden."

29. Yalom, *The American Resting Place*, 46.

30. Ibid., 134.

31. Sappol, *A Traffic of Dead Bodies*, 321.

32. Yalom, *The American Resting Place*, 24.

33. Ramsland, *Cemetery Stories*, 134–35.

34. Yalom, *The American Resting Place*, 91–92.

35. Laderman, *The Sacred Remains*, 48.

36. Jackson, *The Law of Cadavers*, 380.

37. Bernard, *The Law of Death and Disposal of the Dead*, 84–85.

38. Mitford, *The American Way of Death Revisited*, 103.

39. Ramsland, *Cemetery Stories*, 102.

40. Wilkins, *The Bedside Book of Death*, 158; Sappol, *A Traffic of Dead Bodies*, 35.

41. Clark, "Keep Your Hands Off My (Dead) Body," 70.

42. Wilkins, *The Bedside Book of Death*, 131.

43. Richardson, *Death, Dissection and the Destitute*, 273.

44. Yalom, *The American Resting Place*, 65–66, 93.

45. Webster, *Does This Mean You'll See Me Naked?*, 81.

46. Ibid., 83.

47. Brown, "In Death as in Life"; Mitford, *The American Way of Death Revisited*, 35.

48. Wilford, "Stonehenge Used as Cemetery from the Beginning."

49. Brown, "In Death as in Life"; Jean K. Wolf, *Lives of the Silent Stones in the Christ Church Burial Grounds*, 24.

50. Yalom, *The American Resting Place*, 15, 66.

51. Wolf, *Lives of the Silent Stones in the Christ Church Burial Grounds*, 25.

52. Ramsland, *Cemetery Stories*, 86–87; Matson, *Round-Trip to Deadsville*, 27.

53. Wilkins, *The Bedside Book of Death*, 153.

54. Yalom, *The American Resting Place*, 27.

55. Janet Greene, *Epitaphs to Remember*, 78.

56. Ibid., 84–86.

57. Iserson, *Death to Dust*, 541.

58. Yalom, *The American Resting Place*, 160–61.
59. Trebay, "For a Price, Final Resting Places That Even Tut Could Appreciate."
60. Ibid.
61. Larry McShane, "Leona Helmsley Gets a Tomb with a View."
62. Kevin Manahan, "Hit a Fade, a Draw."
63. Laderman, *The Sacred Remains*, 45.
64. Mitford, *The American Way of Death Revisited*, 139.
65. Iserson, *Death to Dust*, 542.
66. Trebay, "For a Price, Final Resting Places That Even Tut Could Appreciate."
67. Cullen, *Remember Me*, 52; Harris, *Grave Matters*, 38–41.
68. Yalom, *The American Resting Place*, 296.
69. Cullen, *Remember Me*, 58.
70. Harris, *Grave Matters*, 167.
71. Ibid., 155, 167.
72. Roach, *Stiff*, 270–72.
73. Ibid., 261.
74. Love, "What a Way to Go (Down the Drain)," 13.
75. Ibid.
76. Roach, *Stiff*, 252–57.
77. Iserson, *Death to Dust*, 319.
78. Ibid., 321.
79. Quigley, *The Corpse*, 95–96.
80. Ibid., 94–95.
81. Fitzpatrick, "Last Voyage."
82. Wilkins, *The Bedside Book of Death*, 245.
83. Quigley, *The Corpse*, 109.
84. Ibid., 97.
85. Diamant, "N.J. Crematory Reflects Shift in Catholic Church."
86. Wilkins, *The Bedside Book of Death*, 174.
87. Prothero, *Purified by Fire*, 9.
88. Ibid., 17.
89. Ibid., 53; Carey, "The Disposition of the Body after Death," 269.
90. Prothero, *Purified by Fire*, 79.
91. Ibid., 15.
92. Ibid., 108.
93. Ibid., 35.
94. Carey, "The Disposition of the Body after Death," 269.
95. Ibid.
96. Ibid.
97. Prothero, *Purified by Fire*, 128.
98. Ibid., 131.
99. Mitford, *The American Way of Death Revisited*, 113–14.

100. Bernard, *The Law of Death and Disposal of the Dead*, 89; Huntington and Metcalf, *Celebrations of Death*, 192.
101. Mitford, *The American Way of Death Revisited*, 112.
102. Prothero, *Purified by Fire*, 10.
103. Trebay, "For a Price, Final Resting Places That Even Tut Could Appreciate."
104. Diamant, "N.J. Crematory Reflects Shift in Catholic Church."
105. Quigley, *The Corpse*, 103.
106. Laderman, *Rest in Peace*, 143, 198.
107. Diamant, "N.J. Crematory Reflects Shift in Catholic Church."
108. Wilkins, *The Bedside Book of Death*, 244.
109. Hatch, *What Happens When You Die*, 75.
110. Prothero, *Purified by Fire*, 149.
111. Bernard, *The Law of Death and Disposal of the Dead*, 88.
112. Webster, *Does This Mean You'll See Me Naked?*, 91.
113. Bass and Jefferson, *Death's Acre*, 268–69.
114. Quigley, *The Corpse*, 98.
115. Carter, *First Cut*, 115.
116. Maples and Browning, *Dead Men Do Tell Tales*, 141–43.
117. Roach, *Stiff*, 82.
118. Bass and Jefferson, *Death's Acre*, 260-61; Bernard, *The Law of Death and Disposal of the Dead*, 87.
119. Ramsland, *Cemetery Stories*, 194–95.
120. Mitford, *The American Way of Death Revisited*, 18.
121. Quigley, *The Corpse*, 102.
122. Mitford, *The American Way of Death Revisited*, 118.
123. Quigley, *The Corpse*, 101.
124. Bass and Jefferson, *Death's Acre*, 262–69.
125. Brown, "In Death as in Life."
126. Ibid.
127. Hatch, *What Happens When You Die*, 67.
128. Iserson, *Death to Dust*, 271.
129. Wilkins, *The Bedside Book of Death*, 177.
130. Diamant, "N.J. Crematory Reflects Shift in Catholic Church."
131. Brown, "In Death as in Life."
132. Finder, "Colleges Offering Campuses as Final Resting Places."
133. Rivenburg, "A Degree of Finality."
134. Ibid.
135. Webster, *Does This Mean You'll See Me Naked?*, 95–96.
136. Laderman, *Rest in Peace*, 205.
137. Mitford, *The American Way of Death Revisited*, 112.
138. Robbins, "Roadblock for Spreading of Human Ashes in Wilderness."
139. Fitzpatrick, "Last Voyage."

140. Ibid.
141. Webster, *Does This Mean You'll See Me Naked?*, 95.
142. Fitzpatrick, "Last Voyage."
143. Cullen, *Remember Me*, 78.
144. Fitzpatrick, "Last Voyage."
145. Josias, "Burying the Hatchet in Burial Disputes," 1146.
146. Wilkins, *The Bedside Book of Death*, 245.
147. Quigley, *The Corpse*, 101.
148. See http://www.celestis.com.
149. Caldwell, "A Space Trek for Scotty's Ashes."
150. Lynch, *The Undertaking*, 88–89.
151. Cullen, *Remember Me*, 22.
152. Webster, *Does This Mean You'll See Me Naked?*, 93.
153. Cullen, *Remember Me*, 66.
154. Chapter 11 analyzes the elements that make certain treatment of cadavers so disrespectful as to be deemed desecration of human remains.
155. Rice, *Funerals Aren't Funny*, 70–71.

## Chapter 6

1. Pringle, *The Mummy Congress*, 268.
2. Lawrence, "Beyond the Grave," 126; Laderman, *The Sacred Remains*, 145.
3. Watson, "Jarred and Jarring," 1.
4. Ediden, "In Search of Answers from the Great Brains of Cornell."
5. Iserson, *Death to Dust*, 152.
6. Lawrence, "Beyond the Grave," 128.
7. Pascoe, "Collect-Me-Nots."
8. Pringle, *The Mummy Congress*, 281.
9. Ramsland, *Cemetery Stories*, 47.
10. Pringle, *The Mummy Congress*, 281.
11. Ibid., 283.
12. Verdery, *The Political Lives of Dead Bodies*, 23–53.
13. Pringle, *The Mummy Congress*, 285.
14. Ramsland, *Cemetery Stories*, 48.
15. Wilkins, *The Bedside Book of Death*, 131; Pringle, *The Mummy Congress*, 246–49.
16. David Raff, "He's Not a Pathologist, He's Pathological."
17. Bahn, *Written in Bones*, 166–68.
18. Wilkins, *The Bedside Book of Death*, 104.
19. Pringle, *The Mummy Congress*, 43
20. Roach, *Stiff*, 176.
21. Quigley, *The Corpse*, 239–40.
22. Pringle, *The Mummy Congress*, 47.
23. Wilkins, *The Bedside Book of Death*, 108.

24. Quigley, *The Corpse*, 240; Pringle, *The Mummy Congress*, 43–47.
25. Iserson, *Death to Dust*, 217–18.
26. Quigley, *The Corpse*, 264–65; Wilkins, *The Bedside Book of Death*, 135.
27. Colman, *Corpses, Coffins, and Crypts*, 53.
28. Pringle, *The Mummy Congress*, 137–38.
29. Iserson, *Death to Dust*, 215.
30. Pringle, *The Mummy Congress*, 119.
31. Iserson, *Death to Dust*, 222.
32. Pringle, *The Mummy Congress*, 263–64.
33. Wilkins, *The Bedside Book of Death*, 117.
34. Laytner, "The Mummy Makers"; Ramsland, *Cemetery Stories*, 74.
35. Cullen, *Remember Me*, 161–62.
36. Laytner, "The Mummy Makers."
37. Pringle, *The Mummy Congress*, 173.
38. Peipert, "The Future Is in Plastics."
39. The company's webpage is http://www.cor-labs.com.
40. Raff, "He's Not a Pathologist, He's Pathological"; Imogen O'Rorke, "Skinless Wonders . . . "
41. Burns, "Gunther von Hagens' BODY WORLDS: Selling Beautiful Education."
42. Weingarten, "Florida Museumgoers Line Up to See Corpses."
43. Peipert, "The Future Is in Plastics"; Burns, "Gunther von Hagens' BODY WORLDS," 11.
44. Raff, "He's Not a Pathologist, He's Pathological."
45. Burns, "Gunther von Hagens' BODY WORLDS," 14.
46. Peipert, "The Future Is in Plastics."
47. Weingarten, "Florida Museumgoers Line Up to See Corpses."
48. Quigley, *The Corpse*, 110.
49. Wilkins, *The Bedside Book of Death*, 144.
50. Iserson, *Death to Dust*, 296.
51. Sandomir, "Please Don't Call the Customers Dead."
52. Ibid.
53. Cullen, *Remember Me*, 121.
54. Wilkins, *The Bedside Book of Death*, 145–46.
55. Best, "Perfusion and Diffusion in Cryonics Protocol."
56. Wilkins, *The Bedside Book of Death*, 144.
57. Foster, "Individualized Justice in Disputes over Dead Bodies," 1354.
58. Quigley, *The Corpse*, 234–35.
59. *Donaldson v. Lungren*, 4 Cal. Reporter 2d 59 (Cal. App. 1992).
60. Lynch, *The Undertaking*, 117.
61. Matson, *Round-Trip to Deadsville*, 78.
62. Iserson, *Death to Dust*, 450.
63. Ibid., 424.
64. Ibid., 425.

65. Colman, *Corpses, Coffins, and Crypts*, 55.
66. The NFDA's webpage is http://www.nfda.org.
67. Lynch, *The Undertaking*, 84.
68. Cullen, *Remember Me*, 208.
69. Pringle, *The Mummy Congress*, 319.
70. Cullen, *Remember Me*, 32–33.
71. Montimurro and Higbie, *Provolone in the Casket*, 121.
72. Mitford, *The American Way of Death Revisited*, 53.
73. Rice, *Funerals Aren't Funny*, 104.
74. Ibid.
75. Yalom, *The American Resting Place*, 20.
76. Laderman, *The Sacred Remains*, 77.
77. Gilbert, *Death's Door*, 220.
78. Ibid., 219.
79. Ibid., 280.
80. Colman, *Corpses, Coffins, and Crypts*, 115; Yalom, *The American Resting Place*, 289.
81. Greene, *Epitaphs to Remember*, 6.
82. Clark, "Keep Your Hands Off My (Dead) Body," 91.
83. Greene, *Epitaphs to Remember*, 60.
84. Sappol, *A Traffic of Dead Bodies*, 37.
85. Koppel, "The Last Gravestone Business Standing."
86. Greene, *Epitaphs to Remember*, 83.
87. Yalom, *The American Resting Place*, 23.
88. Ibid.
89. Colman, *Corpses, Coffins, and Crypts*, 181.
90. Ibid.
91. Greene, *Epitaphs to Remember*, 59.
92. Matson, *Round-Trip to Deadsville*, 95.
93. Ramsland, *Cemetery Stories*, 110.
94. Colman, *Corpses, Coffins, and Crypts*, 184.
95. Ibid.

## Chapter 7

1. Cheney, *Body Brokers*, 168–69.
2. Iserson, *Death to Dust*, 152–53.
3. Emson, "It Is Immoral to Require Consent," 126.
4. Cheney, *Body Brokers*, 170.
5. Colman, *Corpses, Coffins, and Crypts*, 47.
6. Mehlmann, "Presumed Consent to Organ Donation," 45; Orentlicher, "Presumed Consent to Organ Donation," 295.
7. Meyers, *The Human Body and the Law*, 110–12.

8. Fevrier and Gay, "Informed Consent versus Presumed Consent," 10; Bernard, *The Law of Death and Disposal of the Dead*, 57.

9. UAGA Section 5(a) (2007). The UAGA is accessible at http://www.nccusl.org.

10. Reeves et al., "When Is an Organ Donor Not an Organ Donor?," 1260; Schiff, "Arising from the Dead," 929.

11. Reeves et al., "When Is an Organ Donor Not an Organ Donor?," 1261.

12. Ibid.

13. Schiff, "Arising from the Dead," 929.

14. Revised UAGA (2007), accessible at http://www.nccusl.org.

15. Comments by UAGA commissioners accompanying UAGA Sections 8 and 14 (2007), accessible at http://www.nccusl.org.

16. Bray, "Personalizing Personality," 229; *Nichols v. Central Vermont Ry.*, 109 A. 905 (Vt. 1919).

17. *Floyd v. Atlantic Coast Line Ry*, 84 S.E. 12 (N.C. 1914), 12.

18. Schiff, "Arising from the Dead," 926.

19. Quay, "Utilizing the Bodies of the Dead," 891.

20. Cheney, *Body Brokers*, 182; Kittredge, "Black Shrouds and Black Markets."

21. Cheney, *Body Brokers*, 180–82.

22. "Rest in Pieces," *Albany Times-Union*, January 17, 2007.

23. Katz, "The ReGift of Life," 961.

24. Chapter 8 provides more detail about forensic autopsies.

25. Patton, "A Call for Common Sense," 392; Orentlicher, "Presumed Consent to Organ Donation," 300.

26. Matas, "A Gift of Life Deserves Compensation," 604.

27. Shari Roan, "Organ Shortage Has Officials Looking at Presumed Consent"; Organ Procurement and Transplantation Network, http://optn.transplant.hrsa.gov/data/.

28. Truog, "Consent for Organ Donation," 1211.

29. Hill and Anderson, *The Autopsy*, 12.

30. Healy, *Last Best Gifts*, 33.

31. Ibid., 27.

32. Kelso et al., "Palliative Care Consultation in the Process of Organ Donation after Cardiac Death," 124.

33. Reeves et al., "When Is an Organ Donor Not an Organ Donor?," 1261; Burns et al., "Using Newly Deceased Patients to Teach Resuscitation Procedures," 1654.

34. Spital, "Should People Who Commit Themselves to Organ Donation Be Granted Preferred Status to Receive Organ Transplants?," 270.

35. Quante and Wiedebusche, "Overcoming the Shortage of Transplantable Organs," 525.

36. Brody, "The Solvable Problem of Organ Shortages."

37. Truog, "Consent for Organ Donation," 1211; Brody, "The Solvable Problem of Organ Shortages."

38. Kelso et al., "Palliative Care Consultation."

39. Ibid., 122.
40. A sharp differentiation between physicians attending the dying patient and transplant surgeons is maintained to dispel the appearance of divided loyalties on the part of the physicians.
41. Gagandeep et al., "Expanding the Donor Kidney Pool," 1685.
42. Foley et al., "Donation after Cardiac Death," 730.
43. Fidler, "Implementing Donation after Cardiac Death Protocols," 135.
44. Phua et al., "Pro/con Debate," 211.
45. Bernat, "The Boundaries of Organ Donation after Circulatory Death," 670.
46. Professor Norm Fost, in a communication to the Bioethics listserv of the Medical College of Wisconsin, May 18, 2008.
47. Fidler, "Implementing Donation after Cardiac Death Protocols," 129.
48. Ward, "Death's Army."
49. McKinley, "Doctor Cleared of Harming Man to Rush Organ Removal."
50. Cantor and Thomas, "The Legal Bounds of Physician Conduct Hastening Death," 116–19.
51. Revised UAGA Section 14 (2007), accessible at http://www.nccusl.org.
52. See the drafters' summary to the revised UAGA (2007) available at www.http://nccusl.org.
53. Verheijde et al., "The Revised UAGA: New Challenges to Balancing Patient Rights and Physician Responsibilities," *Philos Ethics Humanit Med* 2, no. 19 (September 12, 2007), www.peh-med.com/content/2/1/19.
54. Cantor, *Advance Directives and the Pursuit of Death with Dignity,* 31.
55. Ibid., 72–78.
56. Drafters' comments to revised UAGA Section 14 (2007).
57. Truog, "Consent for Organ Donation," 1209.
58. Verheijde et al., "The Revised UAGA."
59. Magliocca et al., "Extracorporeal Support for Organ Donation after Cardiac Death Effectively Expands the Donor Pool," 1101; Sung and Punch, "Uncontrolled DCDs: The Next Step?," 1506.
60. Bonnie et al., "Legal Authority to Preserve Organs in Cases of Cardiac Death," 746; Childress, "Organ Donation after Circulatory Determination of Death," 767.
61. Bonnie et al., "Legal Authority," 742.
62. Carey, "The Disposition of the Body after Death," 268.
63. Schiff, "Arising from the Dead," 916.
64. Bray, "Personalizing Personality," 223; Miller, "Death and Dead Bodies," 786.
65. Goodwin, "Formalism and the Legal Status of Body Parts," 317.
66. Munson, *Raising the Dead*, 111.
67. Satel and Hippen, "When Altruism Isn't Enough," 194.
68. Bray, "Personalizing Personality," 222; Herring, "Giving, Selling, and Sharing Bodies," 54.
69. Gross, "*E Pluribus UNOS*: The National Organ Transplantation Act," 183.
70. Richardson and Turner, "Bodies as Property," 39; Matas, "A Gift of Life Deserves Compensation," 7.

71. Patton, "A Call for Common Sense," 425.
72. Woan, "Buy Me a Pound of Flesh," 418–20.
73. Volokh, "Medical Self-Defense, Prohibited Experimental Therapies, and Payment for Organs," 29–30.
74. Healy, *Last Best Gifts*, 25–26.
75. Goodwin, "Formalism and the Legal Status of Body Parts," 315; Woan, "Buy Me a Pound of Flesh," 436.
76. Spar, "The Egg Trade—Making Sense of the Market for Human Oocytes," 1289.
77. Healy, *Last Best Gifts*, 21.
78. Katz, "The ReGift of Life," 954–56; Goodwin, *Black Markets*, 174–78; Marchione and Borenstein, "Surgeries Using Cadaver Tissue Pose Risks."
79. Cheney, *Body Brokers*, xv.
80. Calandrillo, "Cash for Kidneys?," 81; When a family member consents to the donation of cadaveric tissue, the immediate recipient is usually a nonprofit charitable tissue bank. But more commercial entities intervene before the tissue reaches the eventual transplant recipient. Tissue processors (for-profit entities) and intermediaries (for-profit brokers) are often involved in financial transactions before such donated tissue reaches transplant recipients in hospitals (Katz, "The ReGift of Life," 974). The processors perform a variety of services in preparing the transplantable tissue—including testing, sterilization, shaping, storage, and shipping. The brokers act as middlemen in the chain of tissue supply. "Even though human organs are not for sale, everything else associated with their transplantation most definitely is" (Calandrillo, "Cash for Kidneys?," ibid.).
81. Katz, "The ReGift of Life," 954, 971–72.
82. Ibid., 976, 1006.
83. Cheney, *Body Brokers*, 8.
84. Katz, "The ReGift of Life," 956, 961; Cohen, "FDA Reviews Cadaver-Tissue Industry"; Cheney, *Body Brokers*, 171.
85. Cohen, "FDA Reviews Cadaver-Tissue Industry."
86. Katz, "The ReGift of Life," 955.
87. Satel and Hippen, "When Altruism Isn't Enough," 196.
88. Calandrillo, "Cash for Kidneys?," 108–9, 115.
89. Healy, *Last Best Gifts*, 128.
90. Ibid., 125.
91. Spital and Taylor, "Routine Recovery of Cadaveric Organs for Transplantation," 301.
92. Jones, "Use of Bequeathed and Unclaimed Bodies in the Dissecting Rooms," 105.
93. Fevrier and Gay, "Informed Consent versus Presumed Consent," 10.
94. Glannon, "Do the Sick Have a Right to Cadaveric Organs?," 155.
95. Spital and Taylor, "Routine Recovery of Cadaveric Organs for Transplantation," 301.
96. Orentlicher, "Presumed Consent to Organ Donation," 300.
97. Ibid., 303, n. 27.
98. See Wis. Statutes Section 157.06(22m); Calif. Health & Safety Code Section 7150.40(a)(10)(A).

99. Mehlmann, "Presumed Consent to Organ Donation," 36; see Fla. Statutes Annotated Section 732.5185; Del. Code Annotated Section 4712.

100. See Orentlicher, "Presumed Consent to Organ Donation," 301, nn. 20, 21; Indiana Code Section 36-2-14-19; Md. Code Section 4-509.1.

101. UAGA Section 9(10) (2006).

102. See the drafters' comments to revised UAGA Section 9(10) (2007).

103. Any proposed statutory scheme for PC—even with an opt-out provision—would face a similar constitutional challenge. For some critics, a PC regime would constitute unconsented government confiscation of organs for transplant. For them, an opt-out provision does not alter the confiscatory nature of PC; they believe either that opting out would not be readily available or that simple inertia of people (in neglecting to opt out) would result in persons becoming unwilling organ donors.

104. *Brotherton v. Cleveland,* 923 F.2d 477 (6th Cir. 1991).

105. Jackson, *The Law of Cadavers,* 128.

106. *Bauer v. North Fulton Medical,* 527 S.E.2d 240 (Ga. App. 1999). But see *George Lanier Hospital v. Andrews,* 901 So.2d 714, 726 (Ala. 2004).

107. Cheney, *Body Brokers,* xv.

108. *State of Florida v. Powell,* 497 So.2d 1188 (Fla. 1986); *Arnaud v. Odom,* 870 F.2d. 304 (5th Cir. 1989); *Newman v. Sathyavaglswaran,* 287 F.3d. 786 (9th Cir. 2001).

109. *Roe v. Wade,* 410 U.S. 113 (1973).

110. *Lawrence v. Texas,* 539 U.S. 558, 574 (2003).

111. Lawrence, "Beyond the Grave," 113; Chadwick, "Corpses, Recycling, and Therapeutic Purposes," 65.

112. *State of Florida v. Powell,* 497 So.2d 1188 (Fla. 1986); *Georgia Lions Eye Bank v. Lavant,* 335 S.E.2d 127 (Ga. 1985) and cases cited in n. 108.

113. *State of Florida v. Powell,* 497 So.2d 1188, 1190 (Fla. 1986).

114. Ibid., 1191.

115. Ibid.

116. *Cruzan v. Missouri Department of Health,* 497 U.S. 261 (1990).

117. Miller, "Death and Dead Bodies," 780; Roan, "Organ Shortage Has Officials Looking at Presumed Consent."

118. Abadie and Gay, "The Impact of Presumed Consent Legislation on Cadaveric Organ Donation," 1, 5.

119. Healey, "Do Presumed-Consent Laws Raise Organ Procurement Rates?," 1042.

120. Liddy, "The New Body Snatchers," 819–20.

121. Orentlicher, "Presumed Consent to Organ Donation," 18, n. 73.

122. *Newman v. Sathyavaglswaran,* 287 F.3d. 786 (9th Cir. 2001).

123. Lawrence, "Beyond the Grave," 113.

124. Ibid., 112.

125. Fevrier and Gay, "Informed Consent versus Presumed Consent," 6; Abadie and Gay, "The Impact of Presumed Consent Legislation on Cadaveric Organ Donation," 5.

126. Childress, "Organ Donation after Circulatory Determination of Death," 768.

## Chapter 8

1. Rodning, "O Death, Where Is Thy Sting?," 281–82.
2. Carlino, *Books of the Body*, 2.
3. Rodning, "O Death, Where Is Thy Sting?," 282.
4. Nelkin and Andrews, "Do the Dead Have Interests?," 262–63; Iserson, *Death to Dust*, 90.
5. Quigley, *The Corpse*, 26.
6. Klaver, *Sites of Autopsy in Contemporary Culture*, 11.
7. Shultz, *Body Snatching*, 5.
8. Carlino, *Books of the Body*, 85.
9. Iserson, *Death to Dust*, 90; Shultz, *Body Snatching*, 13.
10. Iserson, *Death to Dust*, 91.
11. Shultz, *Body Snatching*, 11.
12. Ibid., 6–18.
13. Ibid., 18; Sappol, *A Traffic of Dead Bodies*, 2.
14. Wilkins, *The Bedside Book of Death* 63; Sappol, *A Traffic of Dead Bodies*, 47.
15. Reifler, "Have We Lost Our Heads?," 8.
16. Carter, *First Cut*, 18; Montross, *Bodies of Work*, 7–8.
17. Montross, *Bodies of Work*, 216–17.
18. Carter, *First Cut*, 140.
19. Montross, *Bodies of Work*, 288.
20. Roach, *Stiff*, 52–53.
21. Chung and Lehmann, "Informed Consent and the Process of Cadaver Donation," 964.
22. Cheney, *Body Brokers*, 2, 49.
23. Roach, *Stiff*, 19–24.
24. Carter, *First Cut*, 39.
25. Raff, "He's Not a Pathologist, He's Pathological."
26. Carey, "The Disposition of the Body after Death," 259.
27. Sappol, *A Traffic of Dead Bodies*, 100.
28. Iserson, *Death to Dust*, 462.
29. Quay, "Utilizing the Bodies of the Dead," 920.
30. *Holland v. Metalious*, 198 A.2d 654 (N.H. 1964).
31. Quigley, *The Corpse*, 293.
32. Lawrence, "Beyond the Grave," 122.
33. Krauskopf, "The Law of Dead Bodies," 459.
34. Lawrence, "Beyond the Grave," 122.
35. Carter, *First Cut*, 103, 181, 205; Montross *Bodies of Work*, 69.
36. Iserson, *Death to Dust*, 79.
37. Chung and Lehmann, "Informed Consent and the Process of Cadaver Donation," 966.

38. Hill and Anderson, *The Autopsy*, 13.
39. Chung and Lehmann, "Informed Consent and the Process of Cadaver Donation," 966.
40. Rodning, "O Death, Where Is Thy Sting?," 283.
41. Iserson, *Death to Dust*, 116.
42. Hill and Anderson, *The Autopsy*, 20–21, 37.
43. Klaver, *Sites of Autopsy in Contemporary Culture*, 34.
44. Hill and Anderson, *The Autopsy*, 27.
45. Hoyert, "The Autopsy, Medicine, and Mortality Statistics," 12–13; Hill and Anderson, *The Autopsy*, 4.
46. Quigley, *The Corpse*, 123.
47. Hoyert, "The Autopsy, Medicine, and Mortality Statistics," 13.
48. Webster, *Does This Mean You'll See Me Naked?*, 158.
49. Iserson, *Death to Dust*, 131; Webster, *Does This Mean You'll See Me Naked?*, 160.
50. Hoyert, "The Autopsy, Medicine, and Mortality Statistics," 13.
51. Iserson, *Death to Dust*, 132.
52. Dobbs, "Buried Answers."
53. Hill and Anderson, *The Autopsy*, 127.
54. Ibid., 39, 124.
55. Ibid., 49.
56. Ibid., 14.
57. Ibid., 50–51.
58. Dobbs, "Buried Answers."
59. Quigley, *The Corpse*, 117.
60. Hoyert, "The Autopsy, Medicine, and Mortality Statistics," 39.
61. Hill and Anderson, *The Autopsy*, 11.
62. Ibid., 62.
63. Hoyert, "The Autopsy, Medicine, and Mortality Statistics," 19.
64. Hill and Anderson, *The Autopsy*, 234.
65. Coradazzi et al., "Discrepancies between Clinical Diagnoses and Autopsy Findings," 388.
66. Hill and Anderson, *The Autopsy*, 35; Dobbs, "Buried Answers."
67. Hoyert, "The Autopsy, Medicine, and Mortality Statistics," 1.
68. Hill and Anderson, *The Autopsy*, 164.
69. Ibid., 105.
70. Hoyert, "The Autopsy, Medicine, and Mortality Statistics," 30, 36.
71. Hill and Anderson, *The Autopsy*, 57–59, 234.
72. Savulescu, "Death, Us and Our Bodies," 126.
73. Hill and Anderson, *The Autopsy*, 59.
74. Ibid.
75. Ibid., 196–98.
76. *Burney v. Children's Hospital*, 47 N.E. 401 (Mass 1897); *Coleman v. Sopher*, 499 S.E.2d 592

(W.Va 1997); *Palmquist v. Standard Accident Insurance Co.*, 3 F.Supp. 358 (S.D. Cal. 1933).

77. Nelkin and Andrews, "Do the Dead Have Interests?," 273.

78. Maclean, "Letting Go . . . Parents, Professionals, and the Law," 84; Klaiman, "Whose Brain Is It Anyway?," 475–76.

79. Hill and Anderson, *The Autopsy*, 10.

80. See *Board of Regents v. Oglesby*, 591 S.E.2d 417 (Ga. App. 2003).

81. Iserson, *Death to Dust*, 152–53.

82. Klaiman, "Whose Brain Is It Anyway?," 475–76.

83. *Albrecht v. Treon*, 889 N.E.2d. 120 (Ohio 2008).

84. *Albrecht v. Treon*, 889 N.E.2d. 120, 126–27 (Ohio 2008). A sharp dissent disputed the legality of unannounced retention of the brain—"the source of the deceased's every thought, aspiration, dream, fear, laugh, memory, or emotion." 889 N.E.2d. 120, 134.

85. Sheach Leith, "Consent and Nothing but Consent?," 1032.

86. Klaiman, "Whose Brain Is It Anyway?," 486.

87. Sheach Leith, "Consent and Nothing but Consent?," 1028.

88. Burton, "The Autopsy in Modern Undergraduate Medical Education," 1081.

89. Ely, "In an Age of Images, Teaching Pathology by Hand."

90. Ibid.

91. Quigley, *The Corpse*, 118.

92. Hoyert, "The Autopsy, Medicine, and Mortality Statistics," 17.

93. Long and Reim, *Fatal Facts*, 13.

94. Hill and Anderson, *The Autopsy*, 196–98, 234–36; Miller, "Death and Dead Bodies," 775.

95. Hill and Anderson, *The Autopsy*, 182.

96. Ibid., 158.

97. Hoyert, "The Autopsy, Medicine, and Mortality Statistics," 1.

98. Coradazzi et al., "Discrepancies between Clinical Diagnoses and Autopsy Findings," 388–89.

99. Hoyert, "The Autopsy, Medicine, and Mortality Statistics," 12.

100. Dobbs, "Buried Answers."

101. Hoyert, "The Autopsy, Medicine, and Mortality Statistics," 8, 32.

102. Long and Reim, *Fatal Facts*, 14.

103. Dobbs, "Buried Answers"; Hill and Anderson, *The Autopsy*, 88.

104. Coradazzi et al., "Discrepancies between Clinical Diagnoses and Autopsy Findings," 388–89; Hill and Anderson, *The Autopsy*, 55, 192–94.

105. Hoyert, "The Autopsy, Medicine, and Mortality Statistics," 27.

106. Council on Ethical and Judicial Affairs of the AMA (CEJA), "Performing Procedures on the Newly Deceased," 1212.

107. Morag et al., "Performing Procedures on the Newly Deceased for Teaching Purposes," 92, 94.

108. Schmidt et al., "The Ethical Debate on Practicing Procedures on the Newly Dead," 965.

109. Burns et al., "Using Newly Deceased Patients to Teach Resuscitation Procedures," 1652; Chung and Lehmann, "Informed Consent and the Process of Cadaver Donation," 966.

110. Burns, "Using Newly Deceased Patients to Teach Resuscitation Procedures," 1652–53.

111. Moore, "The Practice of Medical Procedures on Newly Dead Patients—Is Consent Warranted?," 391.

112. Ibid., 390.

113. Morag et al., "Performing Procedures on the Newly Deceased for Teaching Purposes," 95.

114. Schmidt et al., "The Ethical Debate on Practicing Procedures on the Newly Dead," 964.

115. Ibid., 963–64; Morag et al., "Performing Procedures on the Newly Deceased for Teaching Purposes," 95.

116. Nelkin and Andrews, "Do the Dead Have Interests?," 265.

117. Goldblatt, "Don't Ask, Don't Tell," 88; CEJA, "Performing Procedures on the Newly Deceased," 1213.

118. Schmidt et al., "The Ethical Debate on Practicing Procedures on the Newly Dead," 964; Manifold et al., "Patient and Family Attitudes regarding the Practice of Procedures on the Newly Deceased," 112.

119. CEJA, "Performing Procedures on the Newly Deceased," 1213.

120. Morag et al., "Performing Procedures on the Newly Deceased for Teaching Purposes," 92.

121. CEJA, "Performing Procedures on the Newly Deceased," 1214–15.

122. Schmidt et al., "The Ethical Debate on Practicing Procedures on the Newly Dead," 965.

123. Sachs, *Corpse*, 13; Iserson, *Death to Dust*, 138.

124. Hill and Anderson, *The Autopsy*, 108.

125. Sachs, *Corpse*, 15.

126. Burney, *Bodies of Evidence*, 23.

127. Bernard, *The Law of Death and Disposal of the Dead*, 70.

128. Competing coroners sometimes went to great lengths to secure customers for inquests. In New York City, a Brooklyn coroner might pay to have an onlooker push an East River drowning victim toward the Brooklyn side of the river. Or a Brooklyn coroner might fend off a Manhattan coroner with oars while rowing toward a corpse floating in the East River (Quigley, *The Corpse*, 121).

129. Iserson, *Death to Dust*, 140.

130. Ibid., 116.

131. Shultz, *Body Snatching*, 10.

132. Maples and Browning, *Dead Men Do Tell Tales*, 91–92.

133. Sachs, *Corpse,* 23–25.

134. Burney, *Bodies of Evidence,* 115.

135. Iserson, *Death to Dust,* 138.

136. Johnson-McGrath, "Witness for the Prosecution," 185.

137. Webster, *Does This Mean You'll See Me Naked?,* 158.

138. Ibid., 161.

139. Quay, "Utilizing the Bodies of the Dead," 910; Iserson, *Death to Dust,* 126.

140. Quigley, *The Corpse,* 133.

141. Johnson-McGrath, "Witness for the Prosecution," 183.

142. Bass and Jefferson, *Death's Acre,* 33.

143. Iserson, *Death to Dust,* 146–49.

144. Quigley, *The Corpse,* 129.

145. Bahn, *Written in Bones,* 132–33.

146. Sachs, *Corpse,* 4–6.

147. Ibid., 27–28.

148. Ibid., 6–19.

149. Ibid., 18.

150. Ibid., 39.

151. Ibid., 30–31.

152. Ibid., 33.

153. Quigley, *The Corpse,* 124.

154. Sachs, *Corpse,* 256–57.

155. Ibid., 16–17.

156. Ibid., 64–65.

157. Bass and Jefferson, *Death's Acre,* 66–70.

158. Ibid., 95.

159. Bass and Jefferson, *Death's Acre,* 238.

160. Sachs, *Corpse,* 83–84, 107–20.

161. Ibid., 107–13.

162. Ibid., 113–14.

163. Ibid., 192–95.

164. Ibid., 41.

165. Ibid., 257.

166. Roach, *Stiff,* 89–99.

167. Ibid., 150.

168. Cheney, *Body Brokers,* 149.

169. Sachs, *Corpse,* 140.

170. Wikipedia, "The Visual Body Project" accessible at http://en.wikipedia.org/wiki/ Visible_Human_Project.

171. Roach, *Stiff,* 150.

172. Klaver, *Sites of Autopsy,* 33.

173. Matson, *Round-Trip to Deadsville,* 47.

174. Montimurro and Higbie, *Provolone in the Casket*, 57.
175. Hoyert, "The Autopsy, Medicine, and Mortality Statistics," 13–14; Quigley, *The Corpse*, 120.

## Chapter 9

1. Hoffman and Morriss, "Birth after Death," 595–96.
2. Trainor, "Right of Husband, Wife, or Other Party to Custody of Frozen Embryo, Pre-Embryo, or Pre-Zygote in Event of Divorce, Death, or Other Circumstances," Section 2.
3. Zafran, "Dying to Be a Father," 61.
4. Hoffman and Morriss, "Birth after Death," 577.
5. Kahan et al., "Postmortem Sperm Procurement," 1840.
6. Kerr, "Post-Mortem Sperm Procurement," 67–68; Andrews, "The Sperminator."
7. Gilbert, "Fatherhood from the Grave," 545, n. 125.
8. Schiff, "Arising from the Dead," 906–7.
9. Lerner, "In a Wife's Request at her Husband's Deathbed, Ethics Are an Issue."
10. Dwyer, "Dead Daddies," 881.
11. Hoffman and Morriss, "Birth after Death," 599.
12. Katz, "Parenthood from the Grave," 292.
13. Schiff, "Arising from the Dead," 944.
14. Cohen, "The Constitution and the Rights Not to Procreate," 1150–59.
15. Shapiro, "Illicit Reasons and Means for Reproduction," 1129; Robertson, "Posthumous Reproduction," 1031–32, 1042.
16. Cohen, "The Constitution and the Rights Not to Procreate," 1155–59.
17. Kerr, "Post-Mortem Sperm Procurement," 76–77.
18. Andrews, "The Sperminator," 64.
19. Smolensky, "Rights of the Dead," 21.
20. Zafran, "Dying to Be a Father," 62.
21. 59 Cal. Rptr 222 (Cal. App. 1996).
22. *Hall v. Fertility Institute of New Orleans*, 647 So.2d 1348 (La. App. 1994); see also Estate of *Kievernagel*, 83 Cal. Reporter 3d 311 (Cal. App. 2008), upholding a decedent's wish, indicated on a fertility clinic form that his sperm should not be used for reproduction in the event of his death.
23. Kahan et al., "Postmortem Sperm Procurement," 1841.
24. Schiff, "Arising from the Dead," 933.
25. *In re Martin B.*, 841 N.Y.S.2d 207 (N.Y. Surrog. 2007).
26. Zafran, "Dying to Be a Father," 44–45; Kerr, "Post-Mortem Sperm Procurement," 70.
27. Shapiro, "Illicit Reasons and Means for Reproduction," 1130.
28. Schiff, "Arising from the Dead," 949–50.
29. Ibid., 932.
30. Estate of *Kolacy*, 753 A.2d 1257 (N.J. Ch. Div. 2000).

31. Radford, "Post-Mortem Sperm Retrieval and the Social Security Administration," 5.
32. Katz, "Parenthood from the Grave," 293; Strong, "Ethical and Legal Aspects of Sperm Retrieval after Death or Persistent Vegetative State," 347, n. 1.
33. Schiff, "Arising from the Dead," 965; Strong, "Ethical and Legal Aspects of Sperm Retrieval," 349, n. 9.
34. Kahan et al., "Postmortem Sperm Procurement," 1842.
35. Zafran, "Dying to Be a Father," 44.
36. Lerner, "In a Wife's Request at Her Husband's Deathbed, Ethics Are an Issue."
37. Andrews, "The Sperminator," 64.
38. Katz, "Parenthood from the Grave," 301–4.
39. Ibid., 308–9.
40. Ibid., 299.
41. Ibid., 299; Dwyer, "Dead Daddies," 881.
42. Schiff, "Arising from the Dead," 906.
43. Murphy, "Sperm Harvesting and Post-mortem Fatherhood," 384.
44. Spielman, "Post Mortem Gamete Retrieval after Christy."
45. Dwyer, "Dead Daddies," 893–94; Strong, "Ethical and Legal Aspects of Sperm Retrieval," 355; Katz, "Parenthood from the Grave," 306; B. Spielman, "Pushing the Dead into the Next Reproductive Frontier," 334–38.
46. Strong, "Ethical and Legal Aspects of Sperm Retrieval," 355–56.
47. Dwyer, "Dead Daddies," 889.
48. Hansen, "Child Born to Brain-Dead Mother."
49. Jordan, "Incubating for the State," 1107.
50. Sperling, "Maternal Brain Death," 453.
51. Cohen, "The Constitution and the Rights Not to Procreate," 1162.
52. Katz, "Parenthood from the Grave," 291.
53. Jordan, "Incubating for the State," 1108.
54. *University Health Services v. Piazzi*, No. CV86-RCCV-464 (Richmond County, Ga., Aug. 14, 1986), discussed in Jordan, "Incubating for the State," 1109, 1111.
55. Sperling, "Maternal Brain Death," 481–82, 491–92.
56. Ibid., 489–90.
57. Jordan, "Incubating for the State," 1114.
58. Shapiro, "Illicit Reasons and Means for Reproduction,"1133.
59. Schiff, "Arising from the Dead," 964.
60. Sperling, "Maternal Brain Death," 472.
61. Shapiro, "Illicit Reasons and Means for Reproduction," 1188.
62. Robertson, "Posthumous Reproduction," 1033.
63. Bennett, "How Should We Regulate Stored Embryos, Posthumous Pregnancy, Ectogenesis and Male Pregnancy?," 4–6.
64. Cohen, "The Constitution and the Rights Not to Procreate," 1144.
65. *Davis v. Davis*, 842. S.W.2d 588, 597 (Tenn. 1992).
66. Robertson, "Posthumous Reproduction," 1035; Schiff, "Arising from the Dead," 919.

67. Trainor, "Right of Husband, Wife, or Other Party to Custody of Frozen Embryo," Section 4.

68. Robertson, "Posthumous Reproduction," 1067; Cohen, "The Constitution and the Rights Not to Procreate," 1137.

69. *A.Z. v. B.Z.*, 725 N.E.2d 1051 (Mass. 2000); *Kass v. Kass*, 696 N.E.2d 174 (N.Y. 1998); Trainor, "Right of Husband, Wife, or Other Party to Custody of Frozen Embryo," Section 4.

70. *A.Z. v. B.Z.*, 725 N.E.2d 1051 (Mass. 2000).

71. *Kass v. Kass*, 696 N.E.2d 174 (N.Y. 1998).

72. Colman, *Corpses, Coffins, and Crypts*, 88–89, 98.

73. *A.Z. v. B.Z.*, 725 N.E.2d 1051, 1059 (Mass. 2000); *Davis v. Davis*, 842 S.W.2d 588 (Tenn. 1992) at 598.

74. *A.Z. v. B.Z.*, 725 N.E.2d 1051, 1057–58 (Mass. 2000).

75. Ibid.

76. Cohen, "The Constitution and the Rights Not to Procreate," 1164.

77. Colman, *Corpses, Coffins, and Crypts*, 77; *Kass v. Kass*, 696 N.E.2d 174, 179 (N.Y. 1998).

78. La. Revised Statutes, Sections 9:126 and 131.

79. *Nachmani v. Nachmani*, 50(4) Piskei Din 661 (Israel Sup. Ct. 1996).

80. *Davis v. Davis*, 842 S.W.2d 588, 597 (Tenn. 1992).

81. Wright, "Competing Interests in Reproduction," 135.

**Chapter 10**

1. Trope and Echo-Hawk, "NAGPRA," 39.

2. Richardson, *Death, Dissection, and the Destitute*, 76.

3. Ibid., 274.

4. Hodson, "Civil Liability of Undertakers," 374–76.

5. Mackie, "Liability of Funeral Director," 58.

6. Leahy, "Autopsies," 96.

7. Axelrod, "Was Shylock v. Antonio Correctly Decided?," 144.

8. Quigley, *The Corpse*, 278.

9. Schiff, "Arising from the Dead," 924.

10. Kuzenski, "Property in Dead Bodies," 18.

11. Axelrod, "Was Shylock v. Antonio Correctly Decided?," 143.

12. *Gadbury v. Bleitz*, 233 P. 299 (Wash. 1925).

13. Bray, "Personalizing Personality," 230.

14. Carey, "The Disposition of the Body after Death," 262; Sappol, *A Traffic of Dead Bodies*, 122.

15. *Stastny v. Tachovsky*, 132 N.W.2d 317 (Neb. 1964).

16. *Whitehair v. Highland Memory Gardens*, 327 S.E.2d 438 (W.Va. 1985).

17. Sappol, *A Traffic of Dead Bodies*, 112.

18. Tward and Patterson, "From Grave Robbing to Gifting: Cadaver Supply in the United States," 1183.

19. Sappol, *A Traffic of Dead Bodies*, 2.

20. Iserson, *Death to Dust*, 324.

21. Shultz, *Body Snatching*, 15.

22. Iserson, *Death to Dust*, 337.

23. Shultz, *Body Snatching*, ix.

24. Ibid., 27.

25. Iserson, *Death to Dust*, 330.

26. Wilkins, *The Bedside Book of Death*, 64.

27. Quigley, *The Corpse*, 298.

28. Ibid., 295.

29. Duncan, "William Burke and William Hare, 'The Resurrectionists'."

30. Long and Reim, *Fatal Facts*, 15.

31. Iserson, *Death to Dust*, 340.

32. Sappol, *A Traffic of Dead Bodies*, 115.

33. Ibid., 130.

34. Iserson, *Death to Dust*, 339.

35. Cheney, *Body Brokers*, 115.

36. Shultz, *Body Snatching*, 35.

37. Sappol, *A Traffic of Dead Bodies*, 116.

38. Wolf, *Lives of the Silent Stones in the Christ Church Burial Grounds*, 36.

39. Klaver, *Sites of Autopsy*, 21; Wilkins, *The Bedside Book of Death*, 70.

40. Shultz, *Body Snatching*, 44.

41. Quigley, *The Corpse*, 293.

42. Richardson, *Death, Dissection, and the Destitute*, 278.

43. Shultz, *Body Snatching*, 39.

44. Iserson, *Death to Dust*, 435.

45. Wilkins, *The Bedside Book of Death*, 92.

46. Carey, "The Disposition of the Body after Death," 251; Sachs, *Corpse*, 20–21.

47. Laderman, *The Sacred Remains*, 20.

48. Carey, "The Disposition of the Body after Death," 252.

49. Sappol, *A Traffic of Dead Bodies*, 129.

50. Klaver, *Sites of Autopsy*, 21; Sappol, *A Traffic of Dead Bodies*, 81-82.

51. Roach, *Stiff*, 43.

52. Iserson, *Death to Dust*, 336–37.

53. Quigley, *The Corpse*, 297.

54. Iserson, *Death to Dust*, 337.

55. Sappol, *A Traffic of Dead Bodies*, 81–85.

56. Quigley, *The Corpse*, 293.

57. Nelkin and Andrews, "Do the Dead Have Interests?," 263.

58. Ibid., 339.

59. Shultz, *Body Snatching*, 15.

60. Ibid., 61.

61. Shultz, *Body Snatching*, 8; Sappol, *A Traffic of Dead Bodies*, 19.

62. Sappol, *A Traffic of Dead Bodies*, 95.
63. Ibid., 92.
64. Shultz, *Body Snatching*, 23.
65. Iserson, *Death to Dust*, 336.
66. Sappol, *A Traffic of Dead Bodies*, 106.
67. Shultz, *Body Snatching*, 46.
68. Ibid., 48.
69. Ibid.
70. Nelkin and Andrews, "Do the Dead Have Interests?," 264.
71. Krauskopf, "The Law of Dead Bodies," 455.
72. Krauskopf, "The Law of Dead Bodies," 459; Miller, "Death and Dead Bodies," 775.
73. Montross, *Bodies of Work*, 115.
74. Iserson, *Death to Dust*, 340.
75. Carter, *First Cut*, 173; Bouchie, "Parting Gifts," 44.
76. Wilkins, *The Bedside Book of Death*, 94.
77. Kleinknecht, "New Trial Ordered for Leader of Grave-Robbing Cult."
78. Cheney, *Body Brokers*, 7–8, 127–29; Broder, "In Science's Name, Lucrative Trade in Body Parts."
79. Ramsland, *Cemetery Stories*, 195.
80. Cheney, *Body Brokers*, 63.
81. Quigley, *The Corpse*, 298.
82. Cheney, *Body Brokers*, 135–39.
83. *Gudo v. Administrators of Tulane Educational Fund*, 966 So.2d 1069 (La. App. 2007).
84. Ben-Ali, "Grisly Case of Body-Parts Thefts Ends with Guilty Plea," 20; Hays, "Scandal Rocks Human Tissue History."
85. Ben-Ali, "Grisly Case of Body-Parts Thefts Ends with Guilty Plea," 20.
86. Ben-Ali, "Grisly Case of Body-Parts Thefts Ends with Guilty Plea," 20; Kittredge, "Black Shrouds and Black Markets."
87. Cohen, "FDA Reviews Cadaver-Tissue Industry."
88. Brubaker, "Body-Parts Sentence Condemned," 11.

**Chapter 11**

1. Laderman, *The Sacred Remains*, 78.
2. Quigley, *The Corpse*, 179.
3. *New Mexico v. Hartzler*, 433 P.2d 231 (N.M. 1967).
4. Quigley, *The Corpse*, 79.
5. Hart, "Georgia Crematory Manager Pleads Guilty and Gives Apology."
6. *Lott v. State of New York*, 225 N.Y.S.2d 434 (Ct. Cl. 1962).
7. Hodson, "Civil Liability of Undertakers," Section 11.
8. Ibid., Section 7b.
9. Montross, *Bodies of Work*, 28.
10. Quigley, *The Corpse*, 248–49.

11. Iserson, *Death to Dust*, 382.

12. Laderman, *The Sacred Remains*, 100.

13. Iserson, *Death to Dust*, 399.

14. Long and Reim, *Fatal Facts*, 121.

15. Ibid.

16. Bass and Jefferson, *Death's Acre*, 85–87.

17. Quigley, *The Corpse*, 249.

18. O'Rorke, "Skinless Wonders . . ."

19. Roach, *Stiff*, 275.

20. *Maine v. Bradbury*, 9 A.2d 657 (Me. 1939).

21. *Kohn v. United States*, 591 F.Supp. 568 (E.D.N.Y. 1984).

22. Carey, "The Disposition of the Body after Death," 267.

23. Montross, *Bodies of Work*, 288.

24. Ibid., 68.

25. Krauskopf, "The Law of Dead Bodies," 465–66.

26. Lawrence, "Beyond the Grave," 125.

27. *Kohn v. United States*, 591 F.Supp. 568 (E.D.N.Y. 1984); *Gurganious v. Simpson*, 197 S.E. 163 (N.C. 1938).

28. *Epps v. Duke University*, 468 S.E.2d 846, 855 (N.C. App. 1996).

29. Long and Reim, *Fatal Facts*, 20–21.

30. Harold Schechter, "Mourning on the Inside."

31. Long and Reim, *Fatal Facts*, 25.

32. Montross, *Bodies of Work*, 225.

33. Maples and Browning, *Dead Men Do Tell Tales*, 103.

34. Alvarez, "Outrage at Funeral Protests Pushes Lawmakers to Act."

35. Ibid.

36. Wells, "Privacy and Funeral Protests," 184–86.

37. Christensen, "Moral Considerations in Body Donation for Scientific Research," 138–40.

38. Iserson, *Death to Dust*, 400.

39. Quigley, *The Corpse*, 271.

40. Ibid., 249; O'Rorke, "Skinless Wonders . . ."

41. Iserson, *Death to Dust*, 400.

42. Feldman, "Human Dignity as a Legal Value," 697–98; Hennette-Vauchez, "When Ambivilant Principles Prevail," 199–200, 207–8.

43. Clifford and Huff, " Some Thoughts on the Meaning and Scope of the Montana Constitution's Dignity Clause," 329–30; Cantor, "Déjà vu All Over Again: The False Dichotomy Between Sanctity of Life and Quality of Life," 82–83.

44. Clifford and Huff, "Some Thoughts on the Meaning and Scope of the Montana Constitution's Dignity Clause," 303; Englard, "Human Dignity" 1924.

45. Dan-Cohen, "Defending Dignity," 161; Englard, "Human Dignity," 1906.

46. Quigley, *The Corpse*, 168.

47. Sugg, "Corpse Medicine," 2079.

48. Long and Reim, *Fatal Facts*, 128.
49. Ibid.
50. Associated Press, "Richards, Um, Snorted His Dad."
51. Sugg, "Corpse Medicine," 2078; Roach, *Stiff*, 227–32.
52. Quigley, *The Corpse*, 242–43; Lawrence, "Beyond the Grave," 123.
53. Richardson, *Death, Dissection, and the Destitute*, 302.
54. Ochoa and Jones, "Defiling the Dead," 539–40.
55. Rosman and Resnick, "Sexual Attraction to Corpses," 158.
56. Wilkins, *The Bedside Book of Death*, 101.
57. Rosman and Resnick, "Sexual Attraction to Corpses," 161.
58. Ibid., 158.
59. Quigley, *The Corpse*, 300.
60. Ibid.
61. Rosman and Resnick, "Sexual Attraction to Corpses," 158.
62. Ramsland, *Cemetery Stories*, 200–4.
63. Hodson, "Civil Liability of Undertakers," 367.
64. Quigley, *The Corpse*, 299.
65. Ibid., 301.
66. Wilgoren, "In Gory Detail, Prosecution Lays Out Its Case for Tough Sentencing of B. T. K. Killer."

**Chapter 12**

1. Cullen, *Remember Me*, 130–31.
2. Raff, "He's Not a Pathologist, He's Pathological"; Burns, "Gunther von Hagens' BODY WORLDS: Selling Beautiful Education," 13; Hibbs, "Dead Body Porn," 129.
3. Duryea, "Rival Body Show Asserts Rights."
4. Burns, "Gunther von Hagens' BODY WORLDS," 14.
5. Raff, "He's Not a Pathologist, He's Pathological."
6. Peipert, "The Future Is in Plastics, for the Dead"; O'Rorke, "Skinless Wonders . . ."
7. Hibbs, "Dead Body Porn," 129.
8. Burns, "Gunther von Hagens' BODY WORLDS," 16.
9. Duryea, "Rival Body Show Asserts Rights."
10. Weingarten, "Florida Museumgoers Line Up to See Corpses."
11. Quigley, *The Corpse*, 283.
12. Iserson, *Death to Dust*, 512.
13. Berg, "Grave Secrets," 99.
14. Quigley, *The Corpse*, 295.
15. Hodson, "Civil Liability of Undertakers," Section 9(c).
16. *Chesher v. Neyser*, 477 F.3d 784 (6th Cir. 2007).
17. *Board of Regents v. Oglesby*, 591 S.E. 2d 417 (Ga. App. 2003).
18. *Dean v. Chapman*, 556 P.2d 27 (Okla. 1976).
19. Annas, "Family Privacy and Death," 504.

20. Sappol, *A Traffic of Dead Bodies*, 39.
21. Quigley, *The Corpse*, 268.
22. Lawrence, "Beyond the Grave," 125.
23. Sappol, *A Traffic of Dead Bodies*, 91.
24. Quigley, *The Corpse*, 270.
25. Sappol, *A Traffic of Dead Bodies*, 91.
26. Ibid., 95.
27. Pringle, *The Mummy Congress*, 183.
28. Sappol, *A Traffic of Dead Bodies*, 8–12; Lawrence, "Beyond the Grave," 125.
29. Quigley, *The Corpse*, 267.
30. Edidin, "In Search of Answers from the Great Brains of Cornell."
31. Sappol, *A Traffic of Dead Bodies*, 94.
32. Iserson, *Death to Dust*, 396.
33. Gilbert, *Death's Door*, 227.
34. Iserson, *Death to Dust*, 217–18.
35. Montross, *Bodies of Work*, 228.
36. Lawrence, "Beyond the Grave," 138.
37. Ibid., 127.
38. Iserson, *Death to Dust*, 436.
39. Cullen, *Remember Me*, 136.
40. Ibid., 139.
41. Hibbs, "Dead Body Porn," 129.
42. Cullen, *Remember Me*, 132.
43. Ibid.; Burns, "Gunther von Hagens' BODY WORLDS," 7.
44. Burns, "Gunther von Hagens' BODY WORLDS," 30.
45. Klaver, *Sites of Autopsy*, 155.
46. Lawrence, "Beyond the Grave," 128.
47. Ibid., 131–33.
48. *State v. Redd*, 992 P.2d 986 (Utah 1999).
49. Quigley, *The Corpse*, 269–70.
50. Bass and Jefferson, *Death's Acre*, 31–32.
51. Trope and Echo-Hawk, "NAGPRA," 39–40.
52. Ibid., 49.
53. Matson, *Round-Trip to Deadsville*, 49.
54. Lawrence, "Beyond the Grave," 132.
55. Afrasiabi, "Property Rights in Ancient Human Skeletal Remains," 818.
56. Goldberg, "Kennewick Man and the Meaning of Life," 273–75.
57. Afrasiabi, "Property Rights in Ancient Human Skeletal Remains," 805.
58. Bahn, *Written in Bones*, 111–14.
59. Ibid., 85–88.
60. Pringle, *The Mummy Congress*, 17–26.
61. Ibid., 51.
62. Ibid., 53.

**Chapter 13**

1. Yalom, *The American Resting Place*, 24.
2. Sappol, *A Traffic of Dead Bodies*, 135.
3. Mitford, *The American Way of Death Revisited*, 244, 271.
4. Jones and Whitaker, *Speaking for the Dead*, 36.
5. Long, "Chronicle of a Death We Can't Accept."
6. Bouchie, "Parting Gifts," 47.
7. Ibid., 42; Anteby and Hyman, "Entrepreneurial Ventures and Whole-Body Donations," 968.
8. Anteby and Hyman, "Entrepreneurial Ventures and Whole-Body Donations," 964–68; Broder, "In Science's Name, Lucrative Trade in Body Parts," A16.
9. Perhaps this was an adaptation of the precedent set by Diogenes of Sinope, who instructed: "When I die, throw me to the wolves. I'm used to it!"

# Bibliography

Abadie, Alberto, and Sebastien Gay. "The Impact of Presumed Consent Legislation on Cadaveric Organ Donation: A Cross Country Study." Faculty Research Working Paper, John F. Kennedy School of Government, Harvard University, June 2004.

Afrasiabi, Peter R. "Property Rights in Ancient Human Skeletal Remains," 70 *So. Cal. L. Rev.* 805 (1997).

Alvarez, Lizette. "Outrage at Funeral Protests Pushes Lawmakers to Act." *New York Times*, April 17, 2006. www.nytimes.com/2006/04/17/us/17picket.html.

Andrews, Lori B. "The Sperminator." *New York Times Magazine*, March 3, 1999, 62.

Annas, George J. "Family Privacy and Death: Antigone, War, and Medical Research." *N. Engl. J. Med.* 352 (2005): 501–5.

Anteby, Michel, and Mikell Hyman. "Entrepreneurial Ventures and Whole-Body Donations: A Regional Perspective from the United States." *Social Sci. Med.* 66, no. 4 (2008): 963–69.

Associated Press. "Richards, Um, Snorted His Dad." *Trenton Times*, April 4, 2007.

Axelrod, Allan. "Was Shylock v. Antonio Correctly Decided?" 39 *Rutgers L. Rev.* 143 (1986).

Bahn, Paul, ed. *Written in Bones: How Human Remains Unlock the Secrets of the Dead*. New York: Firefly Books, 2003.

Bainham, Andrew, Shelley Day Sclater, and Martin Richards, eds. *Body Lore and Laws*. Portland, OR: Hart Publishing, 2002.

Bass, Bill, and Jon Jefferson. *Death's Acre: Inside the Legendary Forensics Lab: The Body Farm Where the Dead Do Tell Tales*. New York: Penguin Books, 2003.

Bell, M. D. D. "Non-Heart Beating Organ Donation: New Ethical Problems." *J. Med. Ethics* 29 (2003): 176–81.

Ben-Ali, Russell. "Grisly Case of Body-Parts Thefts Ends with Guilty Plea." *Newark Star Ledger*, March 19, 2008, 20.

Bennett, Rebecca. "Is Reproduction Women's Business? How Should We Regulate Stored Embryos, Posthumous Pregnancy, Ectogenesis and Male Pregnancy?" *Studies in Ethics, Law and Technology* 2, no. 3, Article 3, 1–19 (2008).

Berg, Jessica. "Grave Secrets: Legal and Ethical Analysis of Postmortem Confidentiality," 34 *Conn. L. Rev.* 81 (2001).

Berman, Rochel U. *Dignity beyond Death: The Jewish Preparation for Burial*. New York: Urim, 2005.

Bernard, Hugh Y. *The Law of Death and Disposal of the Dead*, 2nd ed. Dobbs Ferry, NY: Oceana Publications, 1979.

Bernat, James L. "The Boundaries of Organ Donation after Circulatory Death." *N. Engl. J. Med.* 359 (2008): 669–71.

Best, Ben. "Perfusion and Diffusion in Cryonics Protocol." www.benbest.com/cryonics/protocol.html.

———. "Vitrification in Cryonics." www.benbest.com/cryonics/vitrify.html.

Bondeson, Jan. *Buried Alive: The Terrifying History of Our Most Primal Fear*. New York: W. W. Norton, 2001.

Bonnie, Richard J., Stephanie Wright, and Kelly K. Deneen. "Legal Authority to Preserve Organs in Cases of Uncontrolled Cardiac Death: Preserving Family Choice," 36 *J. Law, Med. Ethics* 741 (2008).

Bouchie, Robert. "Parting Gifts." *Bostonia* (Fall 2009): 42–47.

Bray, Michelle Bourianoff. "Personalizing Personality: Toward a Property Right in Human Bodies," 69 *Texas L. Rev.* 209 (1990).

Broder, John M. "In Science's Name, Lucrative Trade in Body Parts." *New York Times*, March 12, 2004, A16.

Brody, Jane E. "The Solvable Problem of Organ Shortages." *New York Times*, August 8, 2007. www.nytimes.com/2007/08/28/health/28brod.html?_r=1.

Brooks, David. "A Partnership of Minds." *New York Times*, July 20, 2007. http://select.nytimes.com/2007/07/20/opinion/20brooks.html.

Brooks, Patricia. "The Rich and Famous at Rest in Eden." *New York Times*, October 26, 2008. www.nytimes.com/2008/10/26/nyregion/long-island/26Rburied.html.

Brown, Patricia Leigh. "In Death as in Life, a Personalized Space." *New York Times*, January 18, 2007. www.nytimes.com/2007/01/18/garden/18urns.html.

———. "In Need of Income, Cemeteries Are Seeking Breathing Clientele." *New*

*York Times*, March 25, 2007. www.nytimes.com/2007/05/25/us/25cemetery
.html.

Brubaker, Paul. "Body-Parts Sentence Condemned." *Newark Star Ledger*, June 2, 2009, 11.

Burney, Ian A. *Bodies of Evidence: Medicine and Politics of the English Inquest, 1830–1926*. Baltimore: Johns Hopkins University Press, 2000.

Burns, Jeffrey P., Frank E. Reardon, and Robert D. Truog. "Using Newly Deceased Patients to Teach Resuscitation Procedures." *N. Engl. J. Med.* 331 (1994): 1652–55.

Burns, Lawrence. "Gunther von Hagens' BODY WORLDS: Selling Beautiful Education." *Am. J. Bioethics* 7, no. 4 (2007): 12–23.

Burton, Julian L. "The Autopsy in Modern Undergraduate Medical Education: A Qualitative Study of Uses and Curriculum Considerations." *Med. Education* 37, no. 12 (2003): 1073–81.

Calandrillo, Steve P. "Cash for Kidneys? Utilizing Incentives to End America's Organ Shortage," 13 *Geo. Mason L. Rev.* 69 (2004).

Caldwell, Alicia A. "A Space Trek for Scotty's Ashes." *Newark Star Ledger*, April 26, 2007.

Callahan, Joan C. "On Harming the Dead." *Ethics* 97, no. 2 (1987): 341–52.

Cantor, Norman L. *Advance Directives and the Pursuit of Death with Dignitiy.* Bloomington: Indiana University Press, 1993.

———. "Déjà Vu All Over Again: The False Dichotomy between Sanctity of Life and Quality of Life," 35 *Stetson L. Rev.* 81 (2005).

Cantor, Norman L., and George C. Thomas III. "The Legal Bounds of Physician Conduct Hastening Death," 48 *Buffalo L. Rev.* 83 (2000).

Carey, Francis King. "The Disposition of the Body after Death," 19 *Am. L. Rev.* 251 (1885).

Carlino, Andrea. *Books of the Body*. Translated by John Tedeschi and Anne C. Tedeschi. Chicago: University of Chicago Press, 1999.

Carter, Albert Howard, III. *First Cut: A Season in the Human Anatomy Lab*. New York: Picador USA, 1997.

Chadwick, Ruth F. "Corpses, Recycling, and Therapeutic Purposes." In *Death Rites: Law and Ethics at the End of Life*, edited by Robert Lee and Derek Morgan, 54–71. London: Routledge, 1996.

Chan, Sarah, and John Harris. "Free Riders and Pious Sons—Why Science Research Remains Obligatory." *Bioethics* 22, no. 3 (2008): 161–71.

Cheney, Annie. *Body Brokers: Inside America's Underground Trade in Human Remains*. New York: Broadway Books, 2006.

Childress, James F. "Organ Donation after Circulatory Determination of Death: Lessons and Unresolved Controversies," 36 *J. Law, Med. Ethics* 766 (2008).

Chiong, Winston. "Brain Death without Definitions." *Hastings Center Rep.* 35, no. 6 (2005): 20–30.

Christensen, Angi M. "Moral Considerations in Body Donation for Scientific Research: A Unique Look at the University of Tennessee's Anthropological Research Facility." *Bioethics* 20, no. 3 (2006): 136–45.

Chung, Christine S., and Lisa Soleymani Lehmann. "Informed Consent and the Process of Cadaver Donation." *Arch. Pathol. Lab. Med.* 126, no. 8 (2002): 964–68.

Clark, Mary L. "Keep Your Hands Off My (Dead) Body: A Critique of the Ways in Which the State Disrupts the Personhood Interests of the Deceased," 58 *Rutgers L. Rev.* 45 (2005).

Clifford, Mathew O., and Thomas P. Huff. "Some Thoughts on the Meaning and Scope of the Montana Constitution's Dignity Clause," 61 *Montana L. Rev.* 301 (2000).

Clines, Francis X. "Step Right Up to the Anatomy Lesson." *New York Times*, April 10, 2006. www.nytimes.com/2006/04/10/opinion/10mon4.html?_r=2 &oref=slogin.

Cohen, I. Glenn. "The Constitution and the Rights Not to Procreate," 60 *Stanford L. Rev.* 1135 (2008).

Cohen, Robert. "FDA Reviews Cadaver-Tissue Industry." *Newark Star Ledger*, June 13, 2007.

Colman, Penny. *Corpses, Coffins, and Crypts: A History of Burial.* New York: Henry Holt, 1997.

Coradazzi, A. L., A. Morganti, and M. R. Montenegro. "Discrepancies between Clinical Diagnoses and Autopsy Findings." *Braz. J. Med. Biol. Res.* 36:3 (2003): 385–91.

Council on Ethical and Judicial Affairs of the AMA (CEJA). "Performing Procedures on the Newly Deceased." *Acad. Med.* 77, no. 12 (2002): 1212–16.

Critchley, Simon. "How to Make It in the Afterlife." *New York Times*, June 23, 2009. http://opinionator.blogs.nytimes.com/2009/06/23/how-to-make-it-in-the-afterlife/.

Cullen, Lisa Takeuchi. *Remember Me: A Lively Tour of the New American Way of Death.* New York: Collins, 2007.

Dan-Cohen, Meir. "Defending Dignity." In *Harmful Thoughts: Essays on Law, Self, and Morality*, 150–71. Princeton, NJ: Princeton University Press, 2002.

Daybell, Chad. *One Foot in the Grave: The Strange but True Adventures of a Cemetery Sexton*. Springville, UT: Bonneville Books, 2001.

Dewan, Shaila. "Disasters and Their Dead." *New York Times*, October 16, 2005. www.nytimes.com/2005/10/16/weekinreview/16dewan.html?_r=1&pagewanted=print.

Diamant, Jeff. "N.J. Crematory Reflects Shift in Catholic Church." *Newark Star Ledger*, January 17, 2007.

Dobbs, David. "Buried Answers." *New York Times Magazine*, April 24, 2005. www.nytimes.com/2005/04/24/magazine/24AUTOPSY.html.

Dorff, Elliot N. *Matters of Life and Death: A Jewish Approach to Modern Medical Ethics*. Philadelphia: Jewish Publication Society, 2004.

Dorman, Larry. "Anger over Exhumation in Gipper's Hometown." *New York Times*, November 10, 2007.

Duncan, John, Dan Luginbill, Matthew Richardson, and Robin F. Wilson. "Using Tort Law to Secure Patient Dignity," 40 *Trial* 42 (2004).

Duncan, John A. "William Burke and William Hare, 'The Resurrectionists'." *Scottish History Online*, 2006. www.scotshistoryonline.co.uk/burke.html.

Dunlap, David. "The Life of a Cemetery." *New York Times*, June 16, 2006. http://query.nytimes.com/gst/fullpage.html?res=9F07E3D91130F935A25754C0A9609C8B63.

Duryea, Bill. "Rival Body Show Asserts Rights." *Tampa Bay Buzz*, August 15, 2005. www.sptimes.com/2005/08/15/Tampabay/Rival_body_shows_asse.shtml.

Dwyer, Laura A. "Dead Daddies: Issues in Postmortem Reproduction," 52 *Rutgers L. Rev.* 881 (2000).

Ediden, Peter. "In Search of Answers from the Great Brains of Cornell." *New York Times*, May 24, 2005. www.nytimes.com/2005/05/24/science24brai.html.

Ely, Elissa. "In an Age of Images, Teaching Pathology by Hand." *New York Times*, September 12, 2007. www.nytimes.com/2007/09/11/health/11iht-12prof.7461822.html.

Emson, H. E. "It Is Immoral to Require Consent for Cadaver Organ Donation." *J. Med. Ethics* 29, no. 3 (2003): 125–27.

Engelhardt, H. Tristram, Jr. "Giving, Selling and Having Taken: Conflicting Views of Organ Transfer," 1 *Indiana Health L. Rev.* 31 (2004).

Englard, Ithak. "Human Dignity: From Antiquity to Modern Israel's Constitutional Framework," 21 *Cardozo L. Rev.* 1903 (2000).

Feldman, D. "Human Dignity as a Legal Value." *Public Law* (Winter 1999): 682–702.

Fevrier, Philippe, and Sebastien Gay. "Informed Consent versus Presumed

Consent: The Role of the Family in Organ Donations," 2004. http://ssrn
.com/abstract=572241.

Fidler, Suzanne A. "Implementing Donation after Cardiac Death Protocols." *J. Health Life Sci. Law* 1, no. 123 (2008): 125–49.

Finder, Alan. "Colleges Offering Campuses as Final Resting Places." *New York Times*, May 18, 2007. www.nytimes.com/2007/05/18/education/18campus .html.

Fitzpatrick, Meredith. "Last Voyage." *Boat/US Magazine* (2004).

Foley, David P., Jeffrey T. Cooper, Chin L. Thomas, Nancy R. Krieger, Luis A. Fernandez, Yolanda T. Becker, Jon S. Odorico, Stuart J. Knechtle, Munci Kalayoglu, Hans W. Sollinger, and Anthony M. D'Alessandro. "Donation after Cardiac Death: The University of Wisconsin Experience." *Ann. Surg.* 242, no. 5 (2005): 724–31.

Foster, Frances H. "Individualized Justice in Disputes over Dead Bodies," 61 *Vand. L. Rev.* 1351 (2008).

Frank, Robin Jaffee. *Love and Loss: American Portrait and Mourning Miniatures.* New Haven, CT: Yale University Art Gallery, 2000.

Gagandeep, S., L. Matsuoka, R. Mateo, Y. W. Cho, Y. Genyk, L. Sher, J. Cicciarelli, S. Aswad, N. Jabbour, and R. Selby. "Expanding the Donor Kidney Pool: Utility of Renal Allografts Procured in a Setting of Uncontrolled Cardiac Death." *Am. J. Transplantation* 6, no. 7 (2006): 1682–88.

Gera, Vanessa. "When Matters of the Heart Pain the Soul of a Nation." *Newark Star Ledger*, July 26, 2008.

Giffin, Kenna S., Richard T. Wilbanks, and William J. Winslade. "Autopsy Autonomy: Tradition, Trend, and the Decedent's Last Word." *Health Law News* (1991).

Gilbert, Sandra M. *Death's Door: Modern Dying and the Ways We Grieve: A Cultural Study.* New York: W. W. Norton, 2006.

Gilbert, Sheri. "Fatherhood from the Grave: An Analysis of Postmortem Insemination," 22 *Hofstra L. Rev.* 521 (1993–94).

Glannon, W. "Do the Sick Have a Right to Cadaveric Organs?" *J. Med. Ethics* 29, no. 3 (2003): 153–56.

Goldberg, Steven. "Kennewick Man and the Meaning of Life," 2006 *U. Chi. Legal Forum* 271 (2006).

Goldblatt, A. D. "Don't Ask, Don't Tell: Practicing Minimally Invasive Resuscitation Techniques on the Newly Dead." *Ann. Emerg. Med.* 25, no. 1 (1995): 86–90.

Goodwin, Michele. *Black Markets: The Supply and Demand of Body Parts.* New York: Cambridge University Press, 2006.

———. "Formalism and the Legal Status of Body Parts," 2006 *U. Chi. Legal Forum* 317 (2006).

Greene, Janet. *Epitaphs to Remember*. Chambersburg, PA: Allen C. Hood and Co., 1962.

Gregory, S. Ryan, and Thomas R. Cole. "The Changing Role of Dissection in Medical Education." *JAMA* 287, no. 9 (2002): 1180–81.

Gross, Jed Adams. "*E Pluribus UNOS*: The National Organ Transplantation Act," 8 *Yale J. Health Policy, Law, Ethics* 145 (2008).

Grubb, Andrew. "I, Me, Mine: Bodies, Parts, and Property." *Med. L. Int.* 3, no. 4 (1998): 299–317.

Hamilton, Carey. "Brain Cancer Victim Goes Home to Family." *The Salt Lake Tribune*, October 16, 2004.

Hammond, Norman. "Japanese Team Unlock Sources of Their Ancestors' Cinnabar." *The Times*, February 7, 2005. www.timesonline.co.uk/tol/life_and_style/court_and_social/article511348.ece.

Hansen, Mariann. "Child Born to Brain-Dead Mother." *Los Angeles Times*, July 31, 1986.

Harel, Alon. "Regulating Modesty—Related Practices." *Law Ethics Hum. Rights* 1, no. 1, Article 7, 1–24 (2007).

Harrington, Maxine M. "The Thin Flat Line: Redefining Who Is Legally Dead in Organ Donation after Cardiac Death," 86 *Denver U. L. Rev.* 335 (2009).

Harris, Mark. *Grave Matters: A Journey through the Modern Funeral Industry to a Natural Way of Burial*. New York: Scribners, 2007.

Hart, Ariel. "Georgia Crematory Manager Pleads Guilty and Gives Apology." *New York Times*, November 20, 2004. www.nytimes.com/2004/11/20/national/20cremate.html.

Hatch, Robert T. *What Happens When You Die: From Your Last Breath to Your First Spadeful*. New York: Citadel Press, 1995.

Hays, Tom. "Scandal Rocks Human Tissue Industry." *Associated Press*, June 11, 2006.

Healy, Kieran. *Last Best Gifts: Altruism and the Market for Human Blood and Organs*. Chicago: University of Chicago Press, 2006.

———. "Do Presumed-Consent Laws Raise Organ Procurement Rates?" 55 *DePaul L. Rev.* 1017 (2006).

Hennette-Vauchez, Stephanie, "When Ambivalent Principles Prevail: Leads for Explaining Western Legal Orders' Infatuation with the Human Dignity Principle." *Legal Ethics* 10, no. 2 (2007): 193.

Hernandez, Tanya K. "The Property of Death," 60 *U. Pitts. L. Rev.* 971 (1999).

Herring, Jonathan. "Giving, Selling and Sharing Bodies." In *Body Lore and Laws*, edited by Andrew Bainham, Shelley Day Sclater, and Martin Richards, 43–62. Portland, OR: Hart Publishing, 2002.

Hibbs, Thomas S. "Dead Body Porn." *The New Atlantis* 15 (Winter 2007): 128–31.

Hill, Rolla B., and Robert E. Anderson. *The Autopsy: Medical Practice and Public Policy*. Boston: Butterworths, 1988.

Hodson, John D. "Civil Liability of Undertakers," 53 *Annotated L. Reports* 4th 360 (1987).

Hoffman, Sharona, and Andrew P. Morriss. "Birth after Death: Perpetuities and the New Reproductive Technologies," 38 *Ga. L. Rev.* 575 (2004).

Horton, Richard. "Rediscovering Human Dignity." *The Lancet* 364, no. 9439 (2004): 1081–85.

Hoyert, Donna L. "The Autopsy, Medicine, and Mortality Statistics." National Center for Heath Statistics. *Vital Health Statistics* 3, no. 32 (2001).

Hughes, James J. "The Future of Death: Cryonics and the Telos of Liberal Individualism." *J. Evolution Technol.* 6 (July 2001).

Hughes, Paul M. "Presumed Consent: State Organ Confiscation or Mandated Charity?" *HEC Forum* 21, no. 1 (2009): 1–26.

Huntington, Richard, and Peter Metcalf. *Celebrations of Death: The Anthropology of Mortuary Ritual*. New York: Cambridge University Press, 1979.

Iltis, Ana S., Michael A. Rie, and Anji Wall. "Organ Donation, Patients' Rights, and Medical Responsibility at the End of Life." *Crit. Care Med.* 37, no. 1 (2009): 310–15.

Iserson, Kenneth V. *Death to Dust: What Happens to Dead Bodies*. Tuscon, AZ: Galen Press, 1994.

———. "Law versus Life: The Ethical Imperative to Practice and Teach Using the Newly Dead Emergency Department Patient." *Ann. Emerg. Med.* 25, no. 1 (1995): 91–94.

Jackson, Percival E. *The Law of Cadavers and of Burial and Burial Places*, 2nd ed. New York: Prentice Hall, 1950.

Johnson-McGrath, Julie. "Witness for the Prosecution: Science versus Crime in Twentieth Century America." *Legal Studies Forum* 22 (1998): 183–99.

Jones, D. Gareth. "Use of Bequeathed and Unclaimed Bodies in the Dissecting Room." *Clin. Anat.* 7 (1994): 102–7.

Jones, D. Gareth, and Maja I. Whitaker. *Speaking for the Dead: The Human Body in Biology and Medicine*, 2nd ed. Burlington, VT: Ashgate, 2009.

Jordan, James M., III. "Incubating for the State: The Precarious Autonomy of Persistently Vegetative and Brain-Dead Pregnant Women," 22 *Ga. L. Rev.* 1103 (1988).

Joshi, S. T., and David E. Schultz. *Ambrose Bierce: An Annotated Bibliography.* Westport, CT: Greenwood, 1999.

Josias, Brian L. "Burying the Hatchet in Burial Disputes: Applying ADR to Disputes Concerning the Interment of Bodies," 79 *Notre Dame L. Rev.* 1141 (2004).

Kahan, Steven E., Allen D. Seftel, and Martin I. Resnick, "Postmortem Sperm Procurement: A Legal Perspective." *J. Urology* 161, no. 6 (1999): 1840–43.

Katz, Katheryn D. "Parenthood from the Grave: Protocols for Retrieving and Utilizing Gametes from the Dead or Dying," 2006 *U. Chi. Legal Forum* 289 (2006).

Katz, Robert A. "The ReGift of Life: Can Charity Law Prevent For-Profit Firms from Exploiting Donated Tissue and Nonprofit Tissue Banks?" 55 *DePaul L. Rev.* 943 (Spring 2006).

Kelso, Catharine, Laurie J. Lyckholm, Patrick J. Coyne, and Thomas J. Smith. "Palliative Care Consultation in the Process of Organ Donation after Cardiac Death." *J. Palliative Med.* 10, no. 1 (2007): 118–26.

Keown, John, ed. *Euthanasia Examined: Ethical, Clinical, and Legal Perspectives.* New York: Cambridge University Press, 1995.

Kerr, Susan. "Post-Mortem Sperm Procurement: Is It Legal?" 3 *DePaul J. Health Care L.* 39 (1999).

Kerrigan, Michael. *The History of Death: Burial Customs and Funeral Rites from Ancient to Modern.* Guilford, CT: The Lyons Press, 2007.

Kilgannon, Corey. "Public Lives: Unearthing the Past, Then Burying It with Respect." *New York Times*, October 2, 2003. www.nytimes.com/2003/10/02/nyregion/public-lives-unearthing-the-past-then-burying-it-with-respect.html?pagewanted=1.

Kipnis, Kenneth. "When Are You Dead?" MCW Listserv, March 11, 2005.

Kittredge, Susan Cooke. "Black Shrouds and Black Markets." *New York Times*, March 5, 2006. www.nytimes.com/2006/03/05/opinion/05kittredge.html.

Klaiman, M. H. "Whose Brain Is It Anyway? The Comparative Law of Post-Mortem Organ Retention." *J. Leg. Med.* 26, no. 4 (2005): 474–90.

Klaver, Elizabeth. *Sites of Autopsy in Contemporary Culture.* Albany: SUNY Press, 2005.

Kleinknecht, William. "New Trial Ordered for Leader of Grave-Robbing Cult." *Newark Star Ledger*, April 26, 2007.

Klinkenborg, Verlyn. "Some Thoughts on Seeing the Polymerized Remains of Human Cadavers." *New York Times*, April 6, 2005. www.nytimes.com/2005/04/06/opinion/06wed4.html.

Koppel, Lily. "The Last Gravestone Business Standing." *New York Times*, November 24, 2006. www.nytimes.com/2006/11/24/nyregion/24monuments .html.

Kramer, Matthew H. "Do Animals and Dead People Have Legal Rights?" *Can. J. Law Juris.* 14, no. 1 (2001): 29.

Krauskopf, B. Joan. "The Law of Dead Bodies: Impeding Medical Progress," 19 *Ohio State L. J.* 455 (1958).

Kugel, Seth. "You Can Come and Go, They're Staying Awhile." *New York Times*, November 30, 2008. http://travel.nytimes.com/2008/11/30/travel/30week end.html.

Kuzenski, Walter F. "Property in Dead Bodies," 9 *Marquette L. Rev.* 17 (1924).

Laderman, Gary. *The Sacred Remains: American Attitudes toward Death 1799–1883.* New Haven, CT: Yale University Press, 1996.

———. *Rest in Peace: A Cultural History of Death and the Funeral Home in Twentieth-Century America.* New York: Oxford University Press, 2003.

Lagay, Faith L. "The Living Code: Organ Donation by Anencephalic Neonates." *Virtual Mentor* 6, no. 8 (2004).

Laureys, Steven, and Joseph J. Fins. "Are We Equal in Death? Avoiding Diagnostic Error in Brain Death." *Neurology* 70, no. 4 (2008): 14–15.

Lawrence, Susan C. "Beyond the Grave—The Use and Meaning of Human Body Parts: A Historical Introduction." In *Stored Tissue Samples: Ethical, Legal and Public Policy Implications*, edited by R. E. Weir, 111–42. Iowa City: Iowa University Press, 1998.

Laytner, Ron. "The Mummy Makers." *Edit International*, 2009. www.editinter national.com/read.php?id=47ddcf51d5a3e.

Leahy, Monique C. M. "Autopsies," 87 *Am. Jur. Proof Fact.* 3rd 98 (2008).

Lee, Robert, and Derek Morgan, eds. *Death Rites: Law and Ethics at the End of Life.* New York: Routledge, 1994.

Lerner, Baron H. "In a Wife's Request at Her Husband's Deathbed, Ethics Are an Issue." *New York Times*, September 7, 2004. www.nytimes.com/2004/ 09/07/health/07essa.html.

Leyner, Mark, and Billy Goldberg. *Why Do Men Have Nipples?* New York: Random House, 2005.

Liddy, Maryellen. "The New Body Snatchers: Analysing the Effect of Presumed Consent Organ Donation Laws," 28 *Ford. Urban L. J.* 815 (2001).

Long, Kim, and Terry Reim. *Fatal Facts: A Lively Look at Common and Curious Ways People Have Died.* New York: Arlington House, 1986.

Long, Thomas G. "Chronicle of a Death We Can't Accept." *New York Times*, October 31, 2009. www.nytimes.com/2009/11/01/opinion/01long.html.

Love, Norma. "What a Way to Go (Down the Drain)." *Newark Star Ledger*, May 9, 2008, 13.

Lynch, Thomas. *The Undertaking: Life Studies from the Dismal Trade*. New York: Penguin Books, 1997.

Mackie, Sam A. "Liability of Funeral Director," 53 *Am. Jur. Proof Fact* 3rd 15 (2008).

Maclean, Mavis. "Letting Go . . . Parents, Professionals and the Law." In *Body Lore and Laws*, edited by Andrew Bainham, Shelley Day Sclater, and Martin Richards, 79–90. Portland, OR: Hart Publishing, 2002.

Magliocca J. F., J. C. Magee, S. A. Rowe, M. T. Gravel, R. H. Chenault II, R. M. Merion, J. D. Punch, R. H. Bartlett, and M. R. Hemmila. "Extracorporeal Support for Organ Donation after Cardiac Death Effectively Expands the Donor Pool." *J. Trauma* 58, no. 6 (2005): 1095–1101.

Manahan, Kevin. "Hit a Fade, a Draw." *Newark Star Ledger*, February 23, 2007.

Manifold, Craig A., A. Storrow, and K. Rogers. "Patient and Family Attitudes Regarding the Practice of Procedures on the Newly Deceased." *Acad. Emerg. Med.* 6, no. 2 (1999): 110–15.

Maples, William R., and Michael Browning. *Dead Men Do Tell Tales: The Strange and Fascinating Cases of a Forensic Anthropologist*. New York: Broadway Books, 1994.

Marchione, Marilynn, and Seth Borenstein. "Surgeries Using Cadaver Tissue Pose Risks." *Associated Press*, June 10, 2006.

Matas, Arthur J. "A Gift of Life Deserves Compensation: How to Increase Living Kidney Donation with Realistic Incentives." *Policy Analysis* 604 (Nov. 7, 2007).

Matson, Tim. *Round-Trip to Deadsville: A Year in the Funeral Underground*. White River Junction, VT: Chelsea Green, 2000.

McKinley, Jesse. "Doctor Cleared of Harming Man to Rush Organ Removal." *New York Times*, December 18, 2008.

McShane, Larry. "Leona Helmsley Gets a Tomb with a View." *Newark Star Ledger*, August 22, 2007.

Mehlman, Maxwell J. "Presumed Consent to Organ Donation: A Reevaluation," 1 *Health Matrix* 31 (1991).

Merion, Robert M., Shawn J. Pelletier, Nathan Goodrich, Michael J. Englesbe, and Francis L. Delmonico. "Donation after Cardiac Death as a Strategy to Increase Deceased Donor Liver Availability." *Ann. Surgery* 244, no. 4 (2006): 555–62.

Meyers, David W. *The Human Body and the Law*, 2nd ed. Stanford, CA: Stanford University Press, 1970.

Miller, Franklin G., and Robert D. Truog. "Rethinking the Ethics of Vital Organ Donations." *Hastings Center Rep* 38, no. 6 (2008): 38–46.

Miller, Robert D. "Death and Dead Bodies." In *Problems in Health Care Law*, 9th ed., 765–88. Sudbury, MA: Jones and Bartlett, 2006.

Mitford, Jessica. *The American Way of Death Revisited*. New York: Vintage Books, 2000.

Montimurro, Frank, and William Higbie. *Provolone in the Casket: Memoirs of a Mortician*. Bloomington, IN: Xlibris Corporation, 2001.

Montross, Christine. *Bodies of Work: Meditations on Mortality from the Human Anatomy Lab*. New York: Penguin Press, 2007.

Moore, Charleen M., and C. Mackenzie Brown. "Experiencing Body Worlds: Voyeurism, Education, or Enlightenment." *J. Med. Humanities* 28, no. 4 (2007): 231–54.

Moore, Gregory P. "The Practice of Medical Procedures on Newly Dead Patients—Is Consent Warranted?" *Acad. Emerg. Med.* 8, no. 4 (2001): 389–92.

Morag, Rumm M., Sylvie DeSouza, Petter A. Steen, Ashraf Salem, Mark Harris, Oyvind Ohnstad, Jan T. Fosen, and Barry E. Brenner. "Performing Procedures on the Newly Deceased for Teaching Purposes." *Arch. Intern. Med.* 165, no. 1 (2005): 92–96.

Munson, Ronald. *Raising the Dead: Organ Transplants, Ethics, and Society*. New York: Oxford University Press, 2002.

Murphy, Timothy F. "Sperm Harvesting and Post-mortem Fatherhood." *Bioethics* 9, no. 5 (1995): 380–98.

Murray, Virginia H. "A Right of the Dead and a Charge on the Quick: Criminal Laws Relating to Cemeteries, Burial Grounds, and Human Remains." *J. Mo. Bar* 56 (2000): 115.

National Conference of Commissioners on Uniform State Laws. Comments to the Uniform Anatomical Gift Act (2006). www.nccusl.org.

Nelkin, Dorothy, and Lori Andrews. "Do the Dead Have Interests? Policy Issues for Research After Life," 24 *Am. J. Law Med.* 261 (1998).

Note, "Compulsory Removal of Cadaver Organs," 69 *Columbia L. Rev.* 693 (1969).

Nuland, Sherwin B. *How We Die: Reflections on Life's Final Chapter*. New York: Knopf, 1994.

Nwabueze, Remigius N. "Spiritualising in the Godless Temple of Biotechnology: Ontological and Statutory Approaches to Dead Bodies in Nigeria, England, and the USA," 29 *Manitoba L. J.* 171 (2002).

Ochoa, Tyler Trent, and Christine Newman Jones. "Defiling the Dead: Necrophilia and the Law," 18 *Whittier L. Rev.* 539 (1997).

Orentlicher, David. "Presumed Consent to Organ Donation: Its Rise and Fall in the United States," 61 *Rutgers L. Rev.* 295 (2009).

O'Rorke, Imogen. "Skinless Wonders . . ." *The Observer*, May 20, 2001. www .guardian.co.uk/education/2001/may/20/arts.highereducation.

Paige, Richard. "Post-mortem Pregnancies: A Legal Analysis." *King's College Centre Med. Law Ethics* 9, no. 3 (2000): 2–5.

Partridge, Ernest. "Posthumous Interests and Posthumous Respect." *Ethics* 91, no. 2 (1981): 243–64.

Pascoe, Judith. "Collect-Me-Nots." *New York Times*, May 17, 2007. www .nytimes.com/2007/05/17/opinion/17pascoe.html.

Patton, Laura-Hill M. "A Call for Common Sense: Organ Donation and the Executed Prisoner," 3 *Va. J. Soc. Policy Law* 387 (1996).

Peipert, Thomas. "The Future Is in Plastics, for the Dead." *Newark Star Ledger*, May 20, 2007.

Phua, Jason, Tow Keang Lim, David A. Zygun, and Christopher J. Doig. "Pro/ Con Debate: In Patients Who Are Potential Candidates for Organ Donation after Cardiac Death, Starting Medications and/or Interventions for the Sole Purpose of Making the Organs More Viable Is an Acceptable Practice." *Crit. Care* 11 (2007): 211.

Pringle, Heather. *The Mummy Congress: Science, Obsession, and the Everlasting Dead.* New York: Hyperion, 2001.

Prothero, Stephen. *Purified by Fire: A History of Cremation in America.* Berkeley: University of California Press, 2001.

Pruett, T. L. "Defending Organ Donation." *Los Angeles Times*, August 5, 2007.

Quante, Michael, and Silvia Wiedebusch. "Overcoming the Shortage of Transplantable Organs: Ethical and Psychological Aspects." *Swiss Med. Weekly* 136, no. 33–34 (August 2006): 523–28.

Quay, Paul M. "Utilizing the Bodies of the Dead," 28 *St. Louis U. L. J.* 889 (1984).

Quested, Beverleigh, and Trudy Rudge. "Nursing Care of Dead Bodies: A Discursive Analysis of Last Offices." *J. Adv. Nurs.* 41, no. 6 (2003): 553–60.

Quigley, Christine. *The Corpse: A History.* Jefferson, NC: McFarland, 1996.

Radford, Mary F. "Post-Mortem Sperm Retrieval and the Social Security Administration: How Modern Reproductive Technology Makes Strange Bedfellows." *Texas Southern Univ. Thurgood Marshall School of Law J. of Modern Issues in Estates & Estate Planning.* http://ssrn.com/abstract=1376402 (May 2009).

Rady, Mohamed Y., J. L. Verheijde, and Joan McGregor. "Organ Donation after Circulatory Death: The Forgotten Donor?" *Crit. Care* 10, no. 5 (2006): 166.

Raff, David. "He's Not a Pathologist, He's Pathological." *Haaretz*, May 26, 2006.

Ramsland, Katharine. *Cemetery Stories: Haunted Graveyards, Embalming Secrets, and the Life of a Corpse after Death*. New York: HarperCollins, 2001.

Reeves, Roy R., William S. Agin, Ethyl S. Rose, Marti D. Reynolds, Anthony R. Beazley, and Sharon P. Douglas. "When Is an Organ Donor Not an Organ Donor?" *South. Med. J.* 97, no. 12 (2004): 1259–61.

Reifler, Douglas. "Have We Lost Our Heads?" *Atrium* (Spring 2005): 8.

"Rest in Pieces." *Albany Times-Union*, January 17, 2006.

Rice, J. R. *Funerals Aren't Funny: But Sometimes Funny Things Happen at Funerals*. West Conshohocken, PA: Infinity, 2006.

Richardson, Eileen H., and Bryan S. Turner. "Bodies as Property: From Slavery to DNA Maps. In *Body Lore and Laws*, edited by Andrew Bainham, Shelley Day Sclater, and Martin Richards, 29–42. Portland, OR: Hart Publishing, 2002.

Richardson, Ruth. *Death, Dissection, and the Destitute*, 2nd ed. Chicago: University of Chicago Press, 2000.

Rivenburg, Roy. "A Degree of Finality: Colleges Double as Cemeteries." *Newark Star Ledger*, May 20, 2007.

Roach, Mary. *Stiff: The Curious Lives of Human Cadavers*. New York: W. W. Norton, 2003.

Roan, Shari. "Organ Shortage Has Officials Looking at Presumed Consent." *Chicago Tribune*, December 28, 2005.

Robbins, Jim. "Roadblock for Spreading of Human Ashes in Wilderness." *New York Times*, March 30, 2007. www.nytimes.com/2007/03/30/us/30ashes.html.

Robertson, John A. "Posthumous Reproduction," 69 *Ind. Law J.* 1027 (1994).

Rodning, Charles B. "'O Death, Where Is Thy Sting?' Historical Perspectives on the Relationship of Human Postmortem Anatomy Dissection to Medical Education and Care." *Clinical Anat.* 2, no. 4 (1989): 277–92.

Rogak, Lisa. *Stones and Bones of New England: A Guide to Unusual, Historic, and Otherwise Notable Cemeteries*. Guilford, CT: Globe Pequot Press, 2004.

Rosman, Jonathan P., and Philip J. Resnick, "Sexual Attraction to Corpses: A Psychiatric Review of Necrophilia." *Bull. Am. Acad. Psychiatry Law* 17, no. 2 (1989): 153–63.

Ruggles, Samuel B. "The Law of Burial." *Bradford's Surrogate's Court Reports* 4 (1856): 503.

Sachs, Jessica Snyder. *Corpse: Nature, Forensics, and the Struggle to Pinpoint the Time of Death*. Cambridge, MA: Perseus, 2001.

Sandomir, Richard. "Please Don't Call the Customers Dead." *New York Times,* February 13, 2005. www.nytimes.com/2005/02/13/business/yourmoney/ 13freeze.html.

Sappol, Michael. *A Traffic of Dead Bodies: Anatomy and Embodied Social Identity in Nineteenth-Century America.* Princeton, NJ: Princeton University Press, 2002.

Satel, Sally, and Ben Hippen. "When Altruism Isn't Enough: The Worsening Organ Shortage and What It Means for the Elderly," 15 *Elder L. J.* 153 (2007).

Saulny, Susan. "A Day of Searching, Anger and Renewed Grief in a Desecrated Illinois Cemetery." *New York Times,* July 10, 2009. www.nytimes.com/ 2009/07/11/us/11cemetery.html.

Savulescu, J. "Death, Us and Our Bodies: Personal Reflections." *J. Med. Ethics* 29 (2003): 127–30.

Schechter Harold. "Mourning on the Inside." *New York Times,* April 7, 2007. www.nytimes.com/2007/04/07/opinion/07schechter.html.

Schiff, Anne Reichman. "Arising from the Dead: Challenges of Posthumous Procreation," 75 *N.C. L. Rev.* 901 (1997).

Schmidt, Terri A., Jean T. Abbott, Joel M. Geiderman, Jason A. Hughes, Catherine X. Johnson, Katie B. McClure, Mary P. McKay, Junaid A. Razzak, David Salo, Raquel M. Schears, and Robert C. Solomon. "The Ethical Debate on Practicing Procedures on the Newly Dead." *Acad. Emerg. Med.* 11, no. 9 (2004): 962–66.

Schwarz, Alan. "A Chance for Clues to Brain Injury in Combat Blasts." *New York Times,* June 22, 2009. www.nytimes.com/2009/06/23/health/23brai.html.

Sewell, Peter. "Respecting a Patient's Care Needs after Death." *Nursing Times* 98, no. 39 (2002): 36–37.

Shapiro, Michael H. "Illicit Reasons and Means for Reproduction: On Excessive Choice and Technological Imperatives," 47 *Hastings Law J.* 1081 (1996).

Sheach Leith, Valerie M. "Consent and Nothing but Consent? The Organ Retention Scandal." *Sociology Health Illness* 29, no. 7 (2007): 1023–42.

Shemie, Sam D. "Clarifying the Paradigm for the Ethics of Donation and Transplantation: Was 'Dead' Really So Clear before Organ Donation?" *Phil. Ethics Humanities Med.* 2, no. 18 (September 12, 2007). www.peh-med.com/ content/2/1/18/comments.

Shields, Marjorie A. "Validity and Application of the UAGA," 6 *Annotated Law Reports,* 6th 365 (2005).

Shultz, Suzanne M. *Body Snatching: The Robbing of Graves for the Education of*

*Physicians in Early Nineteenth Century America.* Jefferson, NC: McFarland, 1992.

Smolensky, Kirsten Rabe. "Rights of the Dead," 37 *Hofstra L. Rev.* 763 (2009).

Sneddon, Andrew. "Consent and the Acquisition of Organs for Transplantation." *HEC Forum* 21, no. 1 (2009): 55–69.

Spar, Debora. "The Egg Trade—Making Sense of the Market for Human Oocytes." *N. Engl. J. Med.* 356, no. 13 (2007): 1289–91.

Sperling, Daniel. "Maternal Brain Death," 30 *Am. J. Law Med.* 453 (2004).

Spielman, Bethany. "Post Mortem Gamete Retrieval after Christy." *ABA Health eSource* 5, no. 2 (October 2008). www.abanet.org/health/esource/Volume5/02/spielman.html.

———. "Pushing the Dead into the Next Reproductive Frontier: Post Mortem Gamete Retrieval under the UAGA," 37 *J. Law, Medicine & Ethics* 331 (2009).

Spital, Aaron. "Should People Who Commit Themselves to Organ Donation Be Granted Preferred Status to Receive Organ Transplants?" *Clin. Transplant.* 19, no. 2 (2005): 269–72.

Spital, Aaron, and James Stacey Taylor. "Routine Recovery of Cadaveric Organs for Transplantation: Consistent, Fair, and Life-Saving." *J. Am. Soc. Nephrol.* 2 (2007): 300–303.

Stannard, David E. *The Puritan Way of Death: A Study in Religion, Culture, and Social Change.* New York: Oxford University Press, 1979.

Sterling, Toby. "Netherlands Hospital Euthanizes Babies." *Associated Press*, December 12, 2004.

Strong, Carson. "Ethical and Legal Aspects of Sperm Retrieval after Death or Persistent Vegetative State," 27 *J. Law Med. Ethics* 347 (1999).

Sugg, Richard. "Corpse Medicine: Mummies, Cannibals, and Vampires." *The Lancet* 371, no. 9630 (2008): 2078–79.

Sung, R. S., and J. D. Punch. "Uncontrolled DCDs: The Next Step?" *Am. J. Transpl.* 6, no. 7 (2006): 1505–7.

Surette, Eric C. "Dead Bodies," 25A *Corpus Juris Secondum* Section 1 (2008).

Taylor, R. P. "Right of Sepulture," 53 *Am. L. Rev.* 359 (1919).

Torre, Carlo, and Lorenzo Varetto. "An Exceptional Case of Necrophilia." *Am. J. Forensic Med. Pathol.* 8, no. 2 (1987): 169.

Trainor, Elizabeth. "Right of Husband, Wife, or Other Party to Custody of Frozen Embryo, Pre-Embryo, or Pre-Zygote in Event of Divorce, Death, or Other Circumstances," 87 *Annotated Law Reports* 5th 253 (2001).

Trebay, Guy. "For a Price, Final Resting Places That Even Tut Could Appreciate." *New York Times*, April 17, 2006. www.nytimes.com/2006/04/17/us/17mausoleum.html.

Trope, Jack F., and Walter R. Echo-Hawk. "NAGPRA: Background and Legislative History," 24 *Ariz. St. L. J.* 35 (1992).

Truog, Robert D. "Brain Death—Too Flawed to Endure, Too Ingrained to Abandon," 35 *J. Law Med. Ethics* 273 (2007).

———. "Consent for Organ Donation—Balancing Conflicting Ethical Obligations." *N. Engl. J. Med.* 358 (2008): 1209.

Tward, Aaron D., and Hugh A Patterson. "From Grave Robbing to Gifting: Cadaver Supply in the United States." *JAMA* 287, no. 9 (2002): 1183.

Ungoed-Thomas, Jon. "Dead Organ Donors May Still Feel Pain." *The Sunday Times*, August 20, 2002.

Verdery, Katharine. *The Political Lives of Dead Bodies: Reburial and Postsocialist Change*. New York: Columbia University Press, 1999.

Verheijde, Joseph, Mohamed Rady, and Joan McGregor. "The Revised UAGA: New Challenges to Balancing Patients' Rights and Physician Responsibilities." *Philos. Ethics Humanit. Med.* 2, no. 19 (September 12, 2007). www.pehmed.com/content/2/1/19.

Vinton, Nathaniel. "Ted Williams' Frozen Head for Batting Practice at Cryonics Lab." *New York Daily News*, October 2, 2009.

Volokh, Eugene. "Medical Self-Defense, Prohibited Experimental Therapies, and Payment for Organs," 120 *Harvard L. Rev.* 1813 (2007).

Wagner, Frank D. "Enforcement of Preference Expressed by Decedent as to Disposition of His Body after Death," 54 *Annotated Law Reports* 3d 1037 (1973).

Ward, Geoffrey C. "Death's Army." *New York Times*, January 27, 2008. www.nytimes.com/2008/01/27/books/review/Ward-t.html.

Watson, Katie. "Jarred and Jarring: The Unfolding History of a Museum of Anatomy." *Atrium* (Spring 2005): 1–3.

Webster, Robert D. *Does This Mean You'll See Me Naked? A Funeral Director Reflects on 30 Years of Serving the Living and the Deceased*. Bloomington, IN: Author House, 2006.

Weingarten, Abby. "Florida Museumgoers Line Up to See Corpses." *New York Times*, August 20, 2005. http://travel.nytimes.com/2005/08/20/arts/design/20bodi.html.

Wells, Christina E. "Privacy and Funeral Protests," 87 *N. Carolina L. Rev.* 151 (2008).

Wilford, John Noble. "Stonehenge Used as Cemetery from the Beginning." *New*

*York Times*, May 30, 2008. www.nytimes.com/2008/05/30/science/30stone
henge.html.

Wilgoren, Jodi. "In Gory Detail, Prosecution Lays Out Its Case for Tough Sentencing of B.T.K. Killer." *New York Times*, August, 18, 2005.

Wilkins, Robert. *The Bedside Book of Death: Macabre Tales of Our Final Passage*. New York: Citadel Press, 1990.

Wilkinson, T. M. "Parental Consent and the Use of Dead Children's Bodies." *Kennedy Inst. Ethics J.* 11, no. 4 (2001): 337–58.

Woan, Sunny. "Buy Me a Pound of Flesh: China's Sale of Death Row Organs on the Black Market and What Americans Learn from It," 47 *Santa Clara L. Rev.* 413 (2007).

Wolf, Jean K. *Lives of the Silent Stones in the Christ Church Burial Grounds: 50 Family Profiles*. Darby, PA: Diane, 2003.

Wright, Katharine. "Competing Interests in Reproduction: The Case of Natallie Evans." *King's L. J.* 19, no. 1 (2008): 135–50.

Yalom, Marilyn. *The American Resting Place: Four Hundred Years of History through Cemeteries and Burial Grounds*. Boston: Houghton Mifflin, 2008.

Zafran, Ruth. "Dying to Be a Father: Legal Paternity in Cases of Posthumous Conception," 8 *Houston J. L. Policy* 47 (2008).

Zoloth, Laurie. "The Gaze toward the Beautiful Dead: Considering Ethical Issues Raised by the *Body Worlds* Exhibit." *Atrium* 1 (Spring 2005): 5–6.

# Cases

*Albrecht v. Treon*, 889 N.E.2d 120 (Ohio 2008)

*Arnaud v. Odom*, 870 F.2d 304 (5th Cir. 1989)

*Arthur v. Milstein*, 949 So.2d 1163 (Fla. App. 2007)

*A.Z. v. B.Z.*, 725 N.E.2d 1051 (Mass. 2000)

*Bauer v. North Fulton Medical*, 527 S.E.2d 240 (Ga. App. 1999)

*Board of Regents v. Oglesby*, 591 S.E.2d 417 (Ga. App. 2003)

*Bonnicksen v. U.S. Department of the Army*, 969 F. Supp. 614 (D.Oregon 1997)

*Brotherton v. Cleveland*, 923 F.2d 477 (6th Cir. 1991)

*Burney v. Children's Hospital*, 47 N.E. 401 (Mass. 1897)

*Carney v. Knollwood Cemetery Ass'n*, 514 N.E.2d 430 (Ohio App. 1986)

*Chesher v. Neyser*, 477 F.3d 784 (6th Cir. 2007)

*Cohen v. Cohen*, 896 So.2d 950 (Fla. App. 2005)

*Coleman v. Sopher*, 499 S.E.2d 592 (W.Va. 1997)

*Crocker v. Pleasant*, 778 So.2d 978 (Fla. 2001)

*Cruzan v. Missouri Department of Health*, 497 U.S. 261 (1990)

*Cybart v. Michael Reese Hospital*, 365 N.E.2d 1002 (Ill. App. 1977)

*Davis v. Davis*, 842 S.W.2d 588 (Tenn. 1992)

*Dean v. Chapman*, 556 P.2d 27 (Okla. 1976)

*Donaldson v. Lungren*, 4 Cal. Reporter 2d 59 (Cal. App. 1992)

Matter of *Elman*, 578 N.Y.S.2d 95 (N.Y. Sup. Ct. 1991)

*Enos v. Snyder*, 63 P. 170 (Cal. 1900)

*Epps v. Duke University*, 468 S.E.2d 846, 855 (N.C. App. 1996)

*Fidelity Union Trust v. Heller*, 84 A.2d 485 (N.J. Ch. 1951)

Estate of *Fischer v. Fischer*, 117 N.E.2d 855 (Ill. App. 1954)

*Fitzimmons v. Olinger Mortuary*, 17 P.2d 535 (Colo. 1932)

*Floyd v. Atlantic Coast Line Ry*, 84 S.E. 12 (N.C. 1914)

*Gadbury v. Bleitz*, 233 P. 299 (Wash. 1925)

*Georgia Lions Eye Bank v. Lavant*, 335 S.E.2d 127 (Ga. 1985)

*Gillett-Netting v. Barnhart*, 371 F.3d 593 (9th Cir. 2004)

*Goldman v. Mollen*, 191 S.E. 627 (Va. 1937)

*Graves v. Biomedical Tissue Services*, 488 F.Supp.2d 430 (D.N.J. 2007)

*Grawunder v. Beth Israel Hospital*, 272 N.Y.S. 171 (N.Y. App. Div. 1934)

*Gudo v. Administrators of Tulane Educational Fund*, 966 So.2d 1069 (La. App. 2007)

*Gurganious v. Simpson*, 197 S.E. 163 (N.C. 1938)

*Hall v. Fertility Institute of New Orleans*, 647 So.2d 1348 (La. App. 1994)

*Haney v. Stamper*, 125 S.W.2d 761 (Ky. 1939)

*Hecht v. Superior Ct. of Los Angeles*, 59 Cal. Rptr 222 (Cal. App. 1996)

*Holland v. Metalious*, 198 A.2d 654 (N.H. 1964)

*Infield v. Cope*, 270 P.2d 716 (N.Mex. 1954)

Matter of *Jobes*, 529 A.2d 434 (N.J. 1987)

*Juseinoski v. N.Y. Hosp. Med. Center*, 795 N.Y.S.2d 753 (App. Div. 2005)

*Kass v. Kass*, 696 N.E.2d 174 (N.Y. 1998)

Estate of *Kievernagel*, 83 Cal. Rptr. 3d 311 (Cal. App. 2008)

*Kohn v. United States*, 591 F. Supp. 568 (E.D.N.Y. 1984)

Estate of *Kolacy*, 753 A.2d 1257 (N.J. Ch. Div. 2000)

*Kyles v. Southern Ry Co.*, 61 S.E. 278 (N.C. 1908)

*Larson v. Chase*, 50 N.W. 238 (Minn. 1891)

*Lascurain v. City of Newark*, 793 A.2d 731 (N.J. App. Div. 2002)

*Lavigne v. Wilkinson*, 116 A. 32 (N.H. 1921)

*Lawrence v. Texas*, 539 U.S. 558 (203)

*Leno v. St. Joseph Hospital*, 302 N.E.2d 58 (Ill. 1973)

*Lott v. State of New York*, 225 N.Y.S.2d 434 (N.Y. Ct. Cl. 1962)

*Maine v. Bradbury*, 9 A.2d 657 (Me. 1939)

*In re Martin B.*, 841 N.Y.S.2d 207 (N.Y. Surrog. 2007)

Matter of *Moyer*, 577 P.2d 108 (Utah 1978)

*Nachmani v. Nachmani*, 50(4) Piskei Din 661 (Israel Sup. Ct. 1996)

*National Archives Administration v. Favish*, 541 U.S. 157 (2004)

*Newman v. Sathyavaglswaran*, 287 F.3d 786 (9th Cir. 2001)

*New Mexico v. Hartzler*, 433 P.2d 231 (N.M. 1967)

*Nichols v. Central Vermont Ry.*, 109 A. 905 (Vt. 1919)

*O'Donnell v. Slack*, 55 P. 906 (Cal. 1899)

*Palmquist v. Standard Accident Insurance Co.*, 3 F.Supp. 358 (S.D. Cal. 1933)

*People v. Dlugash*, 363 N.E.2d 1155 (N.Y. 1977)

*Pettigrew v. Pettigrew*, 56 A. 878 (Pa. 1904)

*Pierce v. Proprietors of Swan Point Cemetery*, 10 R.I. 227 (1872)

*Pulsifer v. Douglass*, 48 A. 118 (Me. 1901)

*Roe v. Wade*, 410 U.S. 113 (1973)

*Rosenblum v. New Mount Sinai Cemetery*, 481 S.W.2d 593 (Mo. App. 1972)

*Sacred Heart of Jesus Polish Catholic Church v. Soklowski*, 199 N.W. 81 (Minn. 1924)

*Samsel v. Diaz*, 659 S.W.2d 143 (Tex. App. 1983)

*Silvia v. Helger*, 67 A.2d 27 (R.I. 1949)

*Southern Life & Health Ins. v. Morgan*, 105 So. 161 (Ala. 1925)

*Spiegel v. Evergreen Cemetery*, 186 A. 585 (N.J. 1936)

*Stastny v. Tachovsky*, 132 N.W.2d 317 (Neb. 1964)

*State v. Glass*, 272 N.E.2d 273 (Ohio App. 1971)

*State of Florida v. Powell*, 497 So.2d 1188 (Fla. 1986)

*State of Utah v. Redd*, 922 P.2d 986 (Utah 1999)

*Stewart v. Schwartz Brothers Chapel*, 606 N.Y.S.2d 965 (N.Y. Sup. Ct. 1993)

*Sworski v. B.H. Simons*, 293 N.W. 309 (Minn. 1940)

*Teasley v. Thompson*, 165 S.W.2d 940 (Ark. 1942)

*Thomasits v. Cochise Memory Gardens*, 721 P.2d 1166 (Ariz. App. 1986)

*Thompson v. Deeds*, 61 N.W. 842 (Iowa 1895)

*United States v. Unknown Heirs of All Persons Buried in Post Oak Mission Cemetery*, 152 F.Supp. 452 (W.D. Okla. 1957)

*University Health Services v. Piazzi*, No. CV86-RCCV-464 (Richmond County Ga., Aug. 14, 1986)

*Verein v. Posner*, 4 A.2d 743 (Md. 1939)

*Whaley v. County of Tuscola*, 58 F.3d 1111 (6th Cir. 1995)

*Whitehair v. Highland Memory Gardens*, 327 S.E.2d 438 (W.Va. 1985)

*Whitehurst v. Wright*, 592 F.2d 834 (5th Cir. 1979)

*Woodward v. Comm'r Social Security*, 760 N.E.2d 257 (Mass. 2002)

*Yome v. Gorman*, 152 N.E. 126 (N.Y. 1926)

# Index